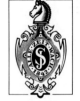

Nuclear Medicine in Clinical Oncology

Current Status and Future Aspects

Edited by Cuno Winkler

With Contributions by
S. J. Adelstein N. C. Armitage J. J. Battermann H. W. Bauer
R. P. Baum H. J. Biersack A. Bischof-Delaloye K. B. Björklund
H. Bockslaff R. C. Brasch U. Büll G. L. Buraggi H. Burrichter
J. H. Clorius H.-J. Correns H. Creutzig V. Diehl P. J. Ell
U. Feine M. Fischer J. Frühling K. Gersonde M. Granowska
C. Gropp S. E. Halpern J. Happ G. Hör G. van Kaick
W. D. Kaplan S. von Kleist W. H. Knapp R. Knopp S. M. Larson
M. Lüthgens J. Mahlstedt R. V. P. Mantravadi V. R. McCready
F. Mundinger G. L. DeNardo P. Oehr E. K. J. Pauwels
A. C. Perkins P. Pfannenstiel Ch. Reiners G. Riccabona
H. Rösler K. Schelstraete O. Schober K. Schomäcker
C. Schümichen R. Schwarzrock R. Senekowitsch B. Shapiro
H.-J. Staab A. Todd-Pokropek H. N. Wellman L. I. Wiebe
B. S. Worthington G. Wunderlich B. H. Zimmermann

With 108 Figures and 132 Tables

Springer-Verlag
Berlin Heidelberg New York Tokyo

CUNO WINKLER, M.D., Ph.D. (hon.)
Professor of Nuclear Medicine
Institute for Clinical and Experimental
Nuclear Medicine
University of Bonn
Sigmund-Freud-Str. 25
D-5300 Bonn-Venusberg

ISBN 3-540-16164-3 Springer-Verlag Berlin Heidelberg New York Tokyo
ISBN 0-387-16164-3 Springer-Verlag New York Heidelberg Berlin Tokyo

The use of registered names, trademarks, etc. in this publication does not imply, even in the absence of
a specific statement, that such names are exempt from the relevant protective laws and regulations and
therefore free for general use.

Product Liability: The publisher can give no guarantee for information about drug dosage and application thereof contained in this book. In every individual case the respective user must check its accuracy
by consulting other pharmaceutical literature.

Typesetting, printing and bookbinding: Konrad Triltsch, Grafischer Betrieb, D-8700 Würzburg
2127/3130-543210

Preface

The introduction of nuclear medicine into oncology dates back to the early 1940s, when Lawrence reported on the tumor retention of ^{32}P-phosphate, von Hevesy and von Euler soon afterwards published their fundamental work on the metabolism of phosphorus in sarcoma cells, and when almost at the same time Keston and his coworkers described their observation of the accumulation of radioactive iodine in metastases of a thyroid carcinoma. Since that time innumerable publications have appeared in oncologic literature which deal with the application of nuclear medical methods in experimental cancer research and also in the diagnosis and treatment of malignant tumors. The significance of some originally very successfully applied clinical methods naturally has changed over the years. For instance, scintigraphy became somewhat less important for the purely morphologic assessment of certain tumors after the introduction of transmission computerized tomography and modern sonographic methods into clinical practice. On the other hand, however, it has also been possible to further develop scintigraphy to a decisive extent, both with reference to the test substances applied and in view of the instrumentation. As far as the scintigraphic equipment is concerned, the introduction of static and sequential digital imaging by means of scintillation camera-computer systems in the mid-1960s represents important progress, as does the recent development of emission computerized tomography with single photon and positron emitters.

Quite a number of tracers which are suited for tumor assessment have been produced and tested, and it has been increasingly possible to use them to localize sites of pathophysiologic changes associated with neoplastic cell growth. The respective methods are based on different mechanisms, including alterations of tissue permeability, metabolic processes, and immunologic reactions. Currently there are strong indications that tumor immunology is undergoing a close amalgamation with oncological nuclear medicine. The latter refers both to the application of radioactive labelled antibodies for immunoscintigraphy and to the assessment of tumor markers in vitro, e.g., in serum and other body fluids.

Another important field of activity for the nuclear physician is the use of nuclear magnetic resonance (NMR) techniques in the form of tomographic imaging as well as in the application of in vivo spectrometry. Rapid progress has already been made in this field lateraly which mainly concerns, the establishment of morphologic structures. Promising experimental approaches, however, seem to indicate that in the future the spectrometric assessment of metabolic changes in neoplastic tissues will also become useful for the diagnosis and differentiation of tumors or for estimating the effects of therapeutic measures. In principle it can be stated that the experience in the field of nuclear medicine available today presents a particularly sound basis for the further development of NMR diagnostics. This applies in general to pathophysiological studies and in particular to contrast media investigations.

Apart from tumor diagnosis, a number of methods have been successfully applied in the therapeutic field for long time, and new possibilities for tumor treatment have been developed in recent years. In this respect the use of ^{131}I-IMBG for treatment of chromaffine tumors, e.g., pheochromocytomas or neuroblastomas, deserves particular mention. In addition, there have been optimistic reports on the possibility of the therapeutic application of radiolabelled antibodies directed against tumor antigens.

In the consideration of the newly developed tumor-affine radiopharmaceuticals, which have already been well tested, it should not be forgotten that nuclear medical methods can, under certain conditions, play an important role in planning the therapeutic approach. This is the case, for instance, in the application of indwelling arterial catheters for high dose delivery of drugs to liver metastases, when the injection of ^{99m}Tc-labelled microspheres portrays the flow distribution; a further example is the assessment of unilateral and global renal function, which permits the preoperative determination of the functional state expected after surgical removal of a tumor-bearing kidney.

With the baffling multiplicity of possibilities which nuclear medicine can contribute to clinical oncology, it is not always easy to correctly assess the practical significance of the respective procedures with regard to application on a broad scale. This is, however, a matter of great urgency in order to ensure that cancer patients receive the best possible treatment and, on the other hand, to avoid unjustified expenses. To achieve this goal, oncologists of every clinical discipline should be as well informed as possible on the often highly specialized methods of nuclear medicine in order to enable them to integrate these methods into their treatment planning in the best manner possible. Nuclear physicians should, on their part, always give careful consideration to the indications for the application of their procedures, taking into account the entire spectrum of diagnostic and therapeutic measures available. This presupposes a dialogue between all clinicians within the field of oncology, and the tumor symposium of the Society of Nuclear Medicine Europe held from May 20−22, 1985 in Bonn, FRG, was intended to establish a comprehensive basis for this purpose in accordance with the current level of knowledge. We have been fortunate in getting internationally renowned experts to speak at this symposium and to present their views on the current importance of nuclear medicine in clinical oncology — both from the point of view of the nuclear physician and from that of other specialists who are involved in the management of cancer. The papers and the lively discussions of the meeting showed the tremendous interest which exists in fully utilizing the possibilities of nuclear medicine in the diagnosis and treatment of cancer. If this present publication of the proceedings can contribute to this, then its purpose will have been fulfilled.

Bonn, February 1986   CUNO WINKLER

Table of Contents

IV. Radioimmunodetection

V. Nuclear Magnetic Resonance Imaging and In Vivo Spectroscopy

IX. Experimental Approaches and Future Aspects

List of Contributors

You will find the addresses of the first authors at the beginning of the respective contribution

I. Introduction and Basic Considerations

Nuclear Oncology:
Current Role and Future Direction

V. Diehl[1] and E. Schell-Frederick[1]

In West Germany there are approximately 250,000 newly diagnosed human malignancies per year, equally divided between males and females. At the time of diagnosis two out of three patients have generalized disease. The tumor will already have undergone 30 cell divisions and thus experienced most of its biological life span in a preclinical phase in which all existing biochemical, morphological, or imaging procedures are too insensitive to detect tumor nests of as few as $10^3 - 10^6$ cells, a magnitude of tumor which might be eliminated by existing methods. This is an "iceberg" situation. The last 10 cell divisions, between $10^9 - 10^{12}$ cells (1 g − 1 kg), give rise to a tumor mass which becomes incompatible with the life of the host [1]. Sensitivity of tumor cells to cytoreductive therapy is dependent on the growth rate and growth fraction of the tumor, both of which are inversely related to total tumor size.

Thus, it is obvious that there is an urgent need to diagnose smaller tumors earlier. Tumor diagnosis involves a multiple-step procedure leading from nonspecific subjective symptoms via noninvasive screening methods to a more or less precise definition of the organ involved, the tissue type, and the biological characterization of the tumor. An oncologist's view of the usefulness of common nuclear medicine imaging techniques is shown in Table 1.

The bone scan is by far the most useful test and plays a role in the evaluation of most tumors. Its extraordinary sensitivity, which allows the detection of possible tumor involvement months before other methods, is highly appreciated and compensates, in variable measure, for its lack of specificity. The rest of the picture appears bleak, with the exception of the unique case of thyroid carcinoma.

However, this is a somewhat overly pessimistic view. The measurement of tumor markers in serum, although as yet only semispecific, is useful. Perhaps more important are the tests reflecting organ function which enter into the planning and evaluation of therapy, e.g., lung perfusion and ventilation, renal clearance, and the determination of cardiac function. Any of the whole range of available nuclear medicine methods can be of real help in specific instances. The use of such tests reflects the interests of individual nuclear medicine departments and underscores the importance of collaboration between oncology and nuclear medicine.

---

1 Medizinische Universitätsklinik I, Joseph-Stelzmann-Str. 9, D-5000 Köln 41

Nuclear Medicine in Clinical Oncology
Ed. by C. Winkler
© Springer-Verlag Berlin Heidelberg 1986

Table 1. Usefulness of Common Nuclear Medicine Imaging Techniques in Oncology

	Bone scan	Brain scan	Cardiac scan	Lung per-fusion	Lung venti-lation	Lympho-scintig-raphy	Renal clear-ance	Thyroid scintig-raphy
Breast	+ + +	0	0	0	0	0	0	0
Gastrointestinal	+ + +	0	0	0	0	0	0	0
gastric								
hepatic	(+)						0	0
pancreatic	(+)						0	0
colon + rectum	+ +						0	0
Genitourinary	+ + +	0	0	0	0	0		0
renal	+ +						+ +	
prostatic	+ + +						0	
Gynecologic	+ + +	0	0	0	0	0	+	0
Head and neck		0	0	0	0	0	0	0
brain	0							
thyroid	+ +							+ + +
Leukemia	+	0	0	0	0	0	0	0
Lung	+ + +	(+)	(+)	+	+	0	0	0
Lymphoma	+ + +	(+)	(+)	0	0	0	0	0
Skin	+ + +	(+)	0	0	0	+	0	0
melanoma	+ +	(+)	0	0	0	+	0	0

The failure of current diagnostic techniques is in general both one of specificity and of sensitivity. The ideal agent would theoretically be 100% tumor specific and sensitive enough to identify all tumor sites, however small and in whatever special tissue environment.

Clearly, one of the most exciting and most promising discoveries in recent years has been that of monoclonal antibodies (MoAb). As the use of radiolabeled MoAb in oncology will be extensively discussed during this symposium, it may be useful to review briefly the potential use of MoAb in oncology and point out some of the problems which may limit their inherent specificity and their sensitivity (see [2]). As shown in Table 2, MoAb may be valuable in many aspects of tumor management. These include detection of circulating tumor-associated antigens, imaging of primary and metastatic tumors via intravenously injected radiolabeled MoAb or lymphoscintigraphy with radiolabeled MoAb and immunohistochemistry on tumor material. The possibilities for tumor therapy are also multiple. Less often mentioned are the experimental aspects which may someday be of real clinical importance (Table 3). For the first time tools other than morphology are available to distinguish between two different tumors or among cell types within a given tumor. One can define the extent of antigenic heterogeneity, study the effects of passage in culture on antigenic phenotype, and determine differences in expressed antigens on primary and metastatic tumors and during the course of the disease. Based on the tumor antigenic phenotype, one can hope to be able to predict the metastatic potential

Table 2. Potential Uses for Monoclonal Antibodies (MoAbs) in the Diagnosis and Treatment of Cancer

Tumor detection and localization
   Circulating tumor associated antigens
   Imaging with radiolabeled MoAbs
      Intravenous
      Lymphoscintigraphy
   Immunhistochemistry
      Aspiration cytology
      Biopsy and surgical material
      Effusions
Treatment
   Drug conjugation
   Toxin conjugation
   Radionuclide conjugation

Table 3. Experimental Aspects of Monoclonal Antibodies in Oncology

Tumor Typing	Ability to distinguish different tumors or cell types within a given tumor
Antigenic Heterogeneity	Extent Effect of extended passage in culture Modulation: Primary vs metastatic tumor during the course of the disease
Antigenic Expression	Definition of determining factors Role in metastasis and eventual response to therapy

of cell populations, favored sites of metastasis, and predict response to specific therapies.

Table 4 summarizes the multiplicity of factors which must be considered in the use of MoAb, factors related to the MoAb themselves, to the tumor in question, and to the interaction between the two. Additional factors involved when MoAb are to be radiolabeled have been purposely left out. When MoAb are destined for use in vivo, immunological problems are likely if mice or rats are used for their preparation. The tissue source of the immunogen is of importance. Different antigens may be expressed on primary and metastatic tumor cells and long-term culture might fundamentally alter the antigenic phenotype. Fab' or F(ab')$_2$ fragments may prove to be more useful than whole immunoglobulins because of possible nonspecific Fc binding to a variety of cells with Fc receptors. Fragments are also more quickly cleared from the body, an advantage with radiolabeled MoAb. It is now clear that one MoAb rarely reacts with all tumors from a particular organ. Thus, the need for cocktails is becoming obvious. MoAb cocktails may also help to overcome the problem raised by the antigenic heterogeneity of tumors, where only some cells express a given antigen or where tumor cells have only a small number of antigenic sites. The size and vascularization of a tumor and the degree of infiltration or necrosis are important determinants of the amount of MoAb reaching the tumor in vivo.

Table 4. Factors in the Use of Monoclonal Antibodies

Monoclonal Ab	*Tumor*
Species	Number of cells expressing the antigen
Tissue source	Number of antigen sites per cell
Whole immunoglobulin or fragments	Size
Dose	Vascularization
Route of inoculation	Infiltration and necrosis
Clearance from the blood	Presence and reactivity of circulating antigen
Cocktails	

Interaction
Avidity of binding
Duration of binding
Fate of antigen-antibody complex

Circulating tumor-associated antigens may compete with tumor tissue for administered monoclonal antibodies.

The second part of this paper concerns specific examples of oncological
problems, some suggestions, and some questions.

Diagnosis, Localization

Oncologists often see patients in whom either the presence of tumor is only suspected or in whom metastatic tumor has been discovered, but the primary tumor is unknown. Presently, such patients are subjected to extensive, often un-
pleasant, costly, and time-consuming tests. It is often emphasized that a tumor-
seeking agent must be highly tumor specific and sensitive enough to identify
even the smallest tumor sites. For these two clinical questions it appears that
the specificity criterion should be modified. Perhaps it is an advantage rather
than a disadvantage here that many MoAb raised against a given tumor have
demonstrated binding to a broad class of carcinomatous tissues. To be useful
clinically, the MoAb must, of course, not react with normal adult tissues. As already mentioned, the use of MoAb cocktails to reveal a specific tissue type of
tumor has been proposed because of the antigenic heterogeneity of many tumors. The development of antibody cocktails based on antigenic characteristics
common to many, perhaps all, tumors or those with common histology could be
of real clinical importance in the detection of unknown tumors. Would there be
an advantage in labeling antibodies in such a cocktail with different radionuclides not only to optimize labeling and retention of functional activity for
each, but also to sharpen the diagnostic possibilities?

Staging

In Hodgkin's disease, verification of tumor extent is of particular importance.
Direct correlation of the staging classification with prognosis has been ex-

tensively proven. Despite optimal utilization of noninvasive procedures, clinical staging of abdominal disease is in error in 20% − 30% of patients, both underestimating and overestimating the extent of disease. The failure of currently available noninvasive techniques is one of both specificity and sensitivity. Thus, a staging procedure which is already long, complicated, and costly usually culminates in exploratory laparotomy and splenectomy in order to exclude abdominal involvement. The mortality rate of the procedure has been reported in one study to be 0.13% and the morbidity 11.7% [3].

In the last 7 years, we have succeeded in establishing five long-term cell cultures from patients with Hodgkin's disease [4]. These in vitro cell lines have been extensively characterized and are now accepted as an in vitro counterpart of the malignant cell of Hodgkin's disease, i.e., Hodgkin's (H-cells) or Sternberg-Reed cells (SR-cells). H- and SR-cells usually constitute less than 10% of tumor mass in biopsied lymph nodes, thus making it very difficult to obtain a pure tumor cell population from patient material. We have therefore used the cell lines for the raising of MoAb.

The first MoAb to show specificity for H- and SR-cells was Ki-1 [5]. Ki-1 has been shown to react with tumor cells in 31/31 biopsy specimens. Ki-1 is, unfortunately, not completely Hodgkin's disease specific. However, Ki-1 shows a much more restricted reactivity in vivo than against in vitro cell lines, suggesting that it may nevertheless be valuable as a diagnostic and/or therapeutic agent. To evaluate its usefulness, we prepared radioiodine-labeled Ki-1 and injected it into nude mice carrying heterotransplanted H-cell line 540. The transplanted Hodgkin's tumor was highly labeled 24 h after injection of radiolabeled Ki-1. In contrast, in a mouse carrying a Jurkat T-cell leukemia transplanted tumor, no radioactivity was observed in the tumor. Activity in the region of the tumor increased up to 50 h, whereas activity in the thorax decreased. The activity in the region of the Jurkat T-cell tumor not only did not increase, but declined slowly with time. Thus, localization in the experimental Hodgkin's tumor cannot be explained by a perfusion effect.

Therapy

The use of radioiodine in thyroid carcinoma is a prime example of nuclear medicine's contribution to clinical oncology. At the same time, it is unfortunately a unique example of the use of a radionuclide for the direct treatment of primary tumor or for the detection and localization of primary and metastatic disease. One could claim with justification that the problem lies with the tumor rather than with nuclear medicine; that, in general, tumors do not differ enough metabolically from normal cells. Will they be antigenically different enough to allow therapy based on MoAb linked to α- or β-emitting radionuclides or conjugated to drugs or toxic substances? The problem of tumor specificity is obviously crucial here. Other considerations relevant to therapy include the problem of immunologic reactions to foreign proteins, i.e., MoAb prepared in mice or rats, particularly if the MoAb has already been used to detect and localize tumor, thus leading to a possible secondary immune reaction.

Clinical trials with MoAb are just beginning. In one such trial involving 20 patients, in which a MoAb directed against colon cancer was used, no adverse effects to an initial injection of $15-1000$ mg IgG_{2a} MoAb per patient were observed. Mouse immunoglobin could be demonstrated in the circulation for various times and was detected in tumor tissue within 1 week. The development of antimouse antibodies in nine patients appeared to be inversely correlated with the dose administered [2].

Follow-up and Complications

As already mentioned, the bone scan is our most valuable tool in nuclear medicine. But we would also wish for an additional new type of bone scan that *selectively* reflects the presence of tumor while retaining the sensitivity of the "classical" bone scan. Is there a future for 99m-Tc labeled MoAb in attempts to solve this problem?

Infection is a major cause of morbidity and mortality in patients with malignant disease. The reasons for the high incidence of infection in this population are multiple, originating in some cases from the underlying disease, but more often from treatment. A number of clinical studies have demonstrated the utility of [111]indium-oxine-labeled leukocytes for the detection and localization of infectious processes not readily revealed by simpler means. However, the use of this technique in patients with malignant disease might be expected to present special problems.

A study of the usefulness of [111]indium-labeled leukocyte scintiscans in 117 patients with cancer has been performed [6]. The specificity (95.4%), sensitivity (86%), and overall accuracy (91.3%) were found to be very similar to previously reported values in patients without tumor. With the exception of accumulation of label at the site of an osteolytic metastasis in one case, no uptake was observed in primary or secondary tumors. Thus, with the [111]indium-labeled leukocyte technique, it is almost always possible to distinguish infection from tumor, an important advantage over [67]gallium in this case. No instances were encountered in which the underlying neoplastic disease could be directly implicated as a cause of a false-negative scan. However, in several patients abnormal distribution of injected cells, as a result of underlying tumor, e.g., uptake by grossly enlarged liver and/or spleen, complicated the interpretation. Five scans were carried out in granulocytopenic patients using AB0-compatible donor leukocytes. All were proven correct, and three were particularly useful in clarifying the clinical situation. This scanning technique thus appears to be a valuable addition to the possibilities for diagnosing and locating infection in patients with cancer.

In conclusion is a list of promising nuclear medicine methods:

1. Use of organic radiopharmaceutical and positron emitting tomography for in vivo assessment of tumor metabolism
2. Evaluation of the role of contrast media in the nuclear magnetic resonance diagnosis of tumor

3. Detection and application of more specific tumor markers for early detection of microtumors
4. Expanded use of radiolabeled monoclonal antibodies for detection and evaluation of micrometastases
5. Therapeutic use of α- and Auger-electron-emitting radionuclides
6. Intravascular administration of yttrium-90 microspheres in the treatment of liver metastases
7. Stereotactic implantation of radionuclides for intracranial tumors
8. Interstitial treatment of local tumors with new radionuclides as adjuvant therapy

We look forward to increasing collaboration between nuclear medicine and medical oncology in tumor research, diagnosis, localization, and therapy.

References

1. Laird AK (1964) Br J Cancer 18:490
2. Schlom J, Colcher D, Hand PH, Greiner J, Wunderlich D, Weeks M, Fisher PB, Noguchi P, Pestka S, Kufe D (1985) Adv Cancer Res 43:143
3. Sterchi JM, Meyers RT (1980) Ann Surg 171:570
4. Diehl V, Kirchner HH, Burrichter H, Stein H, Fonatsch Ch, Gerdes J, Schaadt M, Heit W, Uchanska-Ziegler B, Ziegler A, Heintz F, Sueno K (1982) Cancer Treat Rep 66:615
5. Schwab U, Stein H, Gerdes J, Lemke H, Kirchner H, Schaadt M, Diehl V (1982) Nature (London) 299:65
6. Schell-Frederick E, Frühling J, van der Auwera P, van Laethem Y, Klastersky J (1984) Cancer 54:817

Nuclear Principles of Tumor Detection

U. BÜLL[1]

The goals of diagnostic procedures in oncology are tumor detection and/or tumor evaluation. This differentiation (detection, evaluation) is helpful when classifying the results of a procedure: a tumor may be detected by one method but evaluated according to its type by a second method, or one method may be powerful enough to yield both results. These should lead to a type-specific tumor diagnosis which is the final goal of tumor-seeking procedures. The detection of metastases is of additional help within this frame.

To reach these goals in nuclear oncology, either planar nuclear imaging or SPECT (single-photon emission computed tomography) may be employed. Principles of tumor detection by methods of nuclear medicine are listed in Table 1. Unspecific positive or negative contrasts are still the major criteria in daily routine. For example, the employment of SPECT leads to higher contrasts in either "cold" or "hot" lesions. Thus, the use of SPECT in static imaging considerably improves the delineation of brain tumors or brain metastases (hot) or liver metastases (cold). However, since such criteria do not yield a tumor-specific diagnosis, morphologically focussed methods prevail within this field, since they reveal both the structure of a tumor and its relation to the surroundings. This is demonstrated by the results of a comparative study of imaging procedures employed to detect liver metastases (Table 2).

Transmission computed tomography (TCT), ultrasound, and scintigraphy (planar and SPECT) yield nearly identical diagnostic accuracy. However, since ultrasound and TCT illustrate structures within the lesions, these procedures

Table 1. Principles of tumor detection by methods of nuclear medicine

1. unspecific positive contrast (tumor "affinity")[a]
2. unspecific negative contrast (organ affinity)[b]
3. specific positive contrast (tumor affinity)[c]

[a] bone, brain, skin, prim. liver, lung, lymph
[b] sec. liver, pancreas, kidney, spleen
[c] thyroid, phaeochromocyt., neuroblast., monoclonal AB positive tumor sites

1 Abteilung Nuklearmedizin der Rheinisch-Westfälischen Technischen Hochschule, Pauwelsstr. 1, D-5100 Aachen

Nuclear Medicine in Clinical Oncology
Ed. by C. Winkler
© Springer-Verlag Berlin Heidelberg 1986

Table 2. Diagnostic accuracy and type-specific diagnosis in focal liver disease (metastasis, cyst, abscess, hemangioma) obtained from nuclear imaging (SPECT, Planar Imaging) vs TCT and sonography

	Diagnostic accuracy	Correct type-specific diagnosis
SPECT	92%	50%
Planar imaging	86%	50%
TCT	92%	86%
Sonography	92%	85%

From Buell et al. [1] and Possberg inaugural thesis

Table 3. Criteria for tumor evaluation

→ *Viability*	*perfusion* unspecific/no accumulation of radionuclides or pharmaceuticals
→ *Metabolism*	*specific,* unspecific or no *accumulation* of radionuclides or pharmaceuticals
Lesions defined by site → and *origin*	*blood-brain barrier, differential uptake of iodine,* sec. effects (e.g. ventilation in BC), localization

→ Viability, metabolism, origin govern the term *"Function"*

have been found to be more effective. In some special cases, specific positive contrast (tumor affinity) revealed clinical validity in tumor detection (Table 1) with static nuclear imaging.

Functional Imaging and Nuclear Instrumentation

In a second approach, criteria for nuclear tumor detection and evaluation may be classified according to the scheme in Table 3. To meet such criteria, we employ instruments like probes to measure changed function, gamma cameras to illustrate and measure changed regional function and nuclide distribution or MR to display changed regional proton signals and distribution. Therefore, there is a striking difference between straight imaging and nuclear procedures: classical nuclear procedures are aimed at altered global or regional function, not at morphology. This has led to "functional scintigraphy," for example in three-phase bone scintigraphy (displaying angiographic, blood pool, and bone phases) or cerebral serial scintigraphy (perfusion, blood pool, and disruption of blood-brain barrier).

Moreover, the principles of functional imaging may be used in lung cancer to differentiate between alterations of perfusion and ventilation by bronchial carcinomas. However, the corresponding morphological methods, such as

X-ray (bone tumors), TCT (plain and contrast enhancement), or conventional tomography (bronchial carcinoma) translate the most important data by significant morphological criteria into a result close to the desired type-specific diagnosis. Therefore, one may summarize that, in tumor detection and evaluation (tumor diagnosis), morphological criteria are superior to functional ones. Is this really true?

Radionuclides and Radiopharmaceuticals

Radionuclides and radiopharmaceuticals, which yield by tumor affinity a positive contrast by increased or changed function, may be one step forward (Table 4). Today, the most important precursor is diphosphonate in bone scanning. However, its tumor affinity is a secondary one, since not the tumor but the tumor reaction is labeled. Of the examples given in Table 4, ions are of interest in some special indications. However, we have experienced an uptake of [67]Gallium, ^{201}Tl, or proteins in inflammatory lesions. Iodine only serves as a high specific marker if normal thyreoideal tissue has been removed. Monoclonal antibodies at the moment are the most promising tumor-labeling radiopharmaceuticals. We should, however, bear in mind that false-positives and -negatives may occur with all these radiopharmaceuticals, monoclonal antibodies included.

Morphology or Function?

As yet, tumor- and type-specific tumor diagnoses are mainly performed using noninvasive methods, still aiming at morphology. Table 5 gives an overview of various tumor types and locations, which have been adequately diagnosed by morphologically oriented methods. The proportion of known masses requiring additional nonmorphological methods in order to be evaluated correctly is indeed very small. To detect remote metastases in bone and skin or to check lymphatic drainage of tumors, functional methods are succesfully employed for staging. However, this is not sufficient to employ nuclear medicine methods on a larger basis routinely.

Table 4. Tumor detection: *radionuclides and radiopharmaceuticals*

A. *Tumor affinity* (increased or changed function → positive contrast)
 – radiolabeled precursors (I, MIBG, N-Glu, Iodoquine, Diphosphonates)
 – cytostatics   (Co, In-Bleomycin)
 – proteins   (HSA, fibrinogen, immunoglobulin, MoAB)
 – ions   (Ga, Tl, Se, In, I)

B. *Organ affinity* (decreased or changed function → negative contrast)
 – organ specific radionuclides and pharmaceuticals

From Winkler [2]

Table 5. Known masses (tumor- and type-specific tumor diagnosis)

Noninvasive morphology is to gain high likelihood	sufficient	non sufficient
– intracranial	+	
– thyroid	Ø	adenoma, diff. Ca
– ENT-tumors	+	
– gastrointestinal	+	
– liver	+	FNH, prim. Ca
– pancreas, PTG, AG, NET	+	phaeo, AGC-Tu, neuroblastoma
– urologic	+	
– gynaecologic	+	
– airways, lungs	+	
– prim. bone	+	
– sec. bone	+	osteoblastic metastasis
– lymphatic, spleen	+	
– skin	+	

PTG, parathyroid glands; AG, adrenogenital; NET, neuroepithelioma; FNH, focal nodular hyperplasia

Conclusion

In the present state of tumor detection, morphological principles are superior. Functional principles prevail only in a few special questions. Monoclonal antibodies are, as yet, tumor evaluators. Before they can act as tumor detectors, we need additional specificity and higher photon fluxes.

At the moment, tumors are mainly evaluated on the basis of morphological principles, therefore focussing attention on tumor size, site, or surroundings.

For the future, functional methods, covering functional principles, are well defined and may play an important role (PET, functional MR, monoclonal antibodies and SPECT). We conclude that we are living today in a period in which too much attention is devoted to mere morphological criteria. Therefore, we have degenerated to "imagers." What progress has been made since 1918, when Sir Arthur Keith, the founder of functional anatomy, said, "Structure is a sure guide to function. ..."? In future oncology, we should remember that "structure is a consequence of function" and thus, that "function is the sure guide to early tumor diagnosis."

References

1. Buell U et al. (1983) Fortschr Geb Rontgenstr 138:391
2. Winkler C (1985) Nuklearmedizinische Tumordiagnostik. In: Diethelm L et al. (eds) Nuklearmedizin. Springer, Berlin Heidelberg New York Tokyo (Handbuch der medizinischen Radiologie, vol XV/3, pp 407–463)

Mechanisms Responsible for Radioactive Tracer Uptake in Malignancies

W. D. KAPLAN[1]

Introduction

Tumors, a collection of cells altered so as to reproduce true to type, represent a growth against which the host can demonstrate no adequate control mechanisms. The tumor cell determines its own activities, irrespective of the biologic rules governing the growth of normal cells. Without this single characteristic, there would be no tumors.

Tumor cells are capable of invading adjacent tissue and of metastasizing by blood vessels or lymphatic channels to distant sites, which in turn serve as new centers of tumor cell growth. During these processes of local invasion and subsequent metastasis, tumors alter local blood flow, pH, and tissue permeability, change patterns of amino acid synthesis and local ionic composition, and produce an array of metabolic by-products. Herein lies the strength of nuclear medicine procedures, for it is these very metabolic pertubations which are most readily identified by tracer techniques.

In a discussion of the mechanisms of accumulation of radiopharmaceuticals within sites of neoplastic tissue, one could define an infinite list of radiotracers and their method of localization. In doing so, one could employ a multitude of formulae and clearance curves, punctuated by discussions of single versus multiple compartment distributions. We would suggest, however, that from the point of view of both the oncologist and the practitioner of oncologic nuclear medicine, it would be most appropriate to (a) examine representative radionuclide approaches used to identify the physiologic changes associated with neoplastic cell growth, (b) indicate how the community of radiochemists and nuclear medicine physicians have capitalized upon these changes to allow definition of sites of abnormal tumor growth, and (c) emphasize the clinical relevance of these findings.

For this discussion, we have divided the subject of mechanisms of actions of tumor localization into those which involve indirect and those which involve direct tumor scanning agents.

---

1 Division of Nuclear Medicine, Dana-Farber Cancer Inst., 44 Binney St., Boston, MA 02115, USA

Nuclear Medicine in Clinical Oncology
Ed. by C. Winkler
© Springer-Verlag Berlin Heidelberg 1986

Indirect Imaging Agents

Historically, we are most familiar with the indirect techniques of radionuclide tumor definition. The term "indirect" implies documentation of alterations in blood flow or phagocytosis, for instance, which occur secondary to micro- or macroscopic space-occupying lesions; this documentation is achieved by tracer administration followed by external camera imaging. Let us look at two of the most commonly imaged organ systems, bone and liver, which utilize this indirect approach and explore the details associated with defining the presence of tumor as a manifestation of local biologic alterations.

Chemical Adsorption

Bone Scanning

When we have before us a series of gamma camera images of the skeletal system, it is difficult to perceive of these scintiphotos as anything other than an anatomic depiction of bony structures. However, what in fact we are viewing is a graphic dynamic recording of bone turnover due to bone blood flow and osteoblastic activity.

The commonly used bone agents employ some form of phosphonate labeled with Technetium-99m (Tc-99m), which associates with the bony matrix within minutes of intravenous injection. Although the precise mechanism of action remains undefined, current thinking would suggest that localization in bone is due to adsorption of the phosphonate component in association with the crystalline lattice of the calcium hydroxyapatite [1]. Concentration of tracer is directly related to the degree of regional bone activity.

Consequently, distribution of the radiolabeled phosphonate documents sites of bone blood flow and bone turnover and in doing so defines the earliest alterations due to microscopic bone destruction by metastatic tumor. Indeed, it is not uncommon for the bone scan to define such metastatic sites a year or more preceding the plain radiographic changes of increased or decreased density [2]. This is because functional derangements precede anatomic derangements.

An important diagnostic and interpretive point relates to the fact that there are multiple causes for increased bone turnover. Certainly many benign processes can stimulate such a response; these include trauma, infection, and degenerative change. However, in the tumor population, the manifestation of healing bone following the administration of either chemotherapy or hormonal therapy must also be regarded as a cause of increased bone turnover.

The phenomenon of "clinical flare" following hormonal therapy in patients with breast cancer has been well documented. Such patients report increased bone pain and manifest chemical changes which include elevated serum calcium, alkaline phosphatase, and carcinoembryonic antigen (CEA) values. Indeed, the clinician could erroneously conclude that administration of hormonal therapy is doing little to arrest tumor sites in bone and could be tempted to prematurely discontinue this therapy in favor of another. These clinical manifestations, however, are in fact secondary to changes in bone due to decreased tumor growth and reflect a healing response.

These same manifestations can be noted on bone scan and have been well documented most recently by Rossleigh et al. [3], who showed that in half the patients in their series who responded to therapy, the initial bone scan findings involved either increased tracer uptake in documented sites of disease or the appearance of "new" lesions, later shown to represent subclinical sites of bone metastases only apparent after a healing response was initiated.

This concept is an important one for the clinician to appreciate and demands that these bone scan data be interpreted in the context of the total patient response.

Phagocytosis

Liver Scan

Intravenous administration of radiolabeled colloidal particles on the order of 0.5 μm in diameter has allowed us to map the distribution of the hepatic reticuloendothelial (RE) system. Because functional derangements precede anatomic derangements, deposits of neoplastic cells which have seeded the liver cause local disruption of the RE architecture; this disruption can be defined during radionuclide imaging as areas of diminished radiocolloid deposition.

As with the results of bone scanning, findings of focal derangement are nonspecific; these may be due to benign etiologies including cyst formation, abscess, or hemangioma. It is often necessary to perform a second radiologic study, i.e., either ultrasound or computerized tomographic (CT) evaluation to define the etiology of these focal derangements, particularly if the pattern is one of solitary defect. Drum has shown that although solitary focal defects are commonly associated with malignant causes, many benign entities can present in this manner [4].

A number of neoplasias, such as breast cancer and small-cell carcinoma of the lung, cause no focal derangement of the hepatic parenchyma in their earliest stage of liver metastasis. Rather, they infiltrate the hepatic sinusoids. Because of this growth feature, they may commonly escape detection by either ultrasound or CT examination, both of which in general are modalities which document anatomic alterations. It is the unique ability of the radionuclide liver spleen scan to demonstrate these minute deposits; the scintigraphic manifestations of these early metastases are those of heterogenous distribution of radiocolloid, minimal hepatomegaly, and shift of radiotracer to the extrahepatic RE system [5, 6].

Radionuclide Lymphoscintigraphy

The lymph node is composed in part of RE cells and as such is capable of phagocytosis. With the invasion of sufficient neoplastic metastases, there is ultimately a compromise in the integrity of the nodal tissue and a subsequent decrease in the RE constituents. Consequently, following the interstitial administration of radiocolloids, which normally results in the sequential appearance of radioparticulates along a lymph node chain, we see interrupted lymphatic channels and decreased nodal uptake.

Since the initial studies by Schenk et al. which used Gold-198 colloid [7] the current agent of choice has become a Tc-99m-labeled agent, antimony sulfide colloid. The lymphatics which have received primary attention include those of the internal mammary, iliopelvic, and intradermal systems [8–10]. Data correlating the results of pathologic examination of lymph nodes with those noted by external imaging exist for both the internal mammary and iliopelvic lymphatic chains. Matsuo noted sensitivities and specificities approaching 1.0 during a correlative study of the internal mammary nodes [11]; for the iliopelvic system, sensitivities and specificities centering about 0.80 were described [12].

Of clinical importance, Ege et al. have correlated the results of a positive internal mammary lymph node scan and the incidence of local recurrence and distant metastases from carcinoma of the breast [13]. Compromised phagocytosis resulting in diminished nodal accumulation of radiocolloid was associated with a twofold increase in local recurrence and a threefold increase in the incidence of distant metastases.

An important diagnostic concept is underscored by this technique. Radionuclide lymphoscintigraphy allows the clinician to identify lymph nodes which are normal in size yet involved with tumor; such nodes would routinely escape detection by ultrasound, CT, and contrast lymphangiography.

These indirect radionuclide studies are based on images which delineate alterations in regional physiology, and although sensitive indicators for the presence of disease, they are nonspecific for the diagnosis of cancer. The thrust of clinical nuclear medicine is to develop direct radioindicators which are capable of localizing exclusively within neoplastic tissue such that the physician is able to determine the location and extent of malignant tissue in an individual patient with a primary or recurrent tumor.

Direct Imaging Agents – Simple Ionic Substances

Gallium-67 Citrate Scanning

Perhaps the most widely utilized radiotracer for direct tumor imaging is Gallium 67 citrate (Ga-67), an inorganic cation of Group III_a in the periodic table. Ga-67 has been shown to associate with at least four iron-binding molecules which include transferrin, lactoferrin, ferritin, and siderophores [14].

Larson [15] reported that Ga-67 administered intravenously will rapidly bind to transferrin, resulting in a transferrin complex which in turn is capable of interacting with specific transferrin receptor sites located on the surface of tumor cells. On the other hand, Hayes et al. [16] have shown that Ga-67 is capable of entering tumor tissues in either an unbound or loosely protein-bound form to ultimately become localized in an intracellular location. Radiogallium appears to be concentrated predominantly in the cytoplasm; electron microscopic autoradiography suggests that this site of intracellular concentration is within lysosomes [17].

This relationship to iron metabolism is important clinically. For example, in a patient with elevated levels of serum iron, there will be little available transferrin for Ga-67 transport. Subsequent localization of this radionuclide will therefore be decreased not only in normal tissues, but in sites of tumor cell growth. Consequently, as in our discussion of bone scanning, the clinician must be constantly reminded that the results of nuclear medicine scanning graphically depict *current* metabolic function; the pattern of distribution of these tracers must be interpreted in light of the total clinical status of the patient.

Ga-67 has been shown to be quite avid for a variety of tumors, playing an important role in the follow-up of cancer patients as a metabolic marker of recurrent disease. A common clinical problem, for instance, is that of evaluating the treated lymphoma patient. It is not unusual after therapy for such a patient population to show persistent lymphadenopathy on either ultrasound or CT studies. The clinical question then is whether or not to continue therapy.

Anderson et al. [18] evaluated 52 consecutive patients over a 4-year period to assess the utility of using Ga-67 in the follow-up of Hodgkin's and non-Hodgkin's lymphoma. In these 21 Hodgkin's patients and 31 non-Hodgkins's patients, they obtained a total of 99 scans. To evaluate the data, a retrospective analysis was performed. No gallium scans were reinterpreted in light of new clinical or radiologic findings.

Sensitivity, specificity, and diagnostic accuracy were assessed by the oncology service using the dictated nuclear medicine reports and correlating the Ga-67 scan findings with other radiologic tests and clinical follow-up. Each patient had a median of two other radiologic studies (range, $1-6$ per patient) performed within 3 weeks of the Ga-67 scan. Follow-up information was derived from clinical, surgical, or pathologic data.

When the gallium scan results were compared with 169 contemporaneous radiologic studies, the tests agreed in 147 instances and disagreed in 22. Of the latter group, 18 Ga-67 scans were found to have correctly predicted the course of the disease. Disagreement between the Ga-67 scan data and other radiologic information centered on the results of abdominal CT and ultrasound and chest X-rays. It was found that, in patients with persistently enlarged nodal tissue, the Ga-67 scan was able to differentiate sites of active tumor from residual fibrotic tissue.

When the results of Ga-67 imaging were correlated with clinical course, Anderson's group found a sensitivity of 0.97 and 0.92 for the Hodgkin's and non-Hodgkin's patients respectively. They suggest that Ga-67 imaging should be employed in the post-treatment follow-up in addition to abdominal CT and ultrasound. A positive Ga-67 scan confirms active disease, while a negative one strongly suggests the absence of active disease and residual adenopathy due to a benign cause.

Thallium-201 Chloride Scanning

Thallium 201 chloride (Tl-201), the gamma-emitting radionuclide commonly used for myocardial studies, has been shown to have efficacy in the radionuclide identification of tumors. Specifically, Ancri et al. [19] demonstrated the affinity of this tracer for a variety of cerebral neoplasms, both primary and metastatic. The mechanism of action probably centers on a combination of physiologic factors which include preserved regional cerebral blood flow and integrity of the sodium potassium ATPase membrane pump. By some combination of these factors, intracellular localization of radiothallium occurs and, therefore, delineation of intracerebral tumor is achieved.

Recent experiences in our laboratory [20] gave us the opportunity of studying 29 patients referred for evaluation of their primary gliomas. Difficulties with clinical evaluations centered on a disparity between the patients' functional status and results of CT brain scans. Specifically, CT scans defined persistant and relatively unchanged intracerebral abnormalities following radiation or chemotherapy in patients who at the same time showed marked functional improvement.

A subset of seven of these patients who underwent sequential Tl-201 brain scans had postmortem examinations of their brains. Results of Tl-201 brain scans and CT brain scans were compared with the pathologic information. In each case, Tl-201 accumulation was restricted to sites of active tumor growth; no tracer was localized in sites of necrosis, edema, or infarction. On the other hand, the CT scans in four of the seven patients failed to differentiate critically between active tumor and associated non-neoplastic changes.

Again, a tracer technique capable of delineating metabolic activity, in this case a transport mechanism at the level of the tumor cell membrane, allows the clinician to define the presence of active tumor.

Capillary Blockade

Hepatic Artery Perfusion

A simple yet accurate approach for generating a map of tumor vasculature has evolved from the chemotherapy of intrahepatic neoplasms by arterial perfusion techniques. These patients, selected because their tumor had been shown to be restricted to the liver, were being treated by long-term indwelling hepatic artery catheters; this therapy is predicated on the assumption that there is good blood flow to these tumor sites.

Classical anatomic methods of radiologic estimation of tumor blood flow have relied upon the use of high flow rate intraarterial contrast studies. Unfortunately, this estimate of arterial perfusion does not necessarily predict the pattern of delivery of chemotherapeutic agents which are administered at significantly slower flow rates.

Radionuclide techniques allow for the extremely slow administration of radiolabeled particulates and offer the clinician an opportunity to estimate tumor perfusion at the precise rate of chemotherapeutic delivery. Tc-99m-labeled macroaggregated albumin particles with a mean diameter of 20 µm are administered through the catheter at rates of $10-21$ ml/h. The particles localize within tumor vasculature by capillary blockade; accurate predictions of which patients will respond to the chemotherapy trials can be made based upon whether focal hepatic lesions receive the radioaggregates or not [21].

Metabolite Imaging

With the advent of positron emission tomography (PET), it has become possible to measure a variety of metabolic processes by noninvasive techniques. The positron-emitting radionuclides used are isotopes of common biologic elements such as carbon, oxygen, and nitrogen. These tracers, incorporated into metabolically active substances, will localize within sites of active tumor cell growth. Once within the tumor, they emit their positive electrons. This electron travels a few millimeters in soft tissue and then interacts with a negative electron, only to disappear and be replaced by two 511-KeV photons emitted at an angle of 180° from one another. A coincidence detector records the appearance of these two 511-KeV photons and provides excellent spatial resolution with respect to the three-dimensional location of the initial positron emission (tumor site).

Glucose Utilization

Attempts have been made to identify differences between normal and neoplastic tissue in terms of carbohydrate metabolism. Neoplastic transformation in specific cell lines has been associated with increases in cell membrane transport of glucose [22]. Weber [23] showed that cancer cells have an enzyme composition favoring increased glycolysis.

A method for defining regional cerebral glucose utilization in man has been summarized by Beaney [24]. A glucose analogue 2-deoxy-D-glucose competes with glucose for transport at the cell membrane. When inside the cell, the deoxyglucose competes with glucose for phosphorylation and once this has occurred, it is trapped inside the cell, unavailable for further metabolization.

This glucose analogue has been labeled with fluorine-18, a short-lived (1.8 h) positron emitter. DiChiro et al. [25] examined the correlation between glucose utilization and the grade of primary brain tumor. They found that glucose utilization was significantly greater in high-grade tumors (Grades III and IV) as compared with the lower-grade tumors (Grades I and II). Additionally, they found a regional depression of glucose utilization in tumor-associated edema and in the regions of cortex adjacent to tumor. On a practical and clinical basis, if an intracerebral mass is actively concentrating glucose, therapy is indicated, since active glucose metabolism is characteristic of a growing tumor mass.

Similar studies of glucose metabolism in extracranial tumors have been reported. Beaney et al. [24] have shown a disproportionate increase in F-18 fluorodeoxyglucose uptake in breast tumors when compared with uptake in normal breast tissue. The sensitivity of PET techniques to define differences in regional glucose metabolism or blood flow between normal tissue and neoplastic tissue offers tremendous potential in the evaluation of the cancer patient.

Receptor Imaging

One of the more exciting areas of direct tumor identification, that of utilizing "endocrine analogues" for receptor imaging, involves the use of iodobenzylguanidine (IBG) for defining neuroblastomas. Weiland et al. described a marked adrenomedullary affinity for para-IBG, an analogue of the neuron-blocking agent guanethidine [26]. Use of this radiolabeled agent provided scan data on the adrenal medulla of the dog. These same investigators found, too, that by employing the meta (m) form of IBG they were able to consistently achieve earlier and better adrenal medullary images in an animal model [27].

Measurement of tissue concentrations of m-IBG showed up to six times the adrenal medullary concentration when compared with adrenal cortical levels and even higher concentration ratios for the adrenal medulla when compared with other nonadrenal background organs.

Although this material has been used in patients primarily to image pheochromocytomas [28], Kimmig et al. [29] recently described the scintigraphic identification of an ontogenetically related tumor, the neuroblastoma. Since in more than 90% of cases, this tumor produces homovanillic acid, vanillylmandelic acid, and other catecholamine metabolites, it suggested to the authors that radioiodinated m-IBG should show affinity in the identification of neuroblastomas. This in fact was the case and an elegant delineation of the extent of tumor was achieved. Of major importance, they indicated that, since more than 30% of the injected activity was located in the tumor, the radiation dose normally administered to the neuroblastoma (2000 rads) could be achieved by the administration of approximately 80 mCi of I 131 m-IBG. Additionally, these authors suggest that a broad spectrum of applications exist for this radiodiagnostic agent in the scintigraphic evaluation of other adrenergically innervated organs and tissues.

Immunologic Imaging

Radioimmunoscintigraphy

Development of hybridoma technology by Köhler and Milstein [30] has introduced an array of investigative studies in the techniques of radiolabeled antibody diagnosis and therapy. The importance of hybridoma techniques centers on the ability to generate large quantities (grams) of very pure, monospecific antibody to a tumor-associated antigen.

Antibodies have been labeled primarily with either I 131, using chloramine T or iodogen techniques, or with chelates of indium 111. Both of these gamma emitters have allowed external visualization of sites of radiolabeled antibody accumulation. Whether or not the whole immunoglobulin or its fragments, F (ab')$_2$ or Fab, are utilized, the mechanism of localization is related to the immunologic identification by the antibody of a specific antigen, usually an antigen associated with the cell surface.

A number of practical considerations related to mechanisms of action have dictated the selection of antibodies used for immunoscintigraphy and the form which they take. These include antibody specificity, antigen expression, and the potential for serum-blocking factors.

It is important that the clinician use an antibody which is specific to a tumor antigen. That is, the antibody should not show cross-reactivity with antigens associated with either normal tissues or tumors of a different cell line. If, for instance, an antibody is shown to be relatively specific for breast cancer cells but shows some cross-reactivity with cells of normal ovary, this could lead to significant diagnostic problems. If however, cross-reactivity is demonstrated between breast cancer cells and those from prostate cancer, in a female patient this would obviously be a clinically acceptable scanning situation.

Cell surface antigens may show different intensities of expression within a tumor cell clonal population; this can be related to the phase of cell cycle division. For instance, it may be that a specific cell surface antigen is only expressed during the S or synthesis phase of cell growth. At the time of external imaging, however, it may be that the tumor cells are in the G_0 or G_1 phase of cell growth. Consequently, an attempt to identify tumor cells by immunoscintigraphy at this point in time would yield a false-negative scan. In theory, one needs to ensure enhancement of the expression of these antigens so that they are in a synchronous phase of cell division, leading to more effective tumor detection by immunoscintigraphy.

Assays of circulating serum antigens associated with tumor cells allow clinicians an extremely sensitive in vitro method for monitoring tumor cell growth. Unfortunately, that these antigens are shed from the tumor cell surface and are present in the serum can result in compromised immunoscintigraphic studies. Such is the case for radiolabeled anti-CEA scanning whereby circulating antigen complexes with the intravenously administered radiolabeled antibody. Techniques for blood pool subtraction must be employed in order to allow visualization of tumor cells [31]. Ideally, radiolabeled antibodies to cell surface tumor antigens which are not shed into the circulation will provide the best opportunity for tumor detection by radionuclide techniques.

In spite of these practical considerations, techniques of immunologic imaging have been refined and are moving forward rapidly. Clinical experiences with imaging of malignant melanoma and gastrointestinal and ovarian tumors have provided exciting results and will be covered in greater detail. Suffice it to say that this approach to tumor imaging does work, is in clinical trials at this time, and represents a major diagnostic effort in nuclear medicine laboratories throughout the world.

Conclusions

The radionuclide identification of tumors is based on visualizing either regions of increased or decreased metabolic activity within an organ system or perturbations on a cellular level within the tumor mass per se. In this presentation, we have for the most part expanded upon these principles, using as examples nuclear medicine procedures available in most clinical departments. Receptor imaging and immunoscintigraphy, two developing areas of active clinical investigation, hold promise as providing the most specific and hopefully the most sensitive method of tumor identification.

References

1. Francis MD, Tofe AJ, Benedict JJ et al. (1979) Imaging the skeletal system. Radio Pharm II. Proceedings Second International Symposium on Radiopharmaceuticals, March 19−22, 1979, Seattle, WA. Society of Nuclear Medicine, New York, pp 603−614
2. Arnstein NB, Harbert JC, Byrne PJ (1984) Efficacy of bone and liver scanning in breast cancer patients treated with adjuvant chemotherapy. Cancer 54:2243−2247
3. Rossleigh MA, Lovegrove FTA, Reynolds PM et al. (1984) The assessment of response to therapy of bone metastases in breast cancer. Aust NZ J Med 14:19−22
4. Drum DE (1978) Optimizing the clinical value of hepatic scintiphotography. Semin Nucl Med 8:346−357
5. Drum DE, Beard JM (1976) Scinitgraphic criteria for hepatic metastases from cancer of the colon and breast. J Nucl Med 17:677−680
6. Lin MS, Donati RM (1981) "Mottled" liver scan in giant hepatomegaly due to intrasinusoidal metastasis of small cell lung cancer. Clin Nucl Med 6:496−497
7. Schenk P, zum Winkel K, Becker J (1966) Die Szintigraphie des parasternalen Lymphsystems. Nucl Med 5:388−396
8. Ege GN (1976) Internal Mammary Lymphoscintigraphy − the rationale, technique, interpretation, and clinical application. Radiology 118:101−107
9. Kaplan WD (1983) Iliopelvic Lymphoscintigraphy. Semin Nucl Med 13:42−53
10. Sullivan DC, Croker BP Jr, Harris CC et al. (1981) Lymphoscintigraphy in malignant melanoma: 99m-Tc antimony sulfur colloid. Am J Roentgenol 137:847−851
11. Matsuo S (1974) Studies of the metastasis of breast cancer to lymph nodes − II. Diagnosis of metastasis to internal mammary nodes using radiocolloid. Acta Med Okayama 28:361−371
12. Kaplan WD, Garnick MB, Richie JP (1983) Iliopelvic radionuclide lymphoscintigraphy in patients with testicular cancer. Radiology 147:231−235
13. Ege GN, Clark RM (1980) Internal mammary lymphoscintigraphy in the conservative surgical management of breast carcinoma. Clin Radiol 31:559−563
14. Hoffer P (1980) Gallium: Mechanisms. J Nucl Med 21:282−285
15. Larson SM (1978) Mechanisms of localization of gallium-67 in tumors. Semin Nucl Med 8:193−203
16. Hayes RL, Rafter JJ, Byrd BL et al. (1981) Studies of the in-vivo entry of Ga-67 into normal and malignant tissue. J Nucl Med 22:325−332
17. Swartzendruber DC, Nelson B, Hayes RL (1971) Gallium-67 localization in lysosomal-like granules of leukemic and non-leukemic murine tissues. J Natl Cancer Inst 46:941−952
18. Anderson KC, Leonard RCF, Cannellos GP et al. (1983) High-dose gallium imaging in lymphoma. Am J Med 75:327−331
19. Ancri D, Basset J-Y, Lonchampt MF et al. (1978) Diagnosis of cerebral lesions by thallium-201. Radiology 128:417−422
20. Kaplan WD, Takvorian RW, Morris JH et al. (1985) Thallium-201 brain imaging: A comparative study with pathologic correlation. J Nucl Med 26:P75 (abstr.)
21. Kaplan WD, Ensminger WD, Smith EH et al. (1981) Radionuclide angiography to predict patient response to hepatic artery chemotherapy. Cancer Treat Rep 64:1217−1222
22. Hatanaka M (1974) Transport of sugars in tumor cell membranes. Biochem Biophys Acta 355:77−104
23. Weber G: Enzymology in cancer cells. N Engl J Med 296:486−493
24. Beaney RP (1984) Positron emission tomography in the study of human tumors. Semin Nucl Med 14:324−341

25. DiChiro G, DeLaPaz RL, Brooks RA et al. (1982) Glucose utilization of cerebral gliomas measured by [18]F Fluorodeoxyglucose (18FDG) and positron emission tomography. J Neurol 32:1323−1329
26. Weiland DM, Wu JL, Brown LE et al. (1980) Radiolabeled adrenergic neuron blocking agents: adrenomedullary imaging with 131 I iodobenzylguanidine. J Nucl Med 21:349−353
27. Weiland AM, Brown LE, Tobes MC et al. (1981) Imaging the primate adrenal medulla with I 123 and I 131 meta-iodobenzylguanidine: concise communication. J Nucl Med 22:358−364
28. Lynn MD, Shapiro B, Sisson JC et al. (1984) Portrayal of pheochromocytomas and normal human adrenal medulla by m-123 I iodobenzylguanidine: concise communication. J Nucl Med 25:436−440
29. Kimmig B, Brandeis WE, Eisenhut M et al. (1984) Scintigraphy of neuroblastoma with I 131 meta-iodobenzylguanidine: J Nucl Med 25:773−775
30. Köhler G, Milstein C (1975) Continuous cultures of fused cells secreting antibody of proven defined specificity. Nature 256:495−497
31. Goldenberg DM, DeLand F, Kim E et al. (1978) Use of radiolabeled antibodies to carcinoembryonic antigen for the detection and localization of diverse cancers by external photoscanning. N Engl J Med 298:1384−1386

II. Technical Principles

Gamma Camera Imaging and Single Probe Detection of Tumors

R. KNOPP[1]

Two main methods are available for the detection and differentiation of tumors by means of radioactive test substances: 1) scintigraphic imaging and 2) single probe detection. Since the introduction of digital data processing into nuclear medicine in the mid-60s [3, 11, 15] quite a few procedures have been developed for scintigraphy which have opened up important possibilities for tumor diagnosis, particularly in connection with gamma camera computer systems [4]. Such systems have made it possible to assess data in a digital format for subsequent analysis and thus to obtain through image processing methods quantitative information on the uptake and turnover of gamma emitting tracers in suspicious areas.

Single probes consisting of semiconductor radiation detectors are mainly used for differential diagnostic purposes in superficially localized tumors, e.g. of the eyes or the skin. However, catheter semiconductor detectors have also been developed for insertion into the body [12]. The tumor identification tests are usually performed by using the β-emitter P-32 whose increased selective accumulation in certain malignant tissues is well known since many years [1].

Out of the variety of scintigraphic imaging procedures (use of digital filters etc.), the most important one concerns the contrast enhancement obtained by the subtraction of background activity, resulting in an improved target-to-nontarget ratio. Digital image subtraction techniques have already been described more than 20 years ago for isolated imaging of the pancreas [11]. This was performed by means of a double tracer technique which is, in principle, also suitable for background elimination in the scintigraphic establishment of cancerous lesions [8, 9]. Contrast enhancement has gained particular interest for radioimmunoscintigraphy when the specific uptake for a radiolabelled antibody in the tumor tissue is relatively low. In respective investigations of our own we have used I-131 for labelling the tumor-specific antibody, and In-111 as a label for unspecific gamma globulin. The tracers were i.v. injected simultaneously and after an appropriate period 3 scintigrams were recorded: 1) with spectrometer setting at the iodine peak, 2) with setting of the window at the indium peak, in which case indium activity is recorded together with scattered radiation from radioiodine, and 3) a scattered ray image with a window setting in between the iodine and the indium peaks. The pure scintigraphically detectable

---

1 Institut für klinische und experimentelle Nuklearmedizin, Universität Bonn, Sigmund-Freud-Straße 25, D-5300 Bonn 1

Nuclear Medicine in Clinical Oncology
Ed. by C. Winkler
© Springer-Verlag Berlin Heidelberg 1986

indium distribution is achieved by subtracting the scatter image from the indium scintigram. Subtracting this image from the iodine scintigram leads finally to the presentation of the specific uptake of the I-131-labelled antibody in the tumor without background overlay.

Despite good results achieved using the double tracer subtraction technique in phantom studies the practical application of the method in patients has occasionally proved to be problematic. Artifacts may occur due to the following reasons: 1) the imaging properties of the gamma camera depend to a certain extent on the gamma energies of the radionuclides that are used, both with regard to geometrical resolution and to the influence of scattered rays, 2) the spatial distribution of a background tracer may not always be identical with the background distribution of the tumor specific antibody (which should be mostly the case when only simple blood pool labelling is applied), and 3) changes in the position of the patient during the scintigraphic measurements can lead to an incorrect alignment of the image matrices. The proper and accurate use of geometrical markers is therefore an inevitable prerequisite for the achievement of satisfying results.

Even though the above mentioned problems have to be faced the double tracer technique has proved to be useful in quite a number of investigations [5]. As an example, Fig. 1 represents the scintigraphic demonstration of the recidivation of a testicular teratocarcinoma. Imaging was performed by means of monoclonal β-hCG antibody labelled with I-131 and In-111-labelled unspecific gamma globulin as background tracer. The tumor areas which were confirmed by subsequent surgery are clearly visualized in the immunoscintigram.

Another interesting approach to the assessment of malignant tissue is the kinetic analysis of radioimmunoscintigrams [6]. This method is based on the likelihood that specific uptake increases whereas blood pool and tissue background decreases with time. Computer analysis of serial data obtained at different periods after injection of the labelled antibody gave very promising results in cases of ovarian cancer.

An example for a somewhat more sophisticated evaluation of scintigraphic data is the computer-assisted differential diagnosis of brain lesions [10, 16]. This method requires rapid sequential scintigraphy after bolus injection of Tc-99m-pertechnetate and repeated imaging during a period of 2−3 h. By means of the region-of-interest technique, the focus and also a nonaffected area are selected and the course of the tracer accumulation in these regions is quantita-

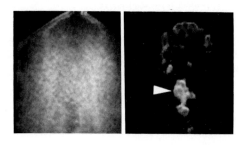

Fig. 1. Immunoscintigraphic assessment of testicular teratocarcinoma recidivation (*arrow*).
Left Image of I-131 β-hCG distribution.
Right Scintigram after background subtraction (see text)

tively assessed. The calculated target-nontarget ratios reflect specific properties of the lesion concerning the perfusion as well as the alteration of the blood-brain barrier.

In view of corresponding differences in various tumors and other lesions of the brain it has been possible to establish typical patterns which were collated in incidence matrices [14] were used in the application of a computer program based on the Bayesian theorem of conditional probabilities [13]. The program has been successfully applied for differentiation of tumors, e.g., meningiomas, gliomas, angiomas, or metastases, and of other organic diseases of the brain.

It might be a matter of interest that the assessment of the course of contrast has lately come to be regarded to be significant when paramagnetic contrast media, e.g., gadolinium-DTPA, are used for tumor diagnosis by NMR imaging [2]. The kinetic behavior of this substance appears to be similar to that of pertechnetate.

As mentioned in the beginning, the use of single probe detectors can be profitable for the evaluation of superficially located tumors. The β-emitter P-32 is most frequently used for this purpose which shows increased uptake in various malignancies, such as melanomas, compared to benign tumors, hematomas or normal tissue [1]. Special miniaturized Geiger probes have formerly been used for the P-32 test. Recent developments of semiconductor detectors, however, have led to considerable progress, particularly in the differential diagnosis of eye tumors. The probe can be shaped in such a way that it is usually possible to place it within the requisite 2–3 mm of the suspected lesion. The application of semiconductor detectors for differentiating of a benign from a malignant intraocular tumor has proved particularly useful when used in conjunction with other ophtalmologic techniques, including computer assisted sonography.

In summing up, it can be stated that scintigraphy and single probe detection offer the unique possibility for assessing functional or pathophysiologic changes indicating malignant tumor growth. This will never be replaced by other diagnostic methods, e.g., computerized tomography, sonography, or even magnetic resonance imaging, in spite of the fact that they are partly superior in view of the delineation of morphological structures. There is no doubt that tumor diagnosis in vivo by means of radioactice tracers will increasingly gain importance in the future, particularly because of the continuing development of new radioimmunological methods and radiopharmaceuticals.

References

1. Biersack HJ, Winkler C (1980) Der Einsatz von Halbleiterzählern zur P-32-Diagnostik von Augen- und Hauttumoren. Nuklearmediziner 4(3):359–366
2. Brasch RC et al. (1984) Contrast-enhanced NMR-imaging – Animal studies using Gadolinium-DTPA complex. Am J Roentgenol 142:625–630
3. Brown DW (1964) Digital computer analysis and display of the radioisotope scan. J Nucl Med 5:802
4. Brownell GL et al. (1971) NUMEDICS – A computer system for processing radioisotope data from multiple sources. USAEC Conf 7-10425:51–60
5. Goldenberg DM (1980) An introduction to the radioimmunodetection of cancer. Cancer Res 40:2957–2959

6. Granowska M et al. (1985) Kinetic analysis of radioimmunoscintigraphy, RIS using probability mapping: comparison with multiple biopsy findings in ovarian cancer. European Nuclear Medicine Congress, London, 1985
7. Kolberg T et al. (1974) Präoperative Artdiagnostik hirnorganischer Prozesse mit Hilfe eines Computerprogramms. Acta Neurochir (Wien) 31:23
8. DeLand FH et al. (1980) Imaging approach in radioimmunodetection. Cancer Res 40:3046–3049
9. Perkins AC et al. (1984) Physical approach for the reduction of dual radionuclide imaging subtraction artifacts in immunoscintigraphy. Nucl Med Comm 5:501–512
10. Rösler H et al. (1972) Type-specific tumor patterns in cerebral sequential scintigraphy. Neuroradiology 3:144
11. Schepers H, Winkler C (1964) An automatic scanning system using a tape perforator and computer techniques. In: Medical Radioisotope Scanning, Wien IAEA
12. Takayanagi SI et al. Miniature semiconductor radiation detectors. In: Hine GJ, Sorenson JA (eds) Instrumentation in nuclear medicine. Academic, New York, p 486
13. Virnich H et al. (1975) CEDI – ein Computerprogramm zur präoperativen Artdiagnostik hirnorganischer Prozesse. Methods Inf Med 14:19–25
14. Winkler C (1973) Computer assisted differential diagnosis of human brain lesions. Int Res Comm Syst 16-23-2:12
15. Winkler C (1963) Neue Methoden in der Szintigraphie. In: Atomstrahlung in der Medizin und Technik. München p 137
16. Winkler C (1985) Nuklearmedizinische Tumordiagnostik. In: Diethelm L et al. (eds) Nuklearmedizin. Springer, Berlin Heidelberg New York Tokyo, pp 407–463 (Handbuch der medizinischen Radiologie, vol 15)

Single Photon and Positron Emission Computerized Tomography in Tumor Diagnosis

A. Todd-Pokropek[1]

Tomographic techniques have now become widely available in diagnostic medicine. In nuclear medicine, the two techniques of single photon and positron emission tomography have been extensively used including, to a limited extent, in the area of tumour diagnosis. While emission computerized tomography usually gives better contrast for 'lesions' than conventional planar imaging, it also permits, within certain limits, the quantitation of uptake of a labeled substance within a given volume. Such quantitation may be either absolute or relative. Relative quantitation is of value in following, for example, tumour response to therapy. Absolute quantitation of uptake may be of value in predicting response to therapy. Volume may easily be estimated accurately, and followed.

In attempting to quantitate, various corrections are required. Correction for attenuation is a problem which is much more severe in the single photon case than for positrons. Additionally, in both techniques, great care needs to be exercised in correction for scattered events and other similar perturbing effects such as the variations in point spread function. The partial volume effect, and loss of contrast for objects similar in size to the resolution of the system, can also be taken into account. All tomographic techniques perform badly when there is a shortage of photons such that data acquisition must be performed over a long time. Cardiac and respiratory gating is not trivial. Thus great efforts have been made in both single and positron tomography to improve both sensitivity and resolution by specially designed detector arrays. It is now possible to achieve 3-mm resolution for positrons, and 7-mm resolution for single photons. Studies can acquired in as little as 2 min, provided there are enough photons. Thus volumes of sizes down to 1 cc can, in theory, be assessed. However, conventional rotating gamma camera SPECT systems often have resolution as poor as 2-cm resolution, resulting in a minimum volume for quantitation of > 10 cc.

In principle, emission tomography is best suited to situations, where uptake occurs within small volumes with a high uptake to background ratio, and performs badly when the uptake of an isotope is extended over a large volume, for example the liver, in which one is looking for cold defects. Labelled mono-

---

1 Dept. of Medical Physics and Bio-Engineering, School of Medicine, University College London, Shropshire House 11 – 20, Capper St., London WC1 E6AJ, UK

Nuclear Medicine in Clinical Oncology
Ed. by C. Winkler
© Springer-Verlag Berlin Heidelberg 1986

clonal antibodies, for example, tend to generate data which falls in this category. While the greatest successes of the use of positrons has been in physiological assessment, for example, of cerebral and cardiac function, in SPECT the use of I 123 as a label, and the likelihood of finding suitable Tc 99m substitutes provides reasonable potential in tumour diagnosis. The use of labels such as In 111 and Ga 67 presents special problems of uniformity and scatter correction, particularly when used with rotating gamma cameras, which will be discussed.

NMR Tomography of Cancer: Technical Considerations

B. H. ZIMMERMANN[1]

It has been shown that MR tomography is a useful tool for demonstrating the presence and location of tumors in the human body. The application of MR imaging for cancer detection is feasible as a result of the extraordinary sensitivity of MR with respect to tissue differentiation. Tumors generally possess T_1 and T_2 relaxation times different from those of equivalent normal tissue. A direct classification of tumors according to these factors, however, has only partially been successful so far, due to MR's lack of specificity.

For the detection of stage 2D tumors, spin echo sequences that simultaneously measure a set of thin contiguous slices are increasingly preferred over inversion recovery sequences. One reason is the much shorter data acquisition time. Direct measurement in the most advantageous orientation obviates the need for secondary reconstruction in MR.

For diagnostic purposes a T_2-weighted and, if necessary, a T_1-weighted image are typically measured by selecting recovery times of about 2 s and 0.3 s respectively. Pure T_2 images can be calculated from a single measurement using multiple echoes. Whenever nonexponential T_2 decay is present, several T_2 components can be extracted for this voxel. The calculation of a pure T_1 image typically requires the measurement of one slice with different recovery times. Measurement sequences for the calculation of T_1 from a single scan have also been demonstrated.

Multiple echo sequences are increasingly used to differentiate between tumor and edema. An echo time on the order of 100 ms in combination with a long recovery time has been found to be optimal.

A powerful method for the detection of lipomas or the differentiation of lipomas from other normal or abnormal tissue has been introduced by Dixon. This method exploits the fact that the resonance frequencies of protons in waterlike and fatlike tissue are separated by 3.5 ppm. In a spin echo sequence, water and fat protons point in the same direction, both at the end of the 90° pulse and, more importantly, at the center of the Hahn spin echo following the 180° pulse. Sampling the signal at the time of the spin echo will provide a conventional (in-phase) water and fat proton image. However, water and fat protons do not stay aligned during the pulse sequence, but rather dephase. Sampling the signal at a particular time interval during dephasing produces a wa-

1 Siemens AG – Bereich Medizinische Technik, Henkestraße 127, D-8520 Erlangen

Nuclear Medicine in Clinical Oncology
Ed. by C. Winkler
© Springer-Verlag Berlin Heidelberg 1986

ter-minus-fat (opposed-phase) image. Once the in-phase and opposed-phase images have been obtained, water proton and fat proton images can be calculated by a simple algorithm.

Characteristically, lipomas are present in the fat image and absent in the water image.

The detection of tumors in the thorax and upper abdomen mostly require cardiac and respiratory gating for reducing motion artifacts. In cardiac gating, the recovery time is typically determined by the average beat-to-beat interval. With respiratory gating data acquisition is typically turned off during respiratory motion, as detected by a sensor connected to the patient. This method, however, prolongs measurement time by up to 200%. More sophisticated respiratory gating techniques are based on the fact that views with small-phase encoding values are more sensitive to motion artifacts than those with high-phase encoding values. By proper organization of the data, acquisition algorithm motion artifacts can be drastically reduced without extending measurement time.

Surface coils are increasingly used to provide high-resolution diagnostic images. Special coils have been developed for the eye, ear, spine, breast, neck, and joints.

Care must be given to the selection of the magnetic field strength of the MR system, as field strength is one of the major factors influencing image quality (contrast) and patient throughput. In analytical MR, which uses small samples and no magnetic field gradients, signal-to-noise increases linearly with the magnetic field strength of the spectrometer. In MR imaging, gradient fields are used to encode spatial information in the slice under investigation. Gradient fields, however, increase the frequency spread of the received radio frequency (rf) signal. By applying a gradient, each voxel of a slice will have a frequency distribution that depends on the size and steepness of the gradient.

When the received signal is decoded, signals in a certain bandwidth can be assigned to a specific voxel. To maintain image fidelity, these gradients must be large enough to override frequency spreads originating from the following sources: natural line width, inhomogeneities of the static magnetic field, and chemical shift of proton Larmor frequencies between waterlike and fatlike chemical compounds. When the field strength is increased, steeper magnetic field gradients are required. Thus, the bandwidth and noise of the received signal increase with magnetic field strength. Therefore, in MR imaging, unlike analytical MR, the signal-to-noise ratio (S/N) increases only by the square root of the magnetic field strength. For typical spin echo pulse sequences used for the detection of tumors, the S/N ratio as opposed to the field strength curve flattens out at higher fields, resulting in diminishing returns as the field strength is increased. The gains in S/N at higher fields are further attenuated by the fact that the full S/N advantage at high fields cannot be realized without increasing the repetition time of the pulse sequence.

How well an MR system can differentiate between adjacent structures like normal and abnormal tissue depends on the contrast-to-noise ratio (C/N), i.e., the signal-to-noise difference between adjacent types of tissue in an image. Certain investigators [1−3] have stated that increases or decreases in C/N for most tissue pairs flatten out at higher field strengths, as compared with low field strengths. At fields over 1 T, contrast depends less on field strength than it does on other factors such as rf system optimization, patient size, and acquisition technique.

References

1. Gore JC (1982) The meaning and significance of relaxation in imaging. In: Witcofski RL, Karstaedt N, Partain CL (eds) Proceedings of International Symposium on NMR Imaging. Winston-Salem, NC: Bowman Gray School of Medicine, 15−23
2. Hart HR, Bottomley PA, Edelstein WA, Karr SG, Leue WM, Mueller O, Redington RW, Schenck JF, Smith LS, Vatis D (1983) Nuclear magnetic resonance imaging: contrast-to-noise ratio as a function of strength of magnetic field. AJR 141:1195−1201
3. Crooks LE, Arakawa M, Hoenninger J, McCarten B, Watts J, Kaufman L (1984) Magnetic resonance imaging: effects of magnetic field strength. Radiology 151:127−133

Parameter-Selective Proton NMR Imaging and Tissue Characterization In Vivo

K. Gersonde[1]

Parameter-selective proton imaging is a new tool for tissue characterization and tissue differentiation based on the non-invasive determination of the relaxation times T_2 and T_1, the partial volume α, the proton density ϱ and the diffusion coefficient D [1, 2, 3]. Essential experimental steps of this imaging method are: Slice selection by selective excitation with narrow-band rf pulses, generating of the complete decay traces of the transverse magnetization by Carr-Purcell-Mciboom-Gill (CPMG) pulse sequences with up to 50 echoes and π pulse distances of $\geqq 6$ ms, setting of a $\pi/2$ pulse immediately after the transverse magnetization has been reached zero for measuring the saturation recovery [3], application of high-power pulses, variation of the strength of the read gradient [4] and image reconstruction from 120 projections by filtered backprojection. All facilities for parameter-selective imaging are realized in the whole-body Bruker Tomograph (Type BNT 1100, Bruker Medizintechnik, Karlsruhe, Germany) employing an air-resistive, four-coil, iron-screened magnet and linear field gradients of about 700 Hz/cm for head and body coils respectively at low magnetic fields of $0.24-0.28$ T. Preprocessing of the raw-echo traces resulting in anatomy-related echo images was performed in the Aspect 3000 computer with the software system TOMIKON (Bruker Medizintechnik, Karlsruhe, Germany) which has been supplemented by algorithms for echo shape analysis and spike removal and for voxel size adjustment [5]. The compact echo image data were transferred to a VAX 11/780 computer for further evaluation and for generation of parameter-selective images. For this purpose, the software system RAMSES [6−8] has been developed which consists of five subsystems: IN-FORMATION [6], EVALUATION [7], PARAMETER SELECTION [8], IMAGE GENERATION, and IMAGE PROCESSING. RAMSES is controlled by a command language as well as by function keys.

Before parameter-selective imaging for tissue analysis is performed, the slice of interest can be identified employing 2D-FT techniques. Thus for screening purposes, interleaved multi-slice imaging (acquisition time of $5-10$ min) or RARE imaging (acquisition time of 4 s) have been used. RARE (rapid acquisition with relaxation enhancement) is a new fast imaging technique which takes the advantage of the multiple echoes of a CPMG sequence [9]. Both screening techniques provide T_2-weighted echo images which indicate, for example, space-occupying processes.

---

1 Abteilung Physiologische Chemie, Rheinisch-Westfälische Technische Hochschule (RWTH), RWTH-Klinikum, D-5100 Aachen

Nuclear Medicine in Clinical Oncology
Ed. by C. Winkler
© Springer-Verlag Berlin Heidelberg 1986

For parameter-selective imaging of discrete slices a combination of a CPMG pulse train with a saturation recovery (SR) pulse sequence has been employed [3]. The decay traces of the transverse magnetization of each volume element (voxel) reflect a sum of mono-exponential functions which is decomposed into its components by applying the "peeling off" method after semilogarithmic linearization [1] or the eigenfunction expansion method [7]. A recently developed algorithm combines the advantages of both evaluation methods, i.e. good-quality starting values for the eigenfunction expansion method are calculated with the very fast "peeling off" method. The mobile, non-exchangeable and "compartmentalized" protons contribute independently to the transverse magnetization decay of each voxel. Up to four T_2 relaxation processes per voxel have been found which are assigned to proton classes, like extra- and intracellular water, lipids, proteins, and subclasses thereof. By extrapolation of the echo traces to the time zero the absolute proton density ϱ_i for each proton class and the total proton density ϱ_0 per voxel can be determined. The partial proton concentrations per voxel α_i are indicators of the partial volumes of a voxel. On the basis of SR with a $\pi/2$-$\pi/2$ distance of 400 ms and with the extrapolated magnetization at the time zero, T_1 values can be calculated assuming a mono-exponential saturation recovery. The diffusion coefficients D_i for proton classes defined by T_2 are determined by varying the strength of the read gradient [4]. Thus, such an NMR imaging experiment provides for each voxel of a 256×256-matrix a multi-dimensional vector with the components $T_{2,i}$, α_i, ϱ_i, ϱ_0, D_i and T_1.

These parameters are arranged in parameter histograms indicating the number of voxels for which a particular value is determined. By defining and selecting socalled parameter windows, i.e. intervals on the parameter axis, proton classes as mentioned above are assigned. The combination of the biochemical with the anatomical information leads then to a spatial assignment of the dysfunctional states of the tissues. The pattern of the parameter histogram is slice- and tissue-specific and therefore itself it is a graphical representation of diagnostic value.

The NMR parameters are representation variables as well as selection variables. Both types of variables are necessary for generating images with selective tissue properties [8]. The representation variable visualizes the selected characteristics of the image, whereas the selection variables define a selection criterion. Any of the representation variables can be used to visualize a particular tissue by employing the following modes of parameter-selective imaging: RESI for T_1 and T_2, ALSI for α, ROSI for ϱ, and DISI for D. For example, a tumor can be classified on the basis of the selection of protons of intracellular water by T_1, T_2 and D. The heterogeneity of the tumor tissue then can be visualized by α representation. Finally, by ϱ representation the proton density can be shown. The selectivity of proton classes and the contrast in parameter-selective images can be improved by employing more than one selection variable. Each selection variable or any combination of them can be used for tissue characterization and are the selection criterion. The above mentioned parameter windows define the range of values for both, the representation and the selection variable.

It has to be mentioned that by only *one* experiment (acquisition time of $5-10$ min) all type of information is available. By defining and setting new parameter windows other molecular species or other tissues can be visualized and analyzed. Thus, it is possible to visualize gray and white matter of the brain respectively according to the remarkable differences in T_2 of the lipid protons. Ependyma, meninge and walls of the vessels can be selectively visualized due to differences in T_2 of the intracellular water. Furthermore, each type of tissue can be visualized on the basis of different proton classes. For example, fat tissue can be visualized by representing T_2 values of triglyceride protons and intracellular water protons respectively. Finally, the quantity of a proton class, i.e. partial volume and proton density, can be specific for a tissue.

Overlay image generation allows the simultaneous visualization of an anatomy-related echo image together with a biochemistry-related parameter-selective image. This technique is of particular diagnostic value as the medical user has an easier access for localizing a functional in the well-known morphological pattern.

As examples for selective tissue representation in parameter-selective head images, meninge, ependyma, CSF, cerebral vessels, gray and white matter and an astrocytoma tumor could be assessed. Fine-differentiation within a particular tissue is also possible by defining secondary parameter windows within a primary parameter window. Furthermore, diffusion images of the human head can be achieved. Recent progress in generating parameter-selective images employing the 2D-FT mode allows the separation of fatty tissues, muscle, urinary bladder and connective tissues in the pelvis.

References

1. Gersonde K, Felsberg L, Tolxdorff T, Ratzel D, Ströbel B (1984) Magn Reson Med 1:463−477
2. Gersonde K, Tolxdorff T, Felsberg L (1985) Magn Reson Med 2:390−401
3. Gersonde K, Felsberg L, Tolxdorff T (1984) Abstracts, XIth International conference on magnetic resonance in biological systems. Goa, pp 33−34
4. Gersonde K, Tolxdorff T, Felsberg L, Ratzel D, Ströbl D (1985) International symposium on magnetic resonance 85, Garmisch-Partenkirchen. Schnetzter, Konstanz
5. Staemmler M, Gersonde K (1986) Magn Reson Med (in press)
6. Felsberg L, Mecking B, Tolxdorff T, Repges R, Gersonde K (1985) Proceedings, International Symposium CAR 85. Springer, Berlin Heidelberg New York Tokyo, pp 9−14
7. Repges R, Tolxdorff T, Felsberg L, Broscio G, Gersonde K (1985) Proceedings, International Symposium CAR 85. Springer, Berlin Heidelberg New York Tokyo, pp 25−29
8. Tolxdorff T, Breuer B, Felsberg L, Repges R, Gersonde K (1985) Proceedings, International Symposium CAR 85. Springer, Berlin Heidelberg New York Tokyo, pp 30−35
9. Hennig J, Nauerth A, Friedburg H, Ratzel D (1984) Radiologe 24:579−580
10. Hennig J, Nauerth A, Friedburg H (1985) Magn Reson Med (in press)

Development of Magnetic Resonance Contrast Media for Tumors

R. C. Brasch[1], H. Paajanen, W. Grodd, D. Revel, and B. Engelstad

Introduction

In view of the outstanding inherent contrast available from magnetic resonance imaging (MRI), contrast-enhancing pharmaceuticals may be used advantageously to expand the diagnostic benefits from this new imaging technique. Diagnostic sensitivity may be improved with contrast agents that distribute differentially to magnetically-identical, but histologically-dissimilar, tissues. For example, it may be difficult or impossible to distinguish meningiomas from surrounding normal brain substance, but a contrast agent that accumulates in the tumor can make lesion identification easy. Contrast agents may also improve the diagnostic specificity of MRI, a primarily chemically-dependent technique, by providing physiologic and functional information. For example, a nonfunctioning kidney may appear normal on the MR image, but a urographic contrast agent can demonstrate the lack of excretory function. Contrast agents may further augment the imaging process if imaging time can be reduced through the use of time-efficient pulsing sequences without loss of diagnostic content.

Although the applications of MRI contrast media may sometimes parallel the use of radiographic, iodinated compounds, there are important differences in the principles of contrast manipulation, relationships of dose and effect, toxicology, and chemistry. These differences as well as information on the potential applications of MRI contrast media will be the focus of this discussion.

Principles of Paramagnetic Contrast Enhancement

The basis of hydrogen MRI relies upon the interaction between radiowaves and the body's protons (1H) in the presence of a strong magnetic field [1]. Atomic nuclei, as in the case of hydrogen, that have an odd number of protons or neutrons, behave like small bar magnets in the external magnetic field. Because of their high abundance in the human body and strong NMR signal, hydrogen protons lend themselves best to functioning as signal probes in MRI. The magnetic moments of individual protons align either parallel to or against an externally imposed magnetic field. When energy in the form of a radiofrequency

1 Contrast Media Laboratory, Department of Radiology, University of California, San Francisco, CA, USA

Nuclear Medicine in Clinical Oncology
Ed. by C. Winkler
© Springer-Verlag Berlin Heidelberg 1986

signal (RF) interacts with such a magnetized sample, the protons begin to resonate in a coherent fashion. The magnetic moments of individual nuclei, and thus the net magnetization of the sample, change depending on the strength and duration of the RF pulse. The time constant which characterizes the re-establishment of net magnetic moment after an RF pulse is called T_1 or spin-lattice relaxation time. Spin-spin relaxation time, or T_2, reflects the loss of spin coherence of individual nuclei following termination of the RF excitation. The contrast between tissues in proton MRI is a direct result of intrinsic differences in proton density and T_1 and T_2 relaxation times in different tissues.

Mathematical relationships between MR intensity (I), T_1, and T_2 shown below help to clarify the influence of relaxation times on image intensity in two of the most commonly used imaging sequences. Intensity determines the shade of gray used to display a particular tissue.

Spin echo: $I = H f (v) [1 - \exp(-TR/T_1) \exp(-TE/T_2)]$
Inversion recovery: $I = H f (v) [1 - 2 \exp(-TI/T_1) + \exp(-TR/T_1)]$

where H is the local hydrogen concentration and $f(v)$ is a function of both proton velocity and the fraction of all protons that are moving. TR is a repetition time of RF pulses and TE is an echo delay time (the interval between RF pulse and the effective sampling of the signal). Both TR and TE are software-controlled parameters.

As seen, the hydrogen density, the relaxation behavior of protons (T_1 and T_2 times), and the blood flow all contribute to the intensity, and thus contrast, in MRI. Importantly to contrast manipulation, the equations also indicate that a decrease of T_1 increases the intensity, and a decrease of T_2 has an opposite effect of decreasing intensity, assuming the other factors remain constant. Paramagnetic compounds used as contrast agents enhance proton relaxation, shortening both T_1 and T_2 [3]. The shortening of T_1 produces the desired contrast effect by increasing intensity (spin echo, inversion recovery), while the same influence on T_2 is competitive, causing a reduction in signal intensity (spin echo).

Fortunately, with relatively low concentrations of a paramagnetic substance, T_1 is considerably shortened, and T_2 is only slightly affected. At higher concentrations, T_2 is also markedly shortened, and this diminishes the image intensity. Thus, optimal tissue concentration of an MR contrast agent is essential for the maximum contrast effect. Increasing the dose does not necessarily improve the contrast-enhancing effect.

The mechanism by which paramagnetic agents provide contrast in MRI is fundamentally different from that of radiographic contrast media. The X-ray contrast media are observed directly on radiographic images because of their tendency to absorb X-rays. The paramagnetics, however, operate in an indirect fashion by altering the local magnetic environment of tissue protons. This phenomenon is called 'proton relaxation enhancement' (PRE) [2]. PRE depends on the concentration and the magnetic moment of paramagnetic species in the sample, their interaction with surrounding water and macromolecules, and finally, the temperature of the sample.

Types of Paramagnetic Contrast Agents

Paramagnetism can be defined as the ability to develop a magnetic moment in the same direction as an applied magnetic field and proportional to the strength of the field. Three general types of paramagnetic pharmaceuticals have been proposed for MR contrast agents: (a) transition and lanthanide metal ions with unpaired electrons, (b) the chelates or metal complexes of these same ions, and (c) nitroxide-stable free radicals. Labeling of specific target molecules with one of these agents offers the potential for tissue-, organ-, or tumor-specific MR contrast enhancement (Table 1).

Paramagnetic pharmaceuticals should ideally be pure, stable, nontoxic, readily available, and inexpensive. They should have a potential to be conjugated to organ-avid biomolecules, and they should undergo efficient renal excretion. Unfortunately, unmodified metal ions are probably too toxic for routine human use. They are typically metabolized and/or stored by the liver and demonstrate very slow biological clearance.

Because of the observed toxicity of free transition and lanthanide metal ions, chelated metal complexes have been proposed [15]. Commonly used chelators for human use include ethylenediaminetetra-acetic acid (EDTA) and diethylenetetraminepenta-acetic acid (DTPA). Metal complexes using EDTA and DTPA are less effective at reducing T_1 values, but better tolerated than the corresponding free metals [15]. Intravascular EDTA and DTPA metal complexes tend to be rapidly distributed in the extravascular space and largely excreted through the kidneys by glomerular filtration like X-ray contrast media. A very promising metal complex is Gd-DTPA, which is currently under clinical investigation in Europe and the U.S.A. [5–7]. Gd-DTPA combines properties of strong PRE, high tolerance, and good stability [15].

Nitroxide spin labels are organic, stable free radicals which have one unpaired electron localized in a nitrogen-oxygen bond. Two major classes of nitroxides tested for MRI are the five-membered ring pyrrolidinyl nitroxide

Table 1. Possible contrast agents for MRI

I. Metallic ions
   Transition metal series: Cr^{+2}, Cr^{+3}, Co^{+3}, Cu^{+2}, Fe^{+2}, Fe^{+3}, Ni^{+2}, Mn^{+2}, Mn^{+3}, Ti^{+3}, V^{+4}
   Lanthanide series: Dy^{+3}, Eu^{+3}, Gd^{+3}, Pr^{+3}
   Actinide series: Pa^{+4}

II. Metallic chelates or complexes
   Cr-EDTA, Fe-EDTA, Gd-EDTA, Gd-DTPA
   Desferrioxamine, glucoheptonic acid complexes,
   Sulfide colloid complexes

III. Stable free radicals
   Pyrrolidine and piperidine derivatives, polyradicals

IV. Tissue-specific contrast agents
   Paramagnetic labeling of monoclonal antibodies, porphyrins, liposomes, hydroxycolloids

---

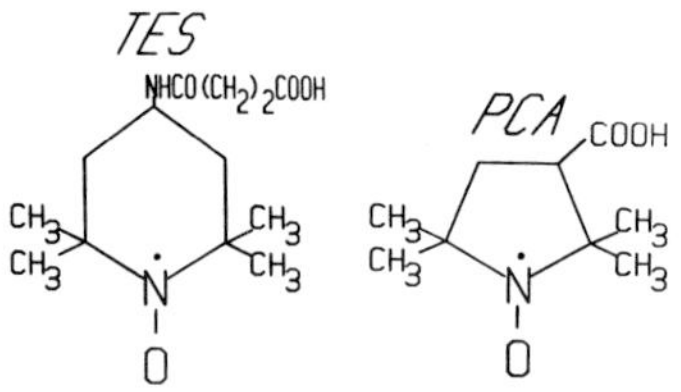

TES

NHCO(CH$_2$)$_2$COOH

PCA COOH

CH$_3$ CH$_3$ CH$_3$ CH$_3$
CH$_3$ CH$_3$ CH$_3$ CH$_3$
         N   N
         | |
         O   O

Fig. 1. Chemical structures of prototype piperidinyl (*TES*) and pyrrolidinyl (*PCA*) nitroxide spin labels used as intravenous MRI contrast media. Both agents are primarily excreted in the urine and have LD$_{50}$ values in mice between 10 and 15 mMol/kg

and the six-membered ring piperidinyl nitroxide (Fig. 1). These chemicals have prolonged stability at varying pH and temperature, long shelf life, chemical versatility for conjugation to biomolecules, and relatively low toxicity [3, 8]. Like Gd-DTPA, nitroxide spin labels are rapidly excreted through the kidneys at the rate of glomerular filtration.

The possibility of chemically combining carrier biomolecules to metal chelates or NSL may allow for the development of organ-specific or function-specific MR contrast media.

MRI Contrast Media Applications

Modern medicine has several precedents for the augmentation of diagnostic imaging examinations with pharmaceutical contrast enhancers. Examples include barium for gastrointestinal examinations, iodinated organic compounds given intravenously for X-ray urography and computed tomography, myelographic contrast media instilled into the subarachnoid space, radiolabelled compounds for nuclear scintigraphy, and, more recently, microsuspensions of air bubbles for echocardiography. With the same intent, researchers are now trying to define pharmaceutical agents which can safely alter the magnetic properties of specific tissues to change the contrast differences for MRI.

Contrast enhancement of the gastrointestinal tract to provide better differentiation of bowel from surrounding abdominal viscera is one of the more obvious pharmaceutical applications in MRI. An orally administered paramagnetic solution, such as ferric ammonium citrate (FAC) in a 1.0 mmol solution, permits delineation of the gastric wall, definition of the duodenal sweep and thus the pancreatic head, and differentiation of bowel loops from contiguous neoplastic and inflammatory masses [16]. These applications closely parallel the use of dilute barium or iodinated solutions used to opacify the bowel in computed tomography. FAC is well tolerated as evidenced by its long-term use as an iron supplement in vitamin preparations, but interestingly this particular form of iron is poorly absorbed when compared with ferrous formulations. Alternative agents for gastrointestinal enhancement might include particulate paramagnetic preparations or solutions of metal chelates such as Gd-DTPA. The latter have the potential disadvantage of absorption by the gastrointestinal tract.

Without the use of contrast agents, MRI provides little direct information about tissue function. For example, an acutely ischemic kidney following renal artery ligation may have the same MRI appearance as a normally functioning kidney. Paramagnetic agents which are administered intravenously and excreted renally, such as Gd-DTPA or NSL, provide a direct measure of renal function on the MR images [3, 15]. It should be possible to measure glomerular filtration rates of the two kidneys or even of different portions of the same kidney using contrast-enhanced MRI. In addition, increasing the intensity of the kidney, ureters, and bladder may help to define contiguous pathologic masses. For example, neuroblastomas and the nonenhanced normal kidney tend to have isomagnetic characteristics: after contrast enhancement, the interface of the kidney with a neuroblastoma could be sharply defined. This application is demonstrated in Fig. 2 of a human renal cell carcinoma implanted in a rat host.

Development of other paramagnetic formulations with a different primary route of excretion, such as the biliary tract, could further expand the abilities of MRI to directly assess tissue function. A paramagnetically labeled HIDA might be used to advantage for this goal [9].

Hepatic contrast enhancement may be achieved by administering a paramagnetic agent which is avidly extracted by the reticuloendothelial system [4]. For example, liposomes, sulfide colloids, and glucoheptonates labeled with paramagnetics could all be used to alter MR characteristics of normally functioning liver and thereby improve the sensitivity of MRI for primary and metastatic hepatic neoplasia.

For MR imaging of the central nervous system, Gd-DTPA and NSL have been shown to be effective for accentuating regions of blood-brain barrier (BBB) disruption. Like conventional radiographic contrast agents used for

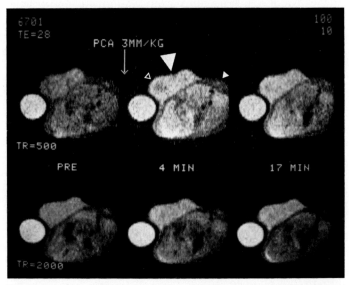

Fig. 2. Spin echo MR images before and after PCA administration in a rat with a renal cell carcinoma implanted in the flank demonstrate a nonspecific enhancement of this relatively vascular tumor. The contrast enhancement is best appreciated in the short TR (500 ms) images

brain computed tomography, these MR contrast agents are excluded by the BBB from normal brain tissue but are permitted into the extracellular fluid space at sites of inflammation and neoplasia. Even a small cerebral lesion induced experimentally with radiation, which could not be detected on multiple spin echo MR images, was easily identified after contrast enhancement. Although neoplastic tissue normally exhibits prolonged T_1 and T_2 relaxation times compared with normal brain tissue, cerebral tumors including meningiomas and metastases may be isomagnetic with normal brain; their detection may depend on contrast enhancement [5]. Use of contrast media may increase diagnostic confidence that a lesion is not being missed, a benefit even when no enhancing lesion is discovered.

For extracerebral tumors, Gd-DTPA and NSL have demonstrated utility in defining and differentiating various histologic zones including edematous, cellular, stromatous, and necrotic elements [10, 13]. For example, experimentally induced breast carcinomas consistently showed a homogeneous appearance on nonenhanced MR images, but after administration of Gd-DTPA the rim of stromatous connective tissue and the cellular zones were enhanced whereas the necrotic zones showed no enhancement.

Targeting

Augmentation of paramagnetic effects has stimulated efforts to chemically incorporate paramagnetic species into carrier molecules that either bind to or enter tumor cells and thereby permit selective enhancement.

Many metal complexes have been studied in the development of tumor-seeking radiopharmaceuticals. Among such agents, porphyrin derivatives appear to exhibit tumor localization, although the mechanism for this is poorly understood. Chen and co-workers compared relaxivities of several paramagnetic porphyrin derivatives and observed that Mn + 3-TPPS4 was quite paramagnetic, more so than the free Mn + 2 salt. Knop and colleagues [11] applied such findings in vivo, reporting preliminary findings of substantial (approximately 50%) T_1 shortening in tumor-bearing athymic mice following infusion of 10 mg manganese-containing porphyrins.

Tumor uptake of monoclonal antibodies has been studied for radioimmunoimaging and more recently for MR imaging [14]. Low tumor uptake as a fraction of total administered dose (typically less than 1% in clinical trials) does not favor application of paramagnetic monoclonal antibodies; however, augmentation of relaxivity due to longer rotational correlation time and field effects (particularly for nitroxides) has stimulated interest in empirically studying the feasibility of such a strategy.

Our group has reported shortened relaxation times and signal enhancement in athymic mice bearing human lymphoma implants using both Gd-DTPA and Gd-DTPA conjugated to an antilymphoma monoclonal antibody. Further study of these initial findings is planned.

A necessary question regarding the development of targeted agents concerns applicability. With the exception of emission computed tomography, there has been relatively little precedent for applying tumor-targeted imaging agents to cross-sectional imaging modalities. Unlike scintigraphy, magnetic resonance imaging is not presently a whole-body screening technology. Consequently, evaluation would appear to require a directed approach. Methods for screening large volumes for contrast enhancement would alter this scenario.

Conclusions

The use of drugs in medical magnetic resonance is in an early stage of development. The present discussion concerning relevance to the cancer problem and the accomplished or ongoing work by several research groups illustrates the diverse diagnostic applications, pharmaceutical considerations, and future directions that contribute to the burgeoning interest and activity in this field.

Summary

Magnetic resonance imaging (MRI) is emerging as a powerful new diagnostic tool for tumors and is valued for its apparent lack of adverse effects. The excellent inherent contrast between biologic tissues and fluids afforded by MRI is one of the foremost characteristics of this technique. Tissue contrast is a multifaceted variable dependent on physicochemical tissue properties such as hydrogen density on T_1 and T_2 relaxation rates, on magnetic field strength, and on operator-chosen factors for MRI signal acquisition. Pharmaceutical contrast-enhancing agents provide a means of limiting the time for the MRI data acquisition with improved sensitivity and diagnostic accuracy. Contrast agents can aid in the evaluations of renal function, blood-brain-barrier integrity, tissue perfusion, and gastrointestinal anatomy. Among the MRI contrast agents that hold promise for clinical use are paramagnetic metal complexes and nitroxide spin labels.

References

1. Bloch F, Hansen WW, Packard M (1946) The nuclear induction experiment. Phys Rev 70:474–485
2. Bloembergen N (1957) Proton relaxation times in paramagnetic solutions. J Chem Phys 27:572–573
3. Brasch RC (1983) Work in progress: methods of contrast enhancement for NMR imaging and potential application. Radiology 147:781–788
4. Burnett KR, Wolf GL, Shumacher HR, Goldstein EJ (1985) Gadolinium oxide: a prototype agent for contrast enhanced imaging of the liver and spleen with magnetic resonance. Invest Radiol 3:65–71
5. Carr DH, Brown J, Bydder GM, Weinmann HJ, Speck U, Thomas DJ, Young IR (1984) Intravenous chelated gadolinium as a contrast agent in NMR imaging of cerebral tumours. Lancet I:484–486
6. Carr DH, Brown J, Bydder GM, Steiner RE, Weinmann HJ, Speck U, Hall AS, Young IR, (1984) Gadolinium-DTPA as a contrast agent in MRI: Initial clinical experience in 20 patients. Am J Roentgenol 143:214–224

7. Carr DH (1985) The use of proton relaxation enhancers in magnetic resonance imaging. Magn Reson Imag 3:17−25
8. Couet WR, Brasch RC, Sosnovsky G, Tozer TN (1985) Factors affecting nitroxide reduction in ascorbate solution and tissue homogenates. Magn Reson Imag 3:83−88
9. Engelstad BE, Brasch RC (1984) Pharmaceutical development of magnetic resonance. In: Margulis AR, James TL (eds) Biomedical magnetic resonance. Radiology Research and Education Foundation, UCSF, San Francisco
10. Ehman RL, Wesbey GE, Moon KL, Williams RD, McNamara MT, Couet WR, Tozer TN, Brasch RC (1985) Enhanced MRI of tumors utilizing a new nitroxyl spin label contrast agent. Magn Reson Imag 3:89−97
11. Knop RH, Patronas NJ, Cohen JS, Dwyer AJ, Anderson AC, Girton M, Colcher D, Lundy J, Mornex F, Myers CE, Doppman JL (1984) In: Proc of Soc. Magn. Reson., 3rd Annual Meeting, pp 423−424
12. Lovin JD, Wesbey GE, Engelstad BL, Sosnovsky G, Moseley M, Tuck DL, Brasch RC (1985) Magnetic field dependence of spin-lattice relaxation enhancement using piperdinyl nitroxyl spin-labels. Magn Reson Imag 3:73−81
13. McNamara MT, Epstein AL, Williams R, Brasch RC (1984) Contrast enhanced MR imaging of tumors using Gd-DTPA. Radiology 153:145
14. McNamara MT, Ehman RL, Quay SC, Epstein AL, Schmidt H, Brasch RC (1984) Alterations of MR tumor relaxation times using a paramagnetically labeled monoclonal antibody. Radiology 153:292 (abstr.)
15. Weinmann HJ, Brasch RC, Press WR, Wesbey GE (1984) Characteristics of gadolinium DTPA complexes: a potential NMR contrast agent. Am J Roentgenol 142:619−624
16. Wesbey GE, Brasch RC, Goldberg HI, Engelstad BL, Moss AA (1985) Dilute oral iron solutions as gastrointestinal contrast agents for magnetic resonance imaging; initial clinical experience. Magn Reson Imag 3:57−64

Computer-Assisted Echographic Tissue Characterization in Tumor Diagnostics

G. van Kaick[1], D. Schlaps, I. Zuna, U. Räth, D. Lorenz, T. Hirning, L. Pickenhan, and W. J. Lorenz

The echographic characterization of tissue is open to three different biophysical approaches:
1. The analysis of the radio-frequency signal (RF-signal)
2. The analysis of the video-A signal
3. The analysis of the B-scan

A hardware-software system for the acquisition and evaluation of ultrasonic data was developed in our institute. This system permitted the quantitative analysis of a series of A-scans by means of distinct statistical parameter sets leading to the differentiation of normal tissue from cirrhotic and metastatic liver [1, 3].

This computer-assisted echographic system was then expanded to permit the generation of a two-dimensional B-scan from the A-scan data. In this way it became possible with the aid of a graphic tablet to define regions of interest within the scan which were then being subject to computer-assisted tissue analysis.

The rapid spread of digital image representation in echography opens up the possibility for a quantitative characterization of the B-scan with the aid of digital image analysis. This procedure of pattern recognition was developed for military purposes within the framework of scientific space programs. For problems investigated with computer-aided echography, two classes of parameters are employed:
1. Parameters describing the overall distribution of gray levels
2. Parameters capable of describing the spatial distribution of gray levels

The various types of parameters are complementary in the description of texture. Therefore, for the quantification of the information in the ultrasonic image, a similar reasonable combination of high information-yield parameters must be found which will make it possible to differentiate the various tissue states. For the B-scan analysis we make use of the same data acquisition and processing system already mentioned (Fig. 1), the only difference being the image evaluation [7].

In the hierarchical procedure used here, the tumours are first differentiated from the overall group. The final differentiation of the subclasses is effected in the final step of the procedure.

---

1 Abteilung Spezielle onkologische Diagnostik und Therapie, Institut für Nuklearmedizin und onkologische Radiologie, Deutsches Krebsforschungszentrum, Im Neuenheimer Feld 280, D-6900 Heidelberg

Nuclear Medicine in Clinical Oncology
Ed. by C. Winkler
© Springer-Verlag Berlin Heidelberg 1986

Data Acquisition

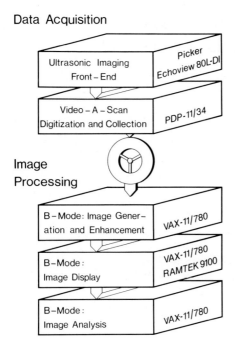

Fig. 1. Schematic representation of the design and function of the ultrasonic data acquisition and processing system

The first step involved checking in a prospective clinical study whether the computer-aided B-scan analysis was comparable with the results obtained from an evaluation of the video-A signal. This study included 40 patients with various liver diseases (normal status, diffuse liver diseases and tumours). The overall accuracy for the analysis of the video-A signal was 83% (Table 1) and 95%, for the computer-aided analysis of the B-scan (Table 2). It was thus demonstrated that the B-scan analysis was actually superior to the analysis of the video-A signal.

The next step undertaken by our working group was a comparative study to correlate the subjective B-scan analysis and the computer-aided B-scan analysis. Three different investigators made a diagnostic evaluation according to the following criteria: echogenicity, attenuation, peripheral blood vessels, portal vein fibrosis, size of the liver, ascites and size of the spleen; and in the case of intrahepatic-space-occupying lesions: localisation, delimitability, size and echo pattern. The mean overall accuracy found in this study was 85% (Table 3). This means that this comparison also revealed the superiority of computer-aided B-scan analysis. Table 4 represents part of the printout of a computer echographic analysis of a patient's liver. Three diagnostic classes are differentiated: normal liver, tumour tissue and diffuse liver diseases. Three areas of interest in the ultrasonic picture are analysed. In the example demonstrated in Table 4 the highest probability is given to the tumour tissue. The result of the computer-assisted tissue characterization was documented by the physician with regard to the findings of the conventional echographic examination.

Table 1. Computer-assisted characterization of liver tissue by video-A-scan analysis

Histology	Ultrasonogram		
	N	D	T
N	9	0	1
D	2	18	0
T	2	2	6

Overall accuracy: 83% ($n = 40$)
N, normal; D, diffuse liver disease; T, tumour

Table 2. Computer-assisted characterization of liver tissue by B-scan analysis

Histology	Ultrasonogram		
	N	D	T
N	10	0	0
D	1	19	0
T	0	1	9

Overall accuracy: 95% ($n = 40$)
N, normal; D, diffuse liver disease; T, tumour

Table 3. Subjective B-scan analysis of ultrasonograms of the liver

Histology	Ultrasonogram		
	N	D	T
N	7	3	0
D	2	17	1
T	0	0	10

Mean overall accuracy: 85% ($n = 40$)
N, normal; D, diffuse liver disease; T, tumour

Computer-aided echography was also applied for the echographic evaluation of space-occupying lesions of the breast [5] in 107 female patients (27 carcinomas, 25 fibroadenomas, 27 cysts and 28 fat lobules). The examinations were carried out at constant system settings with a 5-MHz short focussed probe. For the evaluation, 4 regions of interest were selected from the B-mode images: a) inside the space-occupying lesion, b) next to the lesion, c) immediately below the lesion and d) an additional region next to c). By employing a linear discriminant analysis, an optimum parameter set for the discrimination of the 4 histological classes was selected out of 111 image parameters. This parameter

Table 4. Lower part of the printout of a computer echographic analysis (liver tissue)

Classification of the patient

	1. Classification	2. Classification
1. ROI:	T/P=0.60	N/P=0.22
2. ROI:	T/P=0.54	N/P=0.29
3. ROI:	T/P=0.60	N/P=0.22

Alteration of liver parenchyma indicating a malignant process

Dr. U. RAETH

ROI, region of interest; P, probability; T, tumour; N, normal

Table 5. Computer-assisted B-scan analysis of breast lesions

Histology	Ultrasonogram			
	CA	FA	CYS	FAT
CA	25	2	0	0
FA	0	25	0	0
CYS	0	0	27	0
FAT	0	1	0	27

Rate of reclassification: 97% ($n = 107$)
CA, carcinoma; FA, fibroadenoma; CYS, cyst; FAT, fat lobules

Table 6. Computer-assisted B-scan analysis of thyroid lesions

Histology	Ultrasonogram			
	N	M	B	C
N	8	0	0	0
M	0	10	1	0
B	0	0	21	0
C	0	0	0	7

Rate of reclassification: 97% ($n = 47$)
N, normal; M, malignant; B, benign; C, cyst

set was finally used for reclassification. A hierarchical discriminant analysis, however, resulted in a superior classification rate. By including the regions next to and immediately below the space-occupying lesion, an overall reclassification accuracy of 96% was obtained (Table 5).

Cysts had the highest reclassification rates. As expected from our experience with conventional ultrasound, lower reclassification rates were obtained for the solid lesions. This is probably due to the enormous variation in the tissue structure of these lesions. Because of the echomorphological similarities it was not possible to separate certain benign and malignant solid tumours with our computer-aided system.

Computer-aided echography was also applied to patients with space-occupying lesions of the thyroid [2, 4]. A minimum of 3 sections depicting the lesion was selected for the region-of-interest-based analysis. An optimum parameter set for reclassification was chosen from 109 tissue parameters. A reclassification accuracy of 97% was obtained for the classes malignant and benign tissue changes, cysts and normal tissue (Table 6). Patients with thyroiditis and adenoma were occasionally misclassified as carcinomas. Only 3% of the carcinomas, however, were misclassified into the classes normal or benign tissue changes.

It must be added that these very good reclassification results from the analysis of lesions of the thyroid and breast were obtained in a pilot study; thus, the histological findings were already known and a reclassification was undertaken subsequently. It has to be expected that the overall accuracy will drop about 10% in a repeat application of the system in a prospective clinical study.

A decisive factor for the development in this area is, of course, the cost/benefit ratio. It is, however, to be expected that, in about 3−4 years, computerized systems of the type described here − which can be intergrated into modern real- time ultrasonic equipment − will be available at an acceptable price. Even a critical consideration shows that, as a result, a further improvement and, in particular, an objective approach to the diagnostic possibilities of echography can thus be achieved.

References

1. Geissler M, Lorenz A, Zabel HJ et al. (1982) A computerized echographic data acquisition and evaluation system for tissue characterization. Proc. World Congress Med. Phys. Biomed. Eng., Hamburg
2. Hirning T (1984) Quantifizierung und Klassifizierung echographischer Befunde der Schilddrüse nach objektiven Kriterien mittels rechnergestützter Echographie. Thesis, University of Heidelberg
3. Lorenz WJ, Bihl H, van Kaick G et al. (1981) Methods of image analysis and enhancement. In: Hill CR, Kratochwil A (eds) Medical ultrasonic images: formation, display, and recording. Excerpta Medica, Amsterdam, pp 69−76
4. Lorenz D, Schlaps D, Zuna I, Hirning T, van Kaick G, Lorenz WJ (1983) Computerunterstützte echographische Analyse von szintigraphisch kalten Knoten der Schilddrüse. In: Kratochwil A et al. (eds) Ultraschalldiagnostik 82. Thieme, Stuttgart, pp 405−406
5. Pickenhan L, Teubner J, Schlaps D, Zuna I, van Kaick G, Junkermann H, Lorenz WJ (1984) Computerunterstützte Analyse der Echotextur von raumfordernden Prozessen der Mamma. In: Lutz H, Reichel L (eds) Ultraschalldiagnostik 83. Thieme, Stuttgart, pp 93−95
6. Räth U, Limberg B, Schlaps D et al. (1985) Diagnostic accuracy of computerized B-scan texture analysis and conventional ultrasonography in diffuse parenchymal and malignant liver disease. JCU 13:87−99
7. Schlaps D (1983) Gewebsdifferenzierung durch Computerechographie − Entwicklung eines Verfahrens zur Texturanalyse des Ultraschall-B-Bildes. Thesis, University of Mainz

III. Diagnostic Use of Radiopharmaceuticals

Clinical Aspects of Detection and Imaging of Brain Tumors

P. J. Ell[1]

Introduction

Intracranial tumours comprise about 9% of all primary tumours. About 30% of them are benign, 40% are infiltrating, 5% are of congenital origin and 25% of them are metastatic. A thorough general examination and a recent chest X-ray are a necessary part of investigation of any patient suspected of having a brain tumour [1]. The clinical triad of headache, vomiting and papilloedema is often absent. At admission, one-third of patients with a tumour in the brain have no significant headache and approximately half have no papilloedema. Vomiting occurs in more advanced stages of tumour or if the tumour is within the posterior fossa. With infiltrating tumours, 10 years may elapse between the first fit and the onset of features which prove that a tumour in the brain is the underlying cause. With meningiomas this interval rarely exceeds 5 years [1]. Gliomas are the commonest of brain tumours (about 25%). These comprise of astrocytomas, oligodendrogliomas, ependimomas and medulloblastomas (common in children). Meningiomas occur in about 20% of all brain tumours. Less common tumours include the craniopharyngiomas, pituitary adenomas, neuromas, penealomas, cordoma and the glomus tumour. Cerebral metastases occur relatively frequently and from a variety of primary sources. Parietal and occipital and cerebellar single deposits are often seen, whilst the diagnosis is clear cut when multiple deposits are seen. From the point of view of this review, I will discuss below the role of radionuclide imaging in neoplasms of the brain as far as its detection and its monitoring is concerned.

Detection

In the presence of all available modern technology (ultrasound, X-ray CT, X-ray DSA and NMR) radionuclide imaging of the brain has a limited role to play. CT and NMR are the methods of choice, offering images of unique detail, and the best results in terms of sensitivity and specificity in the detection of primary and secondary neoplasms of the brain. There is a substantial body of literature which confirms the above, but the ultimate role which NMR will play in relation to X-ray CT is still being debated. NMR will detect neoplasia silent

---

1 Institute of Nuclear Medicine, The Middlesex Hospital Medical School, London, UK

Nuclear Medicine in Clinical Oncology
Ed. by C. Winkler
© Springer-Verlag Berlin Heidelberg 1986

on X-ray CT, yet the law of diminishing returns (cost vs. benefits) will be seen to apply. Ever-present all-embracing technology occurs however (even in our Western world) in only the largest and more advanced of medical institutions. A recent survey of equipment in the UK showed the following NMR/X-ray CT/Anger gamma camera ratio: 1:20:30; and the relative costs of these investigations are: 7:5:1.

What can we expect then from modern radionuclide imaging of the brain. With planar imaging, frontal tumours have been detected in 77% of cases, parasagittal tumours in 93%, parietal tumours 89% − 94%, and temporal tumours in 81% of all cases [2]. Invasive procedures, such as arteriography and air encephalography, fare no better in the detection of parasagittal or parietal tumour. In occipital tumours, radionuclide brain scanning and arteriography had similar detection accuracies (92% and 86% respectively). Whilst the highest accuracy of radionuclide brain scanning has been achieved with sphenoid wing meningioma (100%), the worst detection rate is seen in pontine tumours (25%) [2].

With tomographic imaging, several groups have shown an improvement in the detection sensitivity of primary and secondary neoplasms.

In 1980, three interesting reports compared for the first time, SPECT and X-ray transmission computed tomography (CT). The first of these three published studies by Ell et al. [3] compared emission and transmission tomography of the brain in 209 patients. Concordant results were obtained in 169 patients (81%). CT yielded an overall false-positive rate of 0.5% and a false-negative rate of 6%. SPECT yielded a false-positive rate of 0% and a false-negative rate of 2.4% for malignant disease and of 10% for vascular disease (owing to the nonvisualisation of old infarction and cases of non-impaired blood-brain barrier). The rates of detection of recent vascular disease with emission and transmission tomography were identical. For the total population studied, and in comparison with planar scintigraphy, the authors noted an improvement of reporting SPECT data in 20% of all cases, this figure including added sensitivity, improved lesion localisation, and, consequently, reporting performance.

Hill et al. [4] published later in the same year a similar comparison between SPECT and CT. Two hundred patients were investigated, SPECT showing a gain of 10% over and above the sensitivity achieved with planar scintigraphy. Improved specificity was seen with SPECT, often in the indiscrimination with depth of lesions superimposed onto the same planar view.

Surprisingly, Watson et al. [5] in the same year, in a study involving 238 patients, and again comparing SPECT with planar scintigraphy, achieved no significiant improvement with the use of SPECT, although in 80% of all cases there was agreement between these two imaging techniques. In this study only 102 out of the 238 patients had CT data available for comparison. This is the one study where SPECT appeared not to offer a significant and measurable benefit in terms of added sensitivity and specificity. It clearly stands in contrast to the work published by Kuhl, Carril and Ell, and Hill and the experience of most groups working in the field. Biersack et al. [6], utilising a rotating Auger gamma camera system, confirmed the general impression of improvement in reporting performance of brain scintigraphy when section scans were added for inspection.

SPECT of the brain appears to be a promising technique in the investigation of patients with a suspected primary or secondary lesion of this organ. Most centres working in the field have confirmed the merits of section imaging of the brain, with direct improvement on reporting performance. In some centres [3] radionuclide tomography of the brain has replaced conventional planar scintigraphy and has been employed as a routine tool for over 7 years. With the increased availability of tomographic instrumentation, it is predictable that more and more centres will offer this methodology as a clinical service. In the diagnosis of primary or secondary malignant involvement of the brain, SPECT is a definite improvement over planar brain scanning.

Monitoring

New methodologies are emerging with a view to characterise the functional behaviour of an intracranial mass. Positron emission tomography leads in this aim, with a number of interesting observations availabe up to date. In a study involving X-ray CT, C-11-methionine and F-18-fluorodeoxy-glucose, 19 patients were subjected to stereotaxic biopsies to improve localisation and histology assessment [7]. The C-11-methionine scan was superior to all other methods in tumour localisation in almost all patients. Tumour tissue was not found outside the methionine accumulation area in any patient at time of biopsy or surgery. C-11-methionine can show up tumour which is not contrasted or enhanced on CT and hence difficult to distinguish from surrounding oedema (an issue not as yet resolved by NMR CT). C-11-methionine scans appear to reflect more faithfully the true extent of a glioma than X-ray CT. This has been found to be of value in radiotherapy planning of these patients.

Conventional treatment of malignant glioma (surgery and/or irradiation therapy) is remarkably unsuccessful − only 5% of patients are alive after 18

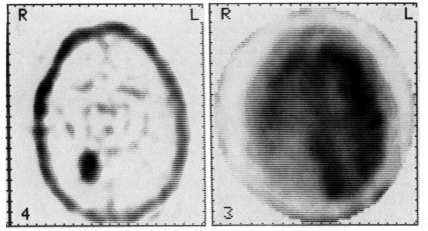

Fig. 1. a ECT Tumor-Delineation with ^{99m}TcO$_4$; **b** ^{123}I-IMP image of this case

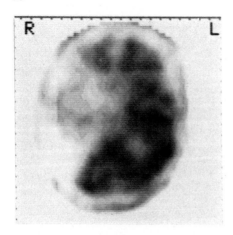

Fig. 2. ECT image performed with ^{99m}Tc-HMPAO (see text)

months. Nitrosurea derivatives such as BCUN have shown promise but its mode of action, breakdown and pharmacokinetics remain largely unknown. Positron emission tomography has a unique place in the investigation of drug behaviour in man and progress is expected in this area [8].

Brain tumours have a profound influence on regional cerebral blood flow (rCBF). In the tumour site, rCBF is generally reduced 20% − 70%. With positron emission tomography, also with the new single photon emission tomographic methodologies, this effect can be identified and measured. A single metastasis in the brain can lead to significant ischaemia in the homolateral cerebrum, and in addition, can cause hyperaemia to the contralateral side of the brain (Fig. 1). Whilst rCBF tomographic maps have been available for some time, it is only now that a truly widely available methodology for rCBF imaging in man is emerging. We demonstrate one of our first 99m-Tc based rCBF studies in man [9] (Fig. 2).

Conclusion

Nuclear medicine continues to provide significant and important information in patients with brain tumours. Nuclear medicine has still a role to play in the detection of this pathology and progress is expected in the general area of monitoring, individual tumour and patient assessment, drug treatment and follow up.

References

1. Weatherall DJ, Ledingham JGG, Warrell DA (eds) (1983) Oxford textbook of medicine, vol 2. Oxford University Press, Oxford, pp 21 − 24
2. George RO, Wagner HN Jr (1975) Ten years of brain tumour scanning at John Hopkins: 1962 − 1972. In: DeBlanc HS, Sorenson JA (eds) Non-invasive brain imaging. Society of Nuclear Medicine

3. Ell PJ, Deacon JM, Ducassou D, Brendel A (1980) Emission and transmission brain tomography. Br Med J 280:438–440
4. Hill T, Lovett RD, McNeil BJ (1980) Observations on the clinical value of emission tomography. J Nucl Med 21:613–616
5. Watson NE, Cowan RJ, Ball MR, Moody DM, Lastee DW, Maynard CD (1980) A comparison of brain imaging with gamma camera, single photon emission computed tomography and transmission computed tomography. J Nucl Med 21:507–511
6. Biersack HJ, Knopp R, Wappenschmidt J, Winkler C (1981) Single photon emission computer-Tomographie des Hirns mit einer rotierenden Gamma Camera – Ergebnisse bei 471 Patienten. Nucl Compact 12:130–134
7. Ericson K, Bergstrom M, Blomquist G, Collins VP, Ehrin E, Eriksson L, von Holst H, Lilja A, Lundquist H, Langstrom B, Mosskin M (1984) Positron emission tomography (PET) using 11-C-Methionine in the examination of intracranial tumours. In: Schmidt, Vauramo (eds) Nuklearmedizin. Schattauer, Stuttgart
8. Yamamoto YL, Diksic M, Sako K, Arita N, Feindel W, Thompson C-J (1983) Pharmacokinetic and metabolic studies in human malignant glioma. In: Magistretti PL (ed) Functional radionuclide imaging of the brain. Raven, New York
9. Ell PJ, Cullum I, Costa DC et al. (1985) Regional cerebral blood flow mapping with a new Tc-99m-labelled compound. Lancet II:50–51

Noncontact Eye Tumor Imaging with a Gamma Camera

H. Bockslaff[1] and D. Ducassou

In diagnostic ophthalmology, the P-32 uptake test is a present standard nuclear procedure to detect intraocular melanoma [1]. However, the physical properties of P-32 present some evident drawbacks, such as counting problems as well as increase of the risk of metastatic spread due to mechanical manipulation of a potentially tumor-bearing eye [2]. Thus, an alternative technique of modern nuclear medicine would be welcome. The use of gamma-emitting labelled compounds affords a noncontact and atraumatic technique for the detection of intraocular tumors [3].

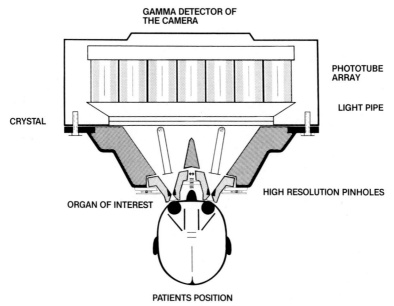

Fig. 1. Cross-section of the twin pinhole eye collimator (TPEC) coupled to a gamma camera detector head. Optimized Mark II/1978 collimator design. Two high-resolution pinholes (*arrow*) close to the objects (*eyes*) project the intraocular structures in magnification technique onto the detector crystal. The distance between the two pinhole planes can be freely adjusted according to the individual interpupillary distance of the patient.

---

1 Städt. Krankenanstalten Bielefeld-Mitte, Röntgen- u. Strahlenklinik, Oelmühlenstraße 26, D-4800 Bielefeld 1

Nuclear Medicine in Clinical Oncology
Ed. by C. Winkler
© Springer-Verlag Berlin Heidelberg 1986

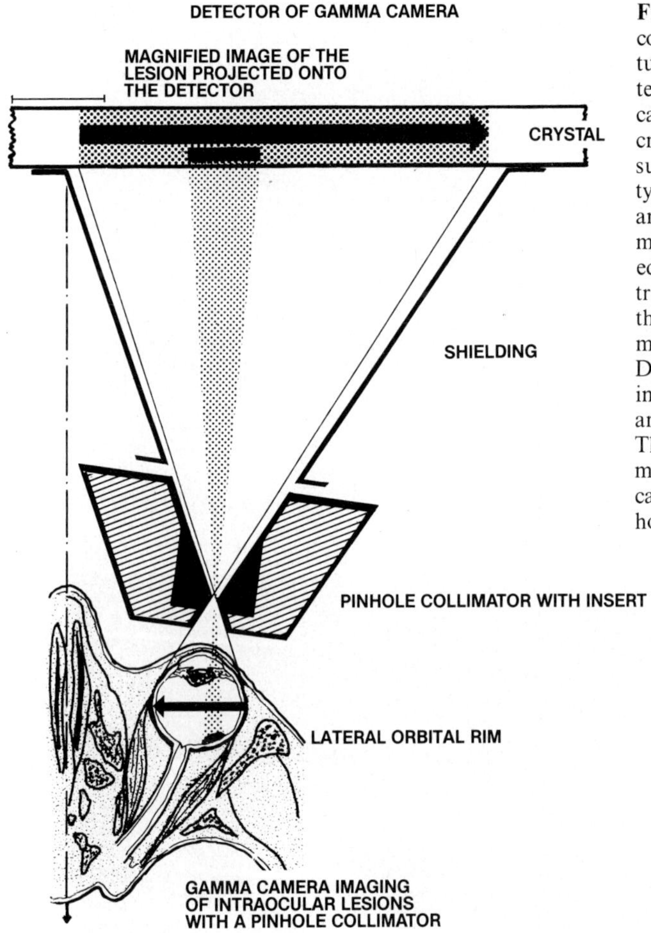

DETECTOR OF GAMMA CAMERA

MAGNIFIED IMAGE OF THE
LESION PROJECTED ONTO
THE DETECTOR

CRYSTAL

SHIELDING

PINHOLE COLLIMATOR WITH INSERT

LATERAL ORBITAL RIM

GAMMA CAMERA IMAGING
OF INTRAOCULAR LESIONS
WITH A PINHOLE COLLIMATOR

Fig. 2. Right eye of a patient with its corresponding pinhole. The eye structures are imaged on one-half the detector crystal. A large field of view camera with its $d = 600$ mm detector crystal gives about 300 mm detector surface for the imaging of each eye. A typical eye globe measures between 28 and 30 mm in diameter. Thus the geometric magnification can be calculated as 1 : 10. The impact of a small intraocular lesion measures 30 mm on the detector crystal if the lesion itself measures only 3 mm in length. Note: Due to pinhole imaging the image is inverted; nasal structures of the eye are imaged laterally and vice versa. This contrast to parallel hole collimator imaging is important for the localisation and interpretation of pinhole images

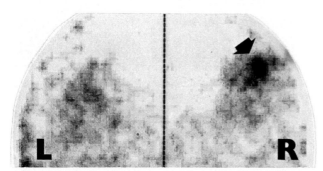

L   R

Fig. 3. Example of a scintiphoto of the eyes imaged with I-131 ICQ (iodochloroquine). Clear accumulation in the right eye (*arrow*). The tumor itself is located in the nasal, caudal segment of the globe. See inversion of scintiphotos by pinhole imaging. The accumulation is situated in the temporal, cranial segment of the scintiphoto. Histologically proven pigmented malignant melanoma of the right eye. (Case study, courtesy Prof. Blanquet, Bordeaux)

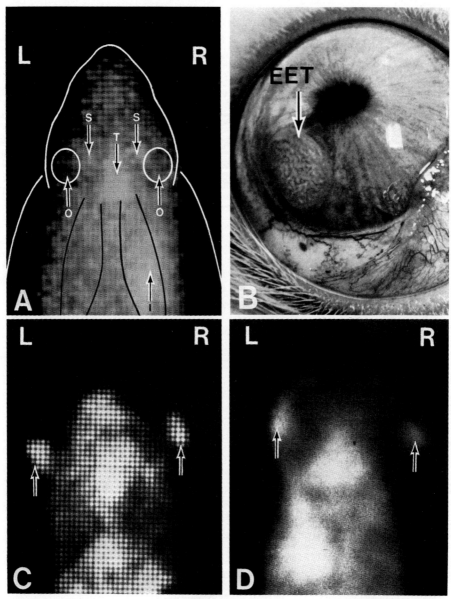

Fig. 4A − D. Evaluation of the imaging potential of the newly designed melanoma seeking compound IMT on experimental eye tumor bearing rabbits [15]. **A** Control. Normal animal, no tumor in the eyes. Rabbits skull imaged in vertex view. Scintiphoto taken with a monopinhole collimator 75 min after i.v. injection of IMT. No accumulation in orbitae. Radioactivity in thyroid, salivary glands and injection site. *I,* injection site, right ear; *O,* orbitae; *S,* salivary gland; *T,* thyroid. **B** Close-up view of rabbit eye. An experimental amelanotic melanoma is implanted into the anterior chamber of the eye. *EET,* experimental eye tumor. **C** K 59-treated scintiphoto of rabbit 90 min after injection. Both tumors clearly visible (*arrows*). Some radioactivity in thyroid and salivary glands (see **A**). Macroscopy, both eyes: Melanoma in the anterior chamber, some necrotic areas and bleedings. Tumor weight right, 750 mg, tumor weight left, 710 mg. **D** K 33-treated scintiphoto of rabbit 60 min after injection. Experimental melanoma in left eye clearly detectable, tumor in right eye slightly (*arrows*). Radioactivity also visible in thyroid and injection site left ear. Necroscopy not performed. Macroscopic inspection before imaging experiment. EET left, about 400 mg; EET right, about 100 mg

Eye scintigraphy (ES) is performed with a special twin pinhole eye collimator coupled to a gamma camera and a data processing device. Pinhole collimators with intrinsic magnification properties provide the best trade-off between geometric resolution (2 mm) and geometric efficiency for small target organs such as eyes [4]. This collimator design is the tool of choice for eye scintigraphy. Since the target structures are extremely small, i.e., eye tumors weighing 50−500 mg, parallel-hole collimators are obsolete [5].

The choice of radiopharmaceuticals for use in nuclear ophthalmology has been oriented by the selectivity of labelled quinoline derivatives for melanin pigment structures of malignant melanoma [6−9]. We have used such labelled compounds for years. The best results in clinical application have been obtained with I-131 or I-123 iodochloroquine (ICQ).

Metal isotopes have also been investigated for application in nuclear ophthalmology. Tc-99m pertechnetate has not been found very useful for eye scintigraphy, with the exception of breast cancer metastasis to the eye [4]. Interesting results came from the studies of Packer and colleagues on Ga-67 citrate and Pb-203 Tris [10]. Here, the laboratory evaluation revealed favorable tumor uptake data and tumor-to-background ratios for eye tumor detection.

Recently, labelled precursors of melanin bioformation have been investigated to develop a new approach for a melanoma-seeking compound, i.e., L-3-I-123-a-methylthyrosine (IMT) [11]. In vivo biodistribution studies on Syrian golden hamsters bearing experimental melanoma showed a rather useful accumulation ratio of 1.6% dose/g tumor tissue for IMT. Another advantage of this compound is its concentration in both pigmented as well as in nonpigmented malignant melanoma tissue. The radiopharmacological behavior of IMT is in striking contrast to that of ICQ, which does not accumulate in amelanotic melanoma [12−14]. In vivo imaging experiments on New Zealand rabbits bear-

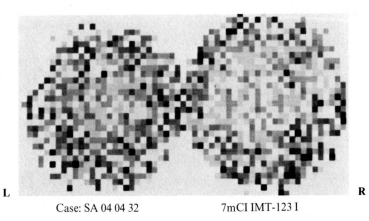

L Case: SA 04 04 32   7mCI IMT-123 I   R

Fig. 5. Normal scintiphotos of the eyes recorded 120 min after i.v. application of 7 mCi IMT. Homogenous distribution of radioactivity in the field of view of each pinhole representing only background radioactivity from adjacent anatomical structures of the skull. Clinically, no evidence of a malignant eye melanoma

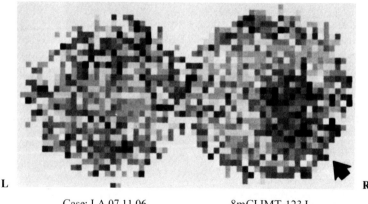

Case: LA 07 11 06   8mCI IMT-123 I

Fig. 6. Abnormal eye scintiphoto. Distinct accumulation of IMT in the caudal, lateral segment of the scintiphoto right eye, i.e., tumor in caudal, nasal segment. Histologically confirmed malignant melanoma of spherical shape in the posterior pole of right eye. Tumor weight, 1200 mg

ing experimental intraocular melanoma of the nonpigmented Greene-Harvey line in the anterior chamber of the rabbit eyes documented the detectability of scant intraocular tumors weighing from 800 mg to 100 mg [15]. A first clinical trial restricted to 10 patients revealed the clinical usefulness of the new compound [16].

Since choroidal melanoma is the most frequently occurring intraocular tumor, a tracer for eye scintigraphy must essentially have melanoma-seeking properties. Up till now, the best radiopharmaceuticals for this purpose seem to be ICQ or IMT. The present state of investigation, especially in the context of clinical application, does not allow final judgement between these two compounds. The choice of an appropriate radiopharmaceutical is still open for discussion. For the near future and depending on the acceptance of ES by eye hospitals, we suggest a consecutive double isotope strategy of:

1. Use of an easily available, more general tumor-seeking compound such as Ga-67 citrate
2. In the case of a positive result of the first diagnostic investigation, a second study with a more specific melanoma-seeking compound such as ICQ or, perhaps better, IMT

In summary, eye scintigraphy (ES) contributes to the atraumatic detection of intraocular tumors and can be proposed as a clinical tool for the management of intraocular lesions such as choroidal melanoma and others. The further use of the radiotracer P-32 for diagnostic purposes must be avoided because of its intolerably high radiation burden to the critical organ, i.e., the bone marrow [17].

References

1. Hagler WS, Jarret WH, Hamphrey WT (1970) Radioactive phosphorus uptake test in the diagnosis of uveal melanoma. Arch Ophthalmol 83:548−557
2. Fraunfelder FT, Boozman FW, Wilson RS, Thomas AH (1977) Notouch technique for intraocular malignant melanoma. Arch ophthalmol 95:1616−1620
3. Safi N, Blanquet P (1973) Apport des molécules marquées au diagnostic et à la surveillance des tumeurs mélaniques. Biomed Express 19:122−125
4. Bockslaff H, Dausch D, Bornemann H, Stöppler L, Hundeshagen H (1979) Noncontact detection of eye melanoma by means of a gamma camera. Graefes Arch Clin Exp Ophthalmol 211:187−203
5. Blanquet P, Safi N (1981) Nuclear medical ophthalmology with special regard to modern test substances − present status and future. In: Schmidt HAE, Wolf F, Mahlstedt J (eds) Nuclear medicine with its interdependencies. Schattauer, Stuttgart, pp 816−839
6. Boyd CM, Beierwaltes H, Liebermann LM, Bergström TJ (1971) I-125 labelled chloroquine analog in the diagnosis of ocular melanoma. J Nucl Med 12:601−605
7. Safi N, Blanquet P, Verin PH (1973) La scintigraphie oculaire. IAEA SM 164/237:497−518
8. Blanquet P, Safi N, Basse-Cathalinat B, Ducassou D, Verin PH (1975) Radionuclidic exploration in ophthalmology. Int J Nucl Med Biol 6:165−173
9. Packer S, Redvanly C, Lamprecht RM, Wolf AP, Atkins HL (1975) Quinoline analog labeled with iodine-123 in melanoma detection. Arch Ophthalmol 93:504−508
10. Packer S, Lamprecht RM, Christman DR, Ansari AN, Wolf AP, Atkins HL (1977) Metal isotopes used as radioactive indicators of ocular melanoma. AM J Ophthalmol 83:80−94
11. Bockslaff H, Kloster G, Stöcklin G, Safi N, Bornemann H (1980) Studies on L-3-I-123-iodo-a-methyltyrosine: a new potential melanoma seeking compound. In: Schmidt HAE, Ricca-Bona C (eds) Clinical significance of nuclear medicine. Schattauer, Stuttgart, pp 179−182
12. Bockslaff H, Kloster G, Safi N, Blanquet P (1980) L-3-I-123-iodo-a-methyltyrosine or 6-I-131/123-iodochloroquine as imaging agents for the detection of malignant melanoma: a comparative study on tumor bearing Syrian golden hamsters. In: Höfer R, Bergmann H (eds) Radioaktive Isotope in Klinik und Forschung. Egermann, Vienna 14:171−178
13. Lindquist NG (1973) Accumulation of drugs on melanin. ACTA Radiol [Suppl] (Stockh) 325:1−92
14. Kloster G, Bockslaff H (1982) L-3-123 I-alpha-methyltyrosine detection: a comparative evaluation. Int J Nucl Med Biol 9:259−269
15. Bockslaff H, Spitznas M, Hahn I, Kloster G (1981) Noncontact detection of small size experimental amelanotic ocular melanoma with L-3-I-123-iodo-methyltyrosine. Albrecht v. Graefes Archiv Klin Exp Ophthalmol 217:255−266
16. Bockslaff H, Kloster G, Dausch D, Schad K, Hundeshagen H, Stöcklin G (1982) IMT as imaging agent for the noncontact detection of intraocular melanoma − a first clinical evaluation. Graefes Archiv Klin Exp Ophthalmol 219:149−154
17. Weinreich R, Bockslaff H (1983) Radiation doses to the eye lens from ocular tumour seeking radiopharmaceuticals. Eur J Nucl Med 8:127−130
18. Bornemann H, Dausch D, Gröne WD, Geisler H, Creutzig B, Knoop W, Michelson H, Bockslaff H, Hundeshagen H (1980) Digitale Sequenz-Szintigraphie bei Augenerkrankungen. In: Schmidt HAE, Riccabona G (eds) Nuklearmedizin. Schattauer, Stuttgart, pp 873−876
19. Gröne WD (1982) Digitale Szintigraphie des Auges, Entwicklung einer Methode. Med. Dissertation, Hannover

Clinical Aspects of Detection and Imaging of Differentiated Thyroid Tumors

J. FRÜHLING[1]

Thyroid cancer, especially the differentiated kind, is one of the most popular subjects in the oncological literature. Moreover, this disease is one of the "favorite children" of nuclear medicine for evident historical reasons: the administration of 131-I for diagnostic and therapeutic reasons has for more than 40 years been strongly involved in the management of thyroid cancer, which therefore is among the first diseases where nuclear medicine has assumed a decisive role as a distinct speciality.

The number of papers concerning differentiated thyroid cancer is rather high, but the results published are often contradictory, and for this reason it is extremely difficult to identify in this material and to extract from it those coherent results which could be considered as something like a "greatest common denominator." This fact is due to the following basic problems:

1. Variation in the histological classification (which has been developing rapidly for the past 15 years)
2. Uncertainty in the field of clinical staging (whenever a system should be considered as recognized definitively by significant groups of clinicians at all)
3. The clinical material exposed is nearly always arranged and analyzed according to different and divergent criteria and principles
4. The representatives of several medical specialties (surgery, endocrinology, radiology, medical oncology, nuclear medicine, radiation therapy) are involved in the management of thyroid neoplasms, with all their often subjective preferences
5. The prognosis of the disease being reasonably good, nearly all published series present survival rates which are satisfactory, despite differences in the diagnostic and therapeutic approach
6. For this last reason, and because the incidence of this neoplastic disease is not very high, there are at present no publications concerning large randomized series which would take into consideration all the important diagnostic and therapeutic variables
7. Our knowledge is developing rapidly (e.g., appearance of new diagnostic methods such as NMR, 201-Tl whole-body scintigraphy, extension of the use of echography, introduction of prognostic factors as guidelines for thera-

---

1 Institut Jules Bordet, Centre des Tumeurs de l'Université Libre de Bruxelles, Brussels, Belgium

Nuclear Medicine in Clinical Oncology
Ed. by C. Winkler
© Springer-Verlag Berlin Heidelberg 1986

Table 1. Differentiated thyroid carcinoma: controversies

- Prognostic factors
- Preoperative evaluation
- Postoperative ablative 131-I-dosis
- Follow-up: – 131-I whole body scintigraphy
  – Use of 201-TL-scintigraphy
  – Role of thyroglobulin
  – T4 withdrawal
- Extent of surgery
- External radiotherapy
- 131-I treatment

Table 2. Use of diagnostic nuclear medicine as function of tumor histology

Histology	Prevalence (%)	Diagnostic Nuclear medicine contribution
A. Differentiated carcinoma	75–80	Preoperative
1. Follicular	15–40	
a) Well-differentiated		Postoperative
b) Moderately differentiated (trabecular)		
2. Papillary	33–80	Follow-up
B. Medullary	5– 6	Pre- and postoperative
C. Anaplastic	± 15	Preoperative
D. Metastatic	<0.1	Preoperative

peutic policy) making more complex the evaluation of old as well as recent data in the literature. (Table 1 demonstrates the most important controversial problems and challenges in the field of diagnosis and treatment of thyroid cancer where the contributions of nuclear medicine are concerned.)

The aim of this paper is to summarize the role of nuclear medical imaging in the diagnostic management of differentiated thyroid cancer according to the different stages of the natural history of this disease: pretreatment diagnosis, post-treatment phase, and follow-up.

The basis of all therapeutic and diagnostic interventions is the histological classification of thyroid tumors. Despite the newest developments in the field of cytochemistry and electron microscopy, the main subdivision into three groups remains without serious contestation (see Table 2). Table 2 also demonstrates that the role of nuclear medicine is determined by the histology of the tumor. This speciality plays a preponderant role in the management of differentiated thyroid carcinoma, but the contribution of isotopic techniques is relatively limited in the case of nondifferentiated tumors (constituting one-sixth of all cases), especially in the postoperative and follow-up phase. For these cancers, the main contribution of nuclear medicine concerns even the preoperative phase, when in

Table 3. Contributions of nuclear medicine in differentiated thyroid carcinoma

A. *Preoperative phase*

  Scintigraphy (123-I, 131-I, 99m-Tc, 201-Tl, 67-Ga)
  Functional test
  RIA

B. *Postoperative Phase*

  Functional test
  Scintigraphy
  Ablative 131-I-therapy

C. *Follow-up*

  Thyroglobulin determination
  131-I-retention measurement
  Whole body scintigraphy (131-I, 201-Tl)
  Bone scintigraphy (99m-Tc-MDP)
  Radioimmunoscintigraphy
  131-I-therapy

Table 4. The thyroid nodule: preoperative evaluation

Mandatory
  1. Clinical history (symptoms, delay)
  2. Physical examination (size, number, consistency)
  3. Scintigraphy: 99m-Tc, 123-I, 131-I, 201-Tl, 67-Ga: size localization, contrast
                 (hypo-, iso-, hyperactive)
  4. Functional evaluation: clinical, biological ("uptake;" RIA)
  5. Sonography (solid or cystic)
  6. Fine-needle aspiration biopsy
  7. CT-scanning
  8. Tentative treatment (T3 or T4)

Table 5. Scintigraphy

Advantages	Disadvantages	Controversies

• Functional imaging
• Physiological tracer
• Dynamic test possible
• Characteristic finding
• ±35 years general experience
	• Resolution
	• Two dimensions only
	• Anatomic localization
	  (moving patient)
	• Radiation exposure
		• Product:
		Thyroid-specific
		  Trapping: 99m-Tc
		  Fixation: iodine
		"Tu-specific:" 201-Tl, 67-Ga
		• Apparatus:
		Rect. scanner
		γ-Camera
		  Collimator (PH, or par.)
		  SPECT
		• Method:
		X-Ray fluorescent scanning

most cases the histological diagnosis and, consequently, the diagnostic policy and prognostic factors are still unknown.

Table 3 summarizes the different interventions of nuclear medicine, particularly in the case of differentiated cancer of the thyroid gland. As shown, these contributions can concern therapeutic and diagnostic problems, in vivo or in vitro techniques, and they can be related to functional evaluation. Some among them are mandatory, some remain optional. In each case, their use must be adapted to the given phase of the cancerous disease.

Table 4 presents the main diagnostic methods which should be used in order to realize the complete evaluation of the thyroid nodule, which is the usual substrate of the nontreated thyroid cancer. The first five points considered as "mandatory" constitute a kind of "greatest common denominator," extracted from the literature. In Table 5, we tried to reassemble the main characteristics of the most important isotopic diagnostic tool in the evaluation of the thyroid nodule, the scintigraphy. The advantages of this diagnostic tool, as indicated in the left column, are generally recognized, the main disadvantages being the limited physical resolution, mainly when nodules of the deeper regions have to be examined. Controversies about scintigraphy are summarized in the right column, and are related to the choice of the isotope, to its specificity, and to the detecting apparatus being used.

As mentioned already, the main or often unique substrate of thyroid cancer is the thyroid nodule, often solitary. As far as the correlation between preoperative scintigraphic findings and postoperative anatomopathologic results is concerned, there is an important scatter in the published values. According to earlier papers (published between 1955 and 1969) 14% to 44% of scintigraphically hypoactive ("cold") nodules corresponded to a verified thyroid cancer. This is presumably due to different clinical selections before the scintigraphic examination and probably to the selective follow-up of the histologically verified cases. We have tried to summarize the most recent results published (or compiled) in the literature [1, 9, 10, 11, 14] and our own observations according to two criteria: 1. Substrate/cancer ratio, meaning what percentage of proven cancerours cases corresponded clinically to a solitary nodule or scintigraphically to a "cold" nodule before surgery 2. Cancer/nodule ratio corresponding to the percentage of nodules which were finally identified as proven cancerous cases. Based on the values obtained on substrate/cancer ratios, the published results are quite homogeneous: 66% to 80.5% of the histologically verified thyroid cancers corresponded before surgery to a clinically solitary nodule, and more than two thirds of these patients presented a scintigraphically hypoactive nodule. The recent results on cancer/nodule ratios confirm the wide distribution of findings encountered in the older papers: 1.3% to 37.5% of the patients presenting a clinically solitary nodule had had thyroid cancer as a final morphological diagnosis and 0.4% to 28.1% among those exhibiting a scintigraphic "cold" nodule. Nevertheless, and our observations also seem to indicate this, when the selection criteria are standardized, the results become more constant and proportional. Thus, the scatter of cancer/nodule ratios is diminished, when only faster growing nodules with high consistency and a diameter greater than 2.5 cm are concerned.

Table 6. Other imaging methods

Echography	CT-Scan	NMR
• Resolution • No radiation exposure • Solid/cystic differences • Real-time exam.	• Resolution • Anatomic image • Morphological referencing technique • True extension, if + for carcinoma	• Imaging + spectrometry unifying the advantages of scingigraphy and CT, moreover in vivo biochemical analysis possible
• No specific carcinoma diagnosis	• Radiation exposure • Contrast product • Social cost	• Common experience still lacking • Technical problems of in vivo spectrometry

Table 7. Differentiated thyroid carcinoma: postoperative evaluation

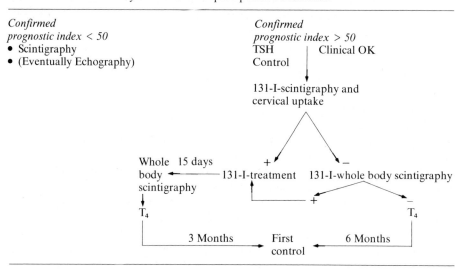

Confirmed prognostic index < 50
• Scintigraphy
• (Eventually Echography)

Confirmed prognostic index > 50
TSH | Clinical OK
Control

131-I-scintigraphy and cervical uptake

Whole 15 days body scintigraphy ← 131-I-treatment   131-I-whole body scintigraphy

T₄   T₄

3 Months   First control   6 Months

Table 8. Differentiated thyroid carcinoma: follow-up

I. Good prognostic index
(no total thyroidectomy, no 131-I treatment!)

Under T_4!

Each 6th, later 12th month: clinical examination, thorax X-ray,
thyroglobuline, complete hematologic examination,
99m Tc-MDP bone scintigraphy
(not mandatory: 201-Tl-scintigraphy)

Until suspicion, or evidence of locoregional nodal relapse,
or metastatic dissemination

Table 6 presents a cursory analysis of the contributions of other medical imaging techniques involved in the evaluation of the thyroid nodule, with their main advantages and disadvantages. Thus, we should keep in mind that ultrasound, currently increasing in popularity, possesses two main advantages (physical resolution, consistency discrimination), but lacks a specific substrate for cancer identification. CT scan is rarely considered as a routine method for thyroid investigation, but nevertheless can often be very useful, especially when preoperative locoregional involvement is suspected. NMR imaging, coupled with spectral analysis will surely be one of the most interesting methods, as soon as industry is able to furnish an apparatus capable of realizing during the same investigation sequence proton imaging and in vivo spectroscopic analysis. Although not a medical imaging technique, fine needle biopsy can play an important role in the preoperative evaluation of thyroid nodules. Responsible for a certain amount of patient discomfort, fine needle biopsy is an extreme method with a high false-negative rate when the findings are negative. On the other hand, positive findings are a proof of the diagnosis [13].

One of the most interesting evolutions in the field of thyroid cancer management is the introduction of the notion of prognostic factors − clinical (age, sex), biological, and histological − as determined by a basic EORTC study [5] and confirmed by some other authors [6, 8, 9, 12]. These factors actually fundamentally influence our therapeutic and diagnostic policy. Thus, as far as the surgical act is concerned these factors determine the choice between total thyroidectomy or limited surgery, the latter being applied in our institution when the prognostic index is inferior to 50. The prognostic index influences diagnostic and therapeutic considerations also after surgery. As demonstrated in Table 7, after restricted surgery the postoperative intervention of nuclear medical imaging is quite minimal, consisting of the evaluation of the remaining thyroid volume. The contrast is important in comparison with the algorithm presented on the right half of the same table. This scheme, compiled from the literature, shows the intensive utilization of nuclear medicine techniques in the diagnostic evaluation and adjuvant therapy of differentiated thyroid carcinoma during the postoperative phase when the prognostic index is equal to or higher than 50 [1−4, 11].

As mentioned already, prognostic factors have a major influence on diagnostic and therapeutic policy during the follow-up period as far as the nature, frequency, and complexity of the different control examinations are concerned. Table 8 presents recommendations for the follow-up when the prognostic index is favorable. In this case, the contribution of nuclear medicine is limited to the use of an in vitro technique (thyreoglobulin RIA) and of a nonthyroid-specific visualization method (99m-Tc-MDP bone scintigraphy). Table 9 summarizes the aspects involved in the follow-up of differentiated thyroid carcinoma, when the prognostic index is considered to be poor. The different control examinations and their relation to nuclear medicine are presented, as well as whether substitutive therapy must be withdrawn or not, which is currently one of the main controversies. Among the investigations cited in this table, radioimmunoscintigraphy is theoretically attractive, but decisive clinical justification for this recently introduced scintigraphic technique is still lacking in daily prac-

Table 9. Differentiated thyroid carcinoma: follow-up

II. Poor prognostic index
(total thyroidectomy followed, or not by 131-I-treatment)

Under T_4!

Control examinations:

Non isotopic	Isotopic, nonspecific			Isotopic, specific
	Mandatory	Optional		
• Clinical evaluation	• TG	• Other tu-	• 201-Tl	• 131-I
• Thorax X-ray	• CEA	markers	whole body	whole body
• Complete hematology	• Bone scan	• Radioimmuno-	scintigraphy	scintigraphy
• Blood chemistry		scintigraphy		• 131-I
• CT-scan				whole body
(optional)				measurement
				(• TG)
	Without T_4 withdrawal			T_4 Withdrawal

tice. 201-Tl whole-body scintigraphy is possibly the most contributive clinical acquisition since the introduction of thyreoglobuline-RIA. This contribution of nuclear medicine [7] offers a valuable alternative to 131-I whole-body scintigraphy with the major advantage that the test can be carried out under substitutive hormone therapy. Nevertheless, we need large confirmative clinical series before recommending 201-T1 whole-body scintigraphy without restriction as a routine replacement for the same examination using radioactive iodine. As far as the 131-I retention measurement by means of a whole-body counter is concerned, its contribution to whole-body scintigraphy in the follow-up is rather complementary. According to our own results, obtained from 100 examinations performed on 40 patients (with 2% retention after 72 h as the normal limit for retention of 131-I in a thyroidectomized patient), in at least 20% of the cases there was a discrepancy in the results of 131-I whole-body scintigraphy and iodine retention measurement, the correction introduced by the morphological technique being more often the correct one.

When the prognostic index is poor, the intervals in the control investigations should be organized according to the following scheme:

1. Three months after postoperative treatment
2. Six months after each therapeutic 131-I-dosis
3. Each 6th month during the first 2 years even in cases of remission
4. Each 12th, later 18th month from the 3rd year of the follow-up in absence of nodal relapse or generalization

Naturally, interval, application of the different examination methods and modification of the treatment are functions of the main clinical situation-possibilities, which can be schematically presented as follows:

1. Remission: see recommendations in the previous paragraph
2. Locoregional relapse: treatment by surgery (neck dissection) and by high dose of 131-I after whole-body scintigraphy, followed by external radiotherapy (if not carried out previously)
3. Metastatic dissemination: treatment by 131-I, if proven, completed by local external radiotherapy, if necessary (bone metastases); chemotherapy, if other therapeutic possibilities are exhausted

As a final conclusion for this so well-known and so controversial field of nuclear medicine, we can only recommend the old latin proverb: *quidquid agis, prudenter agas et respice finem,* which means that instead of presenting a complicated algorithm with strong recommendations, we believe that each specialist should carry out the management of differentiated thyroid cancer according to the best of his conscience and knowledge, the clinical status of the patient, the technical possibilities of his institution, and the recommendations submitted above.

References

1. Altenbrunn H-J (1984) Die nuklearmedizinische Diagnostik der Schilddrüsenmalignome einschließlich der Metastasendiagnostik. In: Altenbrunn H-J (ed) Fortschritte der Onkologie. 12. Nuklearmedizinische Diagnostik maligner Tumoren. Akademie Verlag, Berlin, pp 33−58
2. Beierwaltes WH (1978) The treatment of thyroid carcinoma with radioactive iodine. Semin Nucl Med VIII:79−94
3. Biersack HJ et al. (1981) Zur Behandlung des Schilddrüsenkarzinoms. Dtsch Med Wochenschr 106:350−395
4. Blahd, WH (1979) Treatment of malignant thyroid disease. Semin Nucl Med IX:95−99
5. Byar DP et al. (1979) A prognostic index for thyroid carcinoma. A study of the EORTC Thyroid Cancer Cooperative Group. Eur J Cancer 15:1033−1041
6. Gemsenjäger E et al. (1985) Therapie des differenzierten Schilddrüsenkarzinoms. Schweiz Med Wochenschr 115:153−159
7. Hoefnagel CA et al. (1983) Usefulness of thallium-201 total body scintigraphy in postoperative thyroid carcinoma. In: Carpi A (ed) Clinical and pathological advances in thyroid tumors. ETS, Pisa (in press)
8. Ladurner D, Seeber G (1984) Das follikuläre Schilddrüsenkarzinom. (Eine multivariate Analyse). Schweiz Med Wochenschr 114:1087−1092
9. Mazzaferri EL (1981) Papillary and follicular thyroid cancer. Ann Rev Med 32:73−91
10. Molitch ME et al. (1984) The cold thyroid nodule: an analysis of diagnostic and therapeutic options. Endocr Rev 9:185−199
11. Rösler H, Walther E (1984) Die Strahlentherapie der Struma maligna. In: Heilmann H-P (ed) Radiation therapy of malignant tumors. Springer, Berlin Heidelberg New York Tokyo, Handbuch der medizinischen Radiologie vol 19, part 5, pp 1−87
12. Tubiana M et al. (1985) Long-term results and prognostic factors in patients with differentiated thyroid carcinoma. Cancer 55:794−804
13. Ramacciotti CE et al. (1984) Diagnostic accuracy and use of aspiration biopsy in the management of thyroid nodules. Arch Intern Med 144:1169−1174
14. Werk EE et al. (1984) Cancer in thyroid nodules. A community hospital survey. Arch Intern Med 144:474−476

Clinical Aspects of Detection and Imaging of Lung Tumors

C. SCHÜMICHEN[1]

For practical and logical reasons the imaging of lung tumors will be reviewed separately for primary and secondary lung malignancies.

Primary Lung Malignancy

Diagnosis of Bronchial Carcinoma

Carcinoma of the bronchus is the commonest cancer in men and has recently become the second commonest cancer in women. A tissue diagnosis can usually be made by fibre optic bronchoscopy or sputum cytology. With more peripheral tumors, a direct needle aspiration under fluoroscopy is a satisfactory way of establishing the diagnosis. In some cases, a mediastinoscopy or thoracotomy is required.

Perfusion/Ventilation Scan

Carcinoma of the bronchus may alter both ventilation and perfusion. These tumors appear as defects on perfusion scans. Small tumors less than 2.0 cm in diameter are usually not detected, unless they involve vessels at the hilum. The larger the perfusion defect in relation to the size of the tumor, the greater the involvement of the hilar vessels by tumor. Such involvement may be due to metastatic spread to the lymph nodes, direct invasion of the mediastinum, or, less commonly, invasion and thrombosis of the pulmonary veins or, more rarely still, of the pulmonary arteries. Ventilation defects depend on the degree of bronchial obstruction and are confined to the affected segment, lobe, or whole lung, when the tumor is in a main-stem bronchus. The defect in ventilation is often less than that of perfusion, because there is usually much greater extrabronchial spread of tumor than intrabronchial protrusion. Hence, bronchial carcinoma can produce a ventilation/perfusion mismatch and can thus mimic lung embolism. The results of regional ventilation and perfusion distribution in 1332 patients with suspected lung embolism and in 343 patients with bronchial carcinoma are compared in Tables 1 a + b. A perfusion defect larger than the

---

1 Abt. für klinische Nuklearmedizin, Medizinische Universitätsklinik, Hugstetter Straße 55, D-7800 Freiburg i. Br. 1

Table 1a. Ventilation/perfusion abnormalities in patients with suspected lung embolism. Ventilation measured by radio-aerosol. Results given in percent, n = 1332

		0	I	II	III	IV
	IV	0.05	0.08	0.03	0.18	**1.13**
	III	0.10	0.15	0.08	**1.60**	0.15
Ventilation Defect	II	0.20	0.53	**2.45**	0.05	0
	I	3.95	**20.6**	1.25	0.75	0.38
	0	**54.9**	4.85	3.40	1.85	1.30
		0	I	II	III	IV
				Perfusion Defect		

0, homogeneous; I, inhomogeneous; II, subsegment; III, segment; IV, lobe

Table 1b. Ventilation/perfusion abnormalities in patients with bronchogenic carcinoma. Ventilation measured by radio-aerosol. Results given in percent, n = 342

		0	I	II	III	IV
	IV	0	0.09	0	0.28	**9.05**
	III	0.18	0.38	0.09	**6.03**	0.58
Ventilation Defect	II	0.69	0.69	**3.98**	1.08	0.47
	I	2.91	**22.2**	1.56	1.27	1.17
	0	**42.5**	2.81	0.99	0.48	0.58
		0	I	II	III	IV
				Perfusion Defect		

0, homogeneous; I, inhomogeneous; II, subsegment; III, segment; IV, lobe

corresponding ventilation defect was found in 14% of patients with suspected lung embolism and in 11% of patients with bronchial carcinoma. Consequently, bronchial carcinoma is one of the most important differential diagnoses of lung embolism diagnosed by combined ventilation/perfusion imaging [1]. Occasionally, a ventilation/perfusion scan can localize the site of an otherwise occult carcinoma of the bronchus. The site may be indicated by localized disturbance of perfusion or ventilation or deposition of radioaerosol. Unfortunately the frequent coexistance of chronic bronchitis and emphysema, with their associated abnormalities of ventilation and perfusion, may make it impossible to determine which defect corresponds to the tumor.

Nonspecific Detection

A large number of radionuclides have been investigated in the hope that uptake in the tumor is specific for malignancy. Although a number of these radionuclides are taken up by malignant tissue, they also concentrate in acute inflammatory tissue and granulomatous tissue.

Ga-67 citrate. Positive Ga-67 scans are obtained in up to 96% of patients with untreated bronchial carcinoma (review of literature in [2]). In general, there is no dependence of Ga-67 accumulation on the histomorphological type of tumor. There is an absent or decreased Ga-67 uptake in more or less necrotic tumor masses. The use of Ga-67 as a tumor-imaging agent is limited because of its lack of tumor specificity and its inability to detect tumors smaller than 2 cm in diameter [2]. Ga-67 scanning is also a sensitive but nonspecific indicator of hilar and/or mediastinal spread of pulmonary tumors from the peripheral site. In the case that the primary tumor accummulates Ga-67, an unilateral hilar or mediastinal uptake of Ga-67 has a high specificity for tumor (94%), whereas bilateral hilar uptake is non-specific [3]. A negative Ga-67 study gives only a 67% probability of normal mediastinal nodes [4]. In combination with chest radiography, Ga-67 scanning may be used to select patients for mediastinoscopy [5].

Bleomycin and Others. Bleomycin, the A_2 fraction of choice, can be labeled with Cr-51, Co-57, In-111 (single photon), or with Co-55, Cu-64 (positron), but not with Tc-99m. With Cr-51 bleomycin lung tumors could be diagnosed with a sensitivity of 97% and a specificity of 79% by quantitative evaluation [6]. Sensitivity in detecting primary lung cancer with Tc-99m glucoheptonate was 91%, but detecting of mediastinal spread of lung cancer with Tc-99m glucoheptonate was not recommended because of its unacceptably high false-negative rate [7].

Immunodetection

Radioiodinated antibodies to tumor-associated antigens, such as carcinoembryonic antigen (CEA), alpha fetoprotein (AFP), and human chorionic gonadotropin (HCG), have been used clinically for the radioimmunodetection of lung cancer. However, the tumor to non-tumor ratio was low and the sensitivity of the method below 75% [8]. Tumor-specific monoclonal antibodies against lung cancer are available now [9], but also here new approaches for improving the tumor localization have to be found.

Radioiodinated peanut lectin, which has a strong binding affinity for the Thomsen-Friedenreich (T) antigen, exposed in reactive form on many human adenocarcinomata, proved to be a sensitive and specific agent for immunodetection in animal experiments. However, unsatisfactory results were obtained in humans due to a rapid in vivo breakdown of the agent [10].

A new approach in radioimmunodetection of malignant tumors is Tc-99 IMM (immunomodulator). The immunomodulator is extracted from the nocardia bacteria and can be labeled either with Tc-99m or with In-111. In combination with acetaldehyde, Tc-99m IMM accumulates solely in malignant tumors of various histology, but not in inflammatory diseases. Primary lung tumors and metastatic spread to the hilum or mediastinum can be visualized already 6 h after application of Tc-99m IMM. Sensitivity and specificity of this approach need further clinical investigation.

Prediction of Postoperative Lung Function

Because cigarette smoking is also the major cause of chronic bronchitis and emphysema, many patients with lung cancer have a chronic airflow obstruction and an impaired pulmonary function. When a patient is to have a pneumonectomy, the postoperative reduction in lung function can be predicted with considerable accuracy from a preoperative ventilation/perfusion scan.

Perfusion

The best correlation for the prediction is obtained from a perfusion scan done in the upright position during exertion. In our collective (Table 1b) no ventilation or perfusion abnormalities were noticed in 42.5% of patients with bronchial carcinoma. In 41.2% the perfusion defect was equal to, and in 11.0% larger than, the corresponding ventilation defect.

Consequently, the perfusion scan alone will be sufficient for predicting postoperative lung function in about 95% of cases.

Ventilation

More recent studies have shown that the ventilation values appear to be slightly closer to the postoperative spirometry data [11]. In our data this is definitely true in about 5% of cases (Table 1b).

Inhalation of Radioaerosol

The deposition of radioaerosol in the lung is a less satisfactory method of quantitatively assessing ventilation abnormalities than ventilation imaging with inert gases by principal reasons. On the other hand, certain improvements in aerosol generation have made it possible to replace ventilation studies with inert gases by the radioaerosol technique, provided that all aerosol particles larger than 3 μm in diameter are eliminated before inhalation [12].

Follow-up

Response to therapy

Some return of both ventilation and perfusion is seen after radiotherapy for bronchial carcinoma in 80% of patients with unresectable lung cancer. Quantitative measurements of Ga-67 accumulation in the tumor during chemotherapy or radiotherapy is a more sensitive and accurate method of predicting early tumor response than other techniques currently available [13].

Tumor Marker

In follow-up studies of cancer of the lung, a combined use of CEA and TPA is recommended. At 90% specificity, the sensitivity of CEA alone is 73% and that of TPA 48%, both together 78% [14].

Secondary Lung Malignancy

Early Detection

The early detection of neoplastic disease has been one of nuclear medicine's oldest and major goals. Despite the development of promising new agents for tumor localization, the assigned goal has not been achieved yet, especially in the lung, where most metastases can be easily detected on a routine chest radiograph. The only exception are lung metastases from well-differentiated thyroid carcinoma, which are primarily diagnosed by a positive I-131 scan in a large number of cases (Fig. 1).

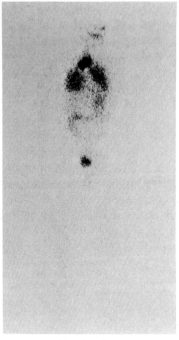

Anterior view

Fig. 1. Diffuse metastatic spread to both lungs of a well-differentiated papillary carcinoma of the thyroid. Clearly visualized on a whole-body scan 48 h after application of 100 mCi I-131, but normal chest radiograph

Differentiation Between Benign and Malignant Lesions

Since Ga-67 localization has been associated with virtually all pulmonary lesions in which inflammation is present as a primary or secondary phenomenon, labeled bleomycin seems to be more suitable for this purpose. Uptake of labeled antibodies is highly specific for malignancy, but even when the tumor histology is known and multiple antibodies against several tumor antigens are used, false-negative results may still be obtained. In conclusion, much has to be done before these new approaches have a substantial impact on the practical management of patients.

References

1. Li DK, Seltzer SE, McNeil BJ (1978) V/Q mismatches unassociated with pulmonary embolism: case report and review of the literature. J Nucl Med 19:1331−1334
2. Kempken K, Langhammer H, Hör G, Pabst HW (1978) Szintigraphische und klinisch-experimentelle Untersuchungen mit ^{67}Ga an 142 Bronchialkarzinomen. Nucl Med 17:47−52
3. Waxman PJ, Komaiko M, Brachman MB, Tanases DE, Wolfstein R, Berman PS (1979) Gallium uptake in hilar and mediastinal structures in patients with pulmonary tumors: the significance of location and cell type on sensitivity and specificity. J Nucl Med 20:645
4. Rezai-Zadeh K, Kirchner PT, DeMeester TR, Colomb H, Cooper M (1979) Gallium-67 scanning in clinical staging of lung cancer. J Nucl Med 20:644
5. Alazraki NP, Ramsdell JW, Taylor A, Friedmann PJ, Peters RM, Tisi GM (1978) Reliability of gallium scan, chest radiography compared to mediastinoscopy for evaluating mediastinal spread in lung cancer. Am Rev Resp Dis 117:415−420
6. Brykalski D, Liniecki J, Dobek J, Pertynski T, Fajndt S, Studniarek M, Durski K, Mussur M (1985) ^{51}Cr-bleomycin in the diagnosis of tumours of the chest. Nucl Med 24:66
7. Passamonte PM, Seger RM, Holmes RA, Hurst DJ (1983) Technetium-99m glucoheptonate imaging in lung cancer and benign lung diseases: concise communication. J Nucl Med 24:997−1000
8. Kim FH, DeLand FH, Domstad PA, Bennett SJ, Simmons GH, Goldenberg DM (1980) Radioimmunodetection of lung cancers using radiolabeled antibodies to carcinoembryonic antigen (CEA), alpha-fetoprotein (AFP) and human chorionic gonadotropin (HCG). J Nucl Med 21:P54
9. Larson SM (1985) Radiolabeled monoclonal anti-tumor antibodies in diagnosis and therapy. J Nucl Med 26:538−545
10. Zabel PL, Noujaim AA, Strysh A, Bray J (1983) Radioiodinated peanut lectin: a potential radiopharmaceutical for immunodetection of carcinoma expressing the T antigen. Eur J Nucl Med 8:250−254
11. Gupta R, Ryo UY, Szidon J, Pinsky SM (1980) Correlation between quantitative radionuclide lung studies and spirometry before and after surgical removal of lung carcinoma. J Nucl Med 21:P12
12. Köhler D, Dolovich M, Goates G, Newhouse M, Matthys H (1983) Können radioaktive Aerosole die radioaktiven Edelgase bei der Ventilationsszintigraphie der Lunge ersetzen? Atemw Lungenkrkh 9:265−270
13. McCready VR, Flower MA, Smythe J (1982) Quantitative studies of Gallium 67 uptake in human lung tumours during chemotherapy. J Nucl Med 23:P96
14. Oehr P, Biersack HJ, Hünermann B, Winkler C (1983) ROC-Analysis of single or combined CEA and TPA determination in a wide spectrum of cancer patients. J Nucl Med 24:P112

Clinical Aspects of Detection and Imaging of Tumors of Liver and Spleen

J. Mahlstedt[1]

Radiocolloidal imaging of liver and spleen was a frequently used diagnostic technique before high-quality sonography and fast transmission computer tomography (TCT) became available. Nowadays, clinical aspects of liver and spleen imaging mainly depend on technical and medical expertise of competing diagnostic disciplines and on the prevalence of the diseases in question. Table 1 gives an overview of the most frequent liver lesions detectable by nuclear medical means. The basic method nearly always concerns the visualization of liver parenchyma using ^{99m}Tc-labelled colloids. Sulfur colloids are cheap and reveal very constant physical properties; phytate is sometimes advantageous when low spleen uptake is wanted. Generally, activity distribution after bolus injection should be analyzed by gamma camera and data processing for the separate evaluation of arterial and portal blood flow.

Although the search for liver metastases in patients with malignant tumors prone to hepatic metastases is more and more covered by sonography and TCT, the results of standard planar liver scintigraphy and emission computer tomography (ECT) are worth comparing. Table 2 shows a statistical analysis of data as published by Strauss et al. [16]. In a definite population of patients (75% bronchogenic carcinoma, 19% gastro-intestinal carcinoma), the prevalence of

Table 1. Space-occupying lesions of the liver

Primary tumors	Secondary tumors	Congenital lesions
Liver cell carcinoma	Metastases	Cysts
Cholangiocarcinoma	Leukemia	Arteriovenous malformations
Sarcoma	Lymphoma	M. Caroli
Angiosarcoma	Carcinoma	
Hepatoblastoma		*Traumatic lesions*
	Inflammatory lesions	
Adenoma		Hematoma
Focal nodular hyperplasia	Abscess	Laceration
Hemartoma	Echinococcus	Spontaneous rupture
Hemangioma		
Angioma		
Lipoma		

1 Institut und Poliklinik für Nuklearmedizin der Universität Erlangen-Nürnberg, Krankenhausstraße 12, D-8520 Erlangen

Nuclear Medicine in Clinical Oncology
Ed. by C. Winkler
© Springer-Verlag Berlin Heidelberg 1986

Table 2. Finding of liver lesions: scintigraphy vs TCT (%)

	Planar scintigraphy	TCT
Sensitivity	81	94
Specificity	85	89
Accuracy	82	92
Prevalence	48	55
Positive predictive value	89	92
Negative predictive value	75	90

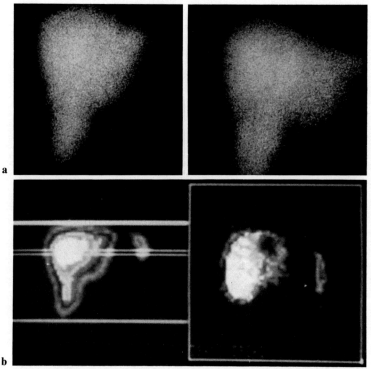

Fig. 1 a,b. Liver metastasis in a patient with mammary cancer. Standard liver scintigraphy using 6 mCi ^{99m}Tc-sulfur colloid. **a** Standard anterior and right anterior oblique projection: no lesion to be seen. **b** Transversal ECT slice: clear-cut lesion in the left liver lobe

liver metastases was around 50%, yielding in a positive predictive value of about 90% by both planar scintigraphy and ECT. However, only 75% was the negative predictive value in planar scintigraphy, compared with 90% in ECT. Other authors [5, 14] find similar results and stress differences with respect to tumor type. Colon cancer will set rather large metastases which can be visualized by planar scintigraphy with 94% accuracy [8], whereas metastases from nongastrointestinal cancers yield only 74% accuracy. This global result

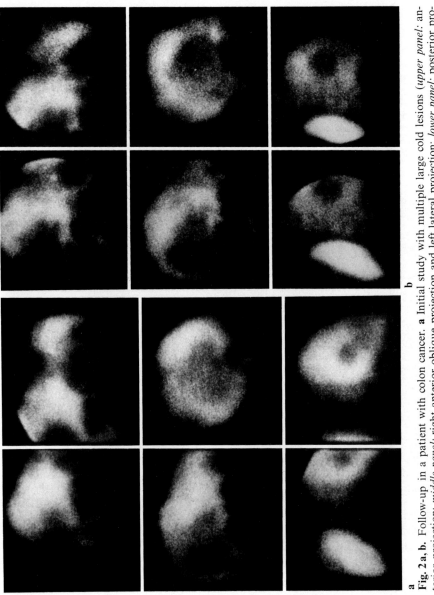

a

b

Fig. 2a, b. Follow-up in a patient with colon cancer. **a** Initial study with multiple large cold lesions (*upper panel*: anterior projection; *middle panel*: right anterior oblique projection and left lateral projection; *lower panel*: posterior projection). **b** Follow-up study 3 months later with clear-cut tumor progression (projections as in **a**)

clearly depends on lesion size and localization, as published by Strauss et al. [16]. Small lesions 1 – 2 cm in diameter are frequently overlooked in the central liver regions, whereas even large lesions are missed by liver scintigraphy when the whole left liver lobe is destroyed. ECT, therefore, often provides diagnostic advantages for excluding metastases in the left liver lobe (Fig. 1a, b). Nevertheless, planar scintigraphy often has clear-cut merits during follow-up for comprehensive visualization of liver metastases and potential progress for clinicians who are not familiar with sonographic documentation (Fig. 2).

Follow-up of liver metastases is of special interest in patients receiving intraarterial chemotherapy for primary or secondary liver cancer. Special advantage can be derived from the use of ^{99m}Tc-labelled microspheres (MS) or macroaggregated albumin (MAA). After transcatheteral injection of these particles, perfused liver tissue, potential extrahepatic flow, arteriovenous shunting to the lungs, or unexpected flow blockade are disclosed. Figure 3a depicts the arterial flow via catheter, whereas Fig. 3b gives evidence that the right liver lobe does not receive any material when injected via catheter. As the catheters are predominantly of the indwelling type, follow-up studies allow monitoring of the effectiveness of chemotherapy and blood flow during the application of vasoconstrictors and starch microspheres of after the application of ^{90}Y-microspheres [20].

Besides finding liver lesions, tumor identification is a diagnostic task much more suitable for nuclear medicine and its implementation of different radionuclides. Table 3 lists the most frequently used radiopharmaceuticals and the corresponding diagnostic patterns occurring in hepatic lesions. Lesion identification is very often possible by using only two or three of the radiopharmaceuticals available.

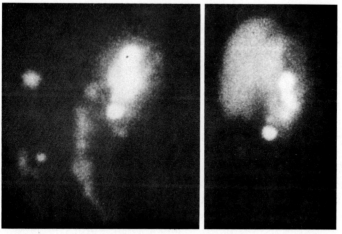

a   b

Fig. 3a,b. Arterial perfusion via indwelling catheter of a patient with liver metastases from colon cancer. **a** *Left side:* visualization of the catheter and the perfused tissue, dominantly the left liver lobe and some extrahepatic regions. At the left side, positive markers of the body surface. **b** *Right side:* additional visualization of the entire liver parenchyma after additional injection of 6 mCi ^{99m}Tc phytate

Table 3. Radiopharmaceuticals and diagnostic patterns in hepatic lesions

	Flow phase	Pool phase	^{99M}Tc S-Colloid	^{99M}Tc HIDA Early phase	^{99M}Tc HIDA Excretion phase	^{67}Ga Citrate	^{111}In Leuko-cytes	^{99M}Ic Erythro-cytes
Liver cyst	Ø	Ø	Ø	Ø	Ø	Ø	Ø	Ø
Bile duct cyst	Ø	Ø	Ø	Ø	+	Ø	Ø	Ø
Metastasis	Ø/=	Ø	Ø	Ø	Ø	Ø	Ø	Ø
Focal nodular hyperplasia	=/+	=	=	Ø	+	Ø	Ø	=
Liver cell adenoma	Ø/=	=	Ø	Ø	Ø	Ø	Ø	=
Hepatoma	Ø/=	=	Ø	Ø	(+)	+	Ø	=
Hemangioma	Ø	+	Ø	Ø	Ø	Ø	Ø	+
Abscess	Ø	Ø	Ø	Ø	Ø	+	+	Ø

Ø, negative contrast ("cold lesion"); =, no contrast; +, positive contrast ("hot lesion")

^{99m}Tc-HIDA is the key pharmaceutical for identification of focal nodular hyperplasia (FNH). In 90% of cases, there is hyperperfusion [1, 6, 9] and more or less normal initial uptake combined with clearly delayed excretion in the late dynamic study. Sulfur colloid is normally handled in FNH, whereas liver adenomas do not contain Kupffer's cells and therefore give negative contrast [13, 18]. Abscesses can be detected by ^{67}Ga citrate or ^{111}In leukocytes in an early stage. Although ^{111}In leukocytes have fewer technical problems of imaging, there are quite a lot of false-positive findings due to ischemic bowel disease, vasculitis, swallowed leukocytes secondary to sinusitis or pneumonia [4, 7], which can be confused with liver abscesses. Hepatomas can be visualized using scintigraphic techniques with varying findings in relation to the histologic type and the stage of the tumor. Typically, hepatic tumors are ^{67}Ga citrate positive [2, 17] and, if they contain bile duct remnants, they are HIDA positive in the late excretion phase (Fig. 4). The amount of HIDA-positive hepatomas in our experience is around 50%, whereas in countries with a high incidence, the amount of HIDA-positive hepatomas is only 4% [19]. These authors do not feel that HIDA scintigraphy is a useful procedure when searching for hepatoma.

Compared with the availability of this focusing technique which uses several pharmaceuticals that are unspecific when used alone, the availability of a specific radiopharmaceutical for a definite tumor is rare. Liver metastases of neuroblastomas or malignant pheochromocytomas can be visualized using ^{131}I-MIBG [11]. Moreover, liver metastases of epithelial thyroid tumors show up with positive contrast, when the thyroid is totally ablated. Further progress is being made due to the availability of specific monoclonal antibodies that bind to specific receptors.

Splenic tumors with clinical significance are listed in Table 4. Lesion finding is again achieved by standard radiocolloids, whereas identification of lesions is

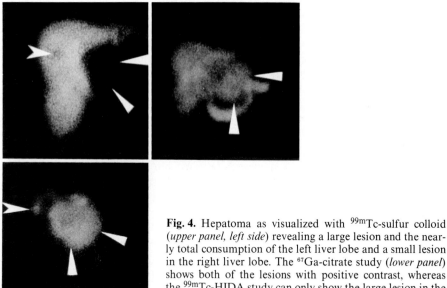

Fig. 4. Hepatoma as visualized with ^{99m}Tc-sulfur colloid (*upper panel, left side*) revealing a large lesion and the nearly total consumption of the left liver lobe and a small lesion in the right liver lobe. The ^{67}Ga-citrate study (*lower panel*) shows both of the lesions with positive contrast, whereas the ^{99m}Tc-HIDA study can only show the large lesion in the left liver lobe with positive contrast in the late excretion phase

Table 4. Space-occupying lesions of the spleen

Primary tumors	Inflammatory lesions	Traumatic lesions
Lymphosarcoma	Abscess	Hematoma
M. Hodgkin	Granulom	Rupture
Reticulum cell carcinoma		Splenosis
	Congenital lesions	
Secondary tumors	Cysts	*Vascular lesions*
Metastases	Accessory spleen	Infarction
	Thesaurosis	Embolism
		Hypoxia (sickle-cell anemia)

possible only to a certain degree by use of heat-damaged ^{99m}Tc-erythrocytes, ^{111}In platelets, or ^{111}In leukocytes. Clinically, it is of interest that radiocolloid follow-up studies can give evidence of complete or partial lesion regression. The spleen can show self-healing after traumata, and tumorous lesions of lymphocytic, histiocytic, and mixed type can show improvement after chemotherapy and/or radiotherapy [15]. After abdominal traumata with spleen rupture, splenosis is a frequent finding. Space-occupying lesions may occur after years, and the positive identification using heat-damaged ^{99m}Tc-erythrocytes is a straightforward approach to solving this diagnostic problem [10]. Analysis of hypersplenism is wanted more often in routine clinical work, as suspected hematologic disorders are not always related to hypersplenism, as expected.

Summary

During clinical work with tumorous lesions of liver and spleen, scintigraphic methods are more and more related to identification of already known space-occupying lesions by functional evaluation. The basic method is visualization of liver and spleen by ^{99m}Tc-labelled colloids. Liver lesion finding is achieved with an accuracy of between 75% and 90% depending on the tumor type. In colorectal tumors with large-sized lesions, the results are better compared to nongastrointestinal tumors. Most of the clinically important liver lesions such as focal nodular hyperplasia, liver adenoma, hemangioma, liver abscess, hepatoma, and cystic lesions of the liver or bile ducts can be identified using two or three scintigraphic investigations with the radiopharmaceuticals: ^{99m}Tc HIDA, ^{67}Ga citrate, ^{111}In leukocytes, ^{99m}Tc erythrocytes, and analysis of activity distribution after bolus injection (flow phase, pool phase). Direct identification of liver lesions is so far possible by ^{131}I MIBG in neuroblastoma metastases, metastases of malignant pheochromocytomas, and liver metastases from epithelial thyroid cancer after ablation of the thyroid. During therapy of liver metastases with indwelling arterial catheters, injection of ^{99m}Tc-labelled microspheres portrays the flow distribution and provides important information with respect to the effectiveness of drug therapy. Primary and secondary splenic tumors are rather infrequent. Cold lesions can be revealed by standard sulfur colloid scintigraphy, follow-up allows discovery of self-healing in post-traumatic situations or normalization of phagocytosis after chemotherapy and/or radiotherapy of lymphocytic/histiocytic splenic lesions. It bears reiterating that functional evaluation of the spleen with respect to perfusion, RES activity, and sequestration of platelets and erythrocytes is invaluable information in hematologic diseases and therefore, too, with regard to predicting the potential benefit of splenectomy.

References

1. Biersack HJ, Thelen M, Torres J et al. (1980) Focal nodular hyperplasia of the liver as established by Tc-99m sulfur colloid and HIDA scintigraphy. Radiology 137:187–190
2. Broderick TW, Gosink B, Menuck L et al. (1980) Echographic and radionuclide detection of hepatoma. Radiology 135:149–151
3. Casarella WJ, Knowles DM, Wolff M et al. (1978) Focal nodular hyperplasia and liver cell adenoma: radiologic and pathologic differentiation. Am J Roentgenol 131:393–402
4. Coleman RE, Welch D (1980) Possible pitfalls with clinical imaging of Indium-111 leukocytes: concise communication. J Nucl Med 21:122–125
5. Frühling J (1980) The role of scintigraphy in the detection of liver metastases in comparison with other techniques. Tumor Diagn 1:32–39
6. Gratz KF, Creutzig H, Brölsch C et al. (1984) Differentialdiagnostik von Lebertumoren mit nuklearmedizinischen Verfahren. In: Höfer R, Bergmann H (eds) Radioaktive Isotope in Klinik und Forschung. Egermann, Wien, pp 297–304
7. Knochel JQ, Koehler PR, Lee TG, Welch DM (1980) Diagnosis of abdominal abscesses with computed tomography, ultrasound, and In-111 leukocyte scans. Radiology 137:425–432
8. Knopf DR, Torres WE, Fajman WJ, Sones PJ Jr (1982) Liver lesions: comparative accuracy of scintigraphy and computed tomography. Am J Radiol 138:623–627

9. König R, Herter M (1983) Zur Differentialdiagnostik benigner intrahepatischer Raumforderungen. Fortschr Geb Röntgenstr 138:1–7
10. Löw A, Tischler E, Meier H, Mahlstedt J, Wolf F (1981) Selektive Milzszintigraphie zur Beurteilung der Splenosishäufigkeit nach posttraumatischer Splenektomie. Nuc Compact 12:210–214
11. Mahlstedt J, Hotze A, Pichl J, Wolf F (1984) Ergebnisse szintigraphischer Untersuchungen mit [131]J-meta-Benzylguanidin (MIBG) bei Raumforderungen neuroektodermaler Herkunft. Nuklearmedizin 5:257–264
12. Marienhagen J, Iro H, Hotze A, König HJ, Mahlstedt J, Wolf F (1985) Zur Darstellung von Thrombozyten-Verteilungsstörungen mit Indium-111-Oxin-markierten heterologen Thrombozyten. Nuc Compact 16:26–29
13. Salvo AF, Schiller A, Athanasoulis C et al. (1977) Hepatoadenoma and focal nodular hyperplasia: pitfalls in radiocolloid imaging. Radiology 125:451–455
14. Scherer U, Büll U, Rothe R et al. (1978) Computerized tomography and nuclear imaging of the liver. Eur J Nucl Med 3:71–80
15. Spencer RP, Mozafareddin K, Sziklas JJ et al. (1982) Radiocolloid studies of the regression of intrasplenic lesions. Clin Nucl Med 7:311–314
16. Strauss L, Bostel F, Clorius JH et al. (1982) Single-photon emission computed tomography (SPECT) for assessment of hepatic lesions. J Nucl Med 23:1059–1065
17. Suzuku T, Matsumoto Y, Manabe T et al. (1974) Serum alpha-fetoprotein and Ga-67 citrate uptake in hepatoma. Am J Roentgenol 120:627–633
18. Tanasescu D, Brachman M, Rigby J et al. (1984) Scintigraphic triad in focal nodular hyperplasia. Am J Gastroenterol 79:61–64
19. Yeh SH, Wang SJ, Chu LS (1981) Sensitivity of technetium-99m HIDA liver scintigraphy for diagnosing hepatoma. J Nucl Med 22:86
20. Ziessman HA, Thrall JH, Yang PJ et al. (1984) Hepatic arterial perfusion scintigraphy with Tc-99m-MAA. Radiology 152:167–172

Use of Scintigraphy for Evaluation of Patients with Renal Malignancies

J. H. Clorius[1], R. Horsch, L. Röhl, and G. Irngartinger

The development of the newer imaging technologies has led to far-reaching changes for evaluating renal masses, reducing scintigraphy's importance. A glance at the literature indicates that ultrasound (US), computed tomography (CT), nuclear magnetic resonance (NMR), and angiography are to be favored for lesion recognition (Table 1). CT permits accurate differentiation of most renal masses [2, 3, 5–7], and determination of the T stage [1, 5, 8]. Initial results for NMR presented by Hricak suggest that lesion recognition and evaluation of tumor extension will be equal to that achieved with CT, while recognition of renal vein involvement will be far improved [6]. Furthermore, Strake reports that 1-cm lesions are easily detected with NMR, and that cyst content will be differentiated [10]. The data presented suggest that scintigraphy can only find limited use when CT and NMR are available. Scintigraphy may however find use in special situations.

Ga-67 Citrate Imaging. Ga-67 citrate has only found limited use for imaging renal malignancies. Kawamura examined 30 renal cell carcinomas [11]. While lesion detectability was poor, the uptake correlated with tumor progression, so that Ga-67 was found to have prognostic value.

Tc-DTPA Imaging. Janowitz examined five avascular and 21 vascular renal cell carcinomas with Tc-DTPA [12]. All vascular tumors demonstrated a "fading blush" sign during serial 1-min images. This sign is due to rapid washout of the tracer compared with the surrounding tissue. The authors did not fail to note that the classical description of the scan of the renal cell carcinoma – hyperperfusion in first-pass images, cold lesion in the delayed scans – is only seen in a minority of tumors. Sachs used the tracer to differentiate the benign mesoblastic nephroma from Wilms' tumors [13]. The mesoblastic nephroma is visualized with DTPA, while the malignant lesion is a nonfunctioning renal mass. The authors suggest that hippurate and DMSA may not be suited for this approach, due to the immaturity of the renal tubular system in the neonate.

Hot Mass Lesions. Renal lesions have at times been imaged as hot spots with various radiopharmaceuticals, resulting in atypical scans. Siddiqui reported

1 Deutsches Krebsforschungszentrum, Institut für Nuklearmedizin, Im Neuenheimer Feld 280, D-6900 Heidelberg

Table 1. Comparison of competitive modalities for tumor imaging (data from [1–10])

	Lesion recognition		Tumor stage	
	(*n*)	(%)	(*n*)	(%)
Scintigraphy	–	85–90	–	–
Ultrasound	157	99	23	70
Angiography	–	–	72	65
Computer tomography	140	100	100	85
Digital subtraction angiography	24	60	24	60
Magnetic resonance	75	100	–	–

that a majority of neuroblastoma show Tc-99m MDP uptake in 3-h images [14]. An occasional Wilms' tumor may however also be visualized with this tracer. Pion noted DMSA uptake in a renal cell carcinoma, resulting in a hot lesion [15]. Cysts have at times been known to fill with tracers, so that these too may result in hot images. At present, these rare hot lesions have no diagnostic consequence.

Initial Lesion Evaluation with Scintigraphy. Numerous reports recommend the combined use of US and scintigraphy for initial evaluation of mass lesions [3, 16]. US identifies the obviously uncomplicated cyst, while solid tumors are referred to scintigraphy. Prominent parenchymal lobulations with normal isotope uptake are clearly separated from malignancies with their cold cortical lesions. I would, however, like to suggest that, with the exception of SPECT, the procedure will result in occasional but unacceptable diagnostic errors. SPECT will improve lesion detectability [17]. Even anterior lesions are easily detected, due to removal of superimposed tissue. While this approach may be acceptable, our experience suggests that SPECT imaging is not used for the initial evaluation of renal lesions when CT is in place. Our urologists will not operate on the basis of US and SPECT. Likewise, they will not discharge patients when SPECT fails to visualize a solid lesion. In our department, SPECT imaging with DMSA has only been requested late in the course of tumor evaluation. The literature contains few data on false-positive and true-negative scan results [16]. This suggests that most other centers may have a similar experience.

Hippurate Renography. Compared with imaging, tracer assessment of renal function may achieve a pivotal position during the therapy-oriented decision process. The importance of the evaluation of renal function with isotopes increases as the complexity of the individual case increases. Moser compared preoperative I-131 hippurate scintigrams with serum creatinine values obtained before and after nephrectomy [18]. He correctly concluded that hippurate scintigrams will not influence the therapeutic approach when the nontumor kidney has a regular morphology, and when there is no evidence of renal insufficiency. When malignancy is complicated by concurrent renal diseases, assessment of regional, unilateral, and global renal function will permit the postoperative determination of renal function prior to surgery. Scintigraphy and clearance, used together, will indicate whether the renal tissue remaining after tumor resection will support life.

Method

We report results obtained in 57 patients referred to hippurate sequential scintigraphy because of renal malignancy. The surgical therapy was complicated since all patients had either bilateral malignancies, unilateral tumors in a solitary organ, or complicating primary or secondary renal disease.

Gamma camera hippurate scintigraphy followed i.v. injection of 6 µCi I-131 hippurate per kg body weight. Serial images were obtained during the 20-min examination. Data were stored on magnetic tape, and were analyzed by minicomputer. Regions of interest were placed over each kidney, to generate renograms and determine single kidney function. Background subtraction of the renogram followed its determination with an ROI placed around the kidney.

Following renography the patients had a single compartment infusion clearance, to determine both effective renal plasma flow (ERPF) und glomerular filtration rate (GFR). To estimate GFR, we injected 200 µCi In-111 DTPA intravenously. This isotope was given with the I-131 hippurate. Thirty min after termination of gamma camera renography we began infusion of both tracers. After reaching steady state, the clearance examination lasted 40 min. A single blood sample was taken at the end of the clearance period.

Thirty patients were evaluated and finally referred to surgery because of a malignant tumor in a solitary kidney. Ten patients had creatinine values above 1.4 mg%, one had a value of 2.4 mg%, at the time of tumor diagnosis. All patients had renography. The relative percentage of each third, and both halves, of the kidney was determined using the ROI technique. Both GFR and ERPF were calculated. The postoperative ERPF remaining after tumor resection was estimated. Six patients required extracorporal tumor resection, 24 had in situ tumor enucleation.

Twenty patients had bilateral renal malignancies. These patients were referred to renography, GFR, and ERPF. Single kidney function, expressed in percent and as ERPF, was determined. The kidney with better function was generally selected for tumor enucleation. Following recovery from surgery, both renography and clearance were repeated. The second examination was to assess whether the tumor-free organ could support life. Adequate function resulted in nephrectomy of the other tumor-carrying organ. Six patients had a creatinine of 1.4 or above at the time of the initial tumor evaluation.

Seven patients had a unilateral malignancy complicated by primary or secondary renal disease. The evaluation of renal function was similar to the approach used in malignant tumors in solitary organs.

Results

Thirty patients were referred to surgery with a malignant tumor in a solitary kidney. Hippurate renography was used to monitor four patients during postoperative acute renal failure. Two patients lost the tumor-resected kidney. All other patients had adequate renal function at the time of discharge (Table 2).

Two patients with bilateral malignancies required bilateral tumor enucleation, since renal function evaluation indicated that neither organ could support life. One patient had bilateral tumor enucleation since the clearance examination could not be obtained prior to surgery. Two patients undergoing tumor resection died without recovering from surgery. The mean creatinine value at discharge was 1.5 mg%, the single most elevated value was 2.9 mg% (Table 3). These data demonstrate that patients having undue risk of postoperative crippling renal insufficiency were identifiable and were excluded from surgical therapy.

Therapy results obtained in patients with malignancy and concurrent renal disease were equally successful. On average, the organ needing tumor resection had 81% of total function and an ERPF of $256 \text{ ml} \times 173 \text{ m}^2$ preceding surgery. The tumor-free kidney had an average ERPF of 52 ml. One patient

Table 2. Summary of results achieved in surgical therapy of 30 malignant tumors in patients with a solitary kidney (two patients died before recovering from surgery)

	Preceding surgery			After surgery	
	(n)	ERPF (ml)	GFR (ml)	(n)	Acute renal failure (n)
In situ	24	276	51	–	2
Extracorporal	6	258	58	–	2
Total	30	273	54	–	4
Creatinine 1.4 or higher	10	–	–	16	–
Creatinine 2.0 or higher	0	–	–	6	–

Mean serum creatinine at time of discharge: 1.9 mg/dl

Table 3. Summary of results obtained in 20 patients examined because of bilateral renal malignancies

	Preoperative function			After tumor resection	Final outcome
n	Creatinine (mg/dl)	Function of organ selected for tumor-resection (%)	ERPF or organ to be retained (ml)	ERPF of tumor-resected organ (ml)	Mean creatinine level at discharge (mg/dl)
20	1.2	68	230	158	1.5

Table 4. Renal malignancy in seven patients with concurrent renal disease (one patient died postoperatively)

n	Preoperative			Postoperative	
	Mean function of the tumor kidney (%)	Mean ERPF of the tumor kidney (ml)	Mean ERPF of the non-tumor kidney (ml)	Total ERPF (ml)	Mean creatinine (mg/dl)
7	81	256	52	281	2.1

died during the postoperative period. Following tumor resection, three patients had a serum creatinine level of 1.0−1.1 mg%, while three others had values of 1.7, 2.3, and 5.7 mg% (Table 4).

Summary

It has been our experience that referral for static renal imaging will be the exception when CT is available. Renal function evaluation does, however, have an important place in therapy planning, particularly when renal function of one or both kidneys is compromised.

References

1. Mitsuhashi K, Kashiwagi A, Kumagai A et al. (1984) Preoperative staging of renal cell carcinoma. Comparison with operative or pathologic finding. Hinyokika Kiyo 30:1379−1386
2. Lang EK (1984) Comparison of dynamic and conventional computed tomography, angiography and ultrasonography in the staging of renal cell carcinoma. Cancer 54:2205−2214
3. O'Reilly PH, Osborn DE, Testa HJ et al. (1981) Renal imaging: a comparison of radionuclide, ultrasound, and computed tomographic scanning in investigation of renal space occupying lesions. Br Med J 282:943−945
4. Freitag J, Otto HJ, Freitag G et al. (1981) Diagnostik raumfordernder Prozesse der Niere mit Sequenzszintigraphie und Renovasographie. Z Urol Nephrol 74:1−11
5. Jaschke W, van Kaick G, Palmtag H et al. (1981) Stadieneinteilung von Nierentumoren mit Hilfe der Computertomographie. Strahlentherapie 157:94−98
6. Hricak H, Demas BE, Williams RD et al. (1985) Magnetic resonance imaging in the diagnosis and staging of renal and perirenal neoplasms. Radiology 154:709−715
7. Engelmann U, Schaub T, Schweden F et al. (1984) Digital subtraction angiography in staging renal cell carcinoma: Comparison with computed tomography and histopathology. J Urol 132:1093−1096
8. Cronan JJ, Zeman RK, Rosenfield AT (1982) Comparison of computed tomography, ultrasound and angiography in staging renal cell carcinoma. J Urol 127:712−714
9. Jaschke W, van Kaick G, Palmtag H (1980) Vergleich der Wertigkeit von Echographie und Computertomographie bei der Diagnostik raumfordernder Prozesse der Niere. RÖFO 132:145−151
10. Strake L, van der Hem GK, Hooijkaas JA et al. (1984) Nuclear magnetic resonance imaging of the kidney. Diagn Imag Clin Med 53:198−202

11. Kawamura J, Itoh H, Yoshida O et al. (1984) "Hot Spot" on Gallium-67-citrate scan in renal cell carcinoma. Clinicopathologic and biochemical correlation. Urology 24:250−254
12. Janowitz WR, Smoak WM, Cuadra AV et al. (1982) Scintigraphic spectrum of renal cell carcinoma. J Nucl Med 23:111
13. Sachs G, Mitchell M, Fleischer AC et al. (1983) Scintigraphic and sonographic diagnosis of neonatal mesoblastic nephroma. Case Report. Clin Nucl Med 8:252−253
14. Siddiqui AR, Cohen M, Moran DP (1982) Enhanced differential diagnosis of abdominal masses using inferior vena cava, renal and bone imaging with single foot injection of Tc-99m methylene diphosphonate (MDP) in children. J Nucl Med 23:P7
15. Pion SJ, Staab EV, Stevens PS (1976) Increased activity in a renal cell carcinoma imaged using 2,3-Dimercaptosuccinic acid. J Urol 116:512−513
16. Older RA, Korobkin M, Workman J et al. (1980) Accuracy of radionuclide imaging in distinguishing renal masses from normal variants. Radiology 136:443−448
17. Teates CD, Croft BY, Brenbridge NA et al. (1983) Emission tomography of the kidney. South Med J 76:1499−1502
18. Moser E, Hahn D, Wieland W et al. (1982) Ergebnisse der Funktionsszintigraphie mit [131]J-Hippuran in der präoperativen Diagnostik von Nierentumorpatienten. Einfluß auf operatives Vorgehen und Vorhersagewert für das Retentionsverhalten. Urologe [A] 21:190−194

Scintigraphy of Lymphokinetics and Lymphatic Neoplasia

G. Hör[1], D. L. Munz, I. Brandhorst, F. D. Maul, H. Holzmann, P. Altmeyer, and R. P. Baum

Lymph node (LN) concentration of radioactive colloidal gold was first detected some decades ago [40, 66, 70]. Clinical applications were promoted by zum Winkel [72−74]. The original concepts to scan (metastatic) LN, control the radiation field, and stage malignant lymphonodular diseases [10, 15, 24, 26, 32, 36, 38, 45, 46, 52, 59, 67, 71−74] were partly replaced [2, 23, 36, 38, 54−56]. The change in indications was induced by the development of new radiopharmaceuticals, high-resolution gamma cameras, and computers, which paved the way for visualizing lymphokinetics, and thus improving the detection of lymphatic malignancies.

This review outlines the progress in radiopharmacy and techniques, presents our own clinical results as well as those of other multicenter studies, and summarizes clinical indications with an outlook on future.

Scintigraphy of Lymphokinetics

Radiopharmacy

The barrier function of LN has been studied for many years [1, 25, 26, 29, 44, 59, 60]: labeled erythrocytes, and extravascular albumin as an index of lymph transport and, further, dextran undergoing rapid clearance through the peripheral afferent lymphatic vessels were used. The velocity of lymph transport ranges between 5 and 10 cm/min and blood flow to (sheep) LN was determined as being around 24 ml/h [52]. Colloids or particles are trapped by phagocytes ("attachment") within LN allowing the documentation of lymphodynamic and lymphostatic phases − "lymphangio-adenoscintigraphy". Radiation exposure at the injection site is between 11 mGy/MBq and 81 mGy/MBq and below 1.1 mGy/MBq at the primary lymphonodular drainage site [55]. The high photon flux results in excellent imaging quality of both dynamic and static lymphatic scans making it possible to visualize even lymph flow in distinct lymphatic collectors.

In Table 1, radiopharmaceuticals which were used in nuclear lymphology and oncology (lymphatic malignancies) are listed.

---

1 Zentrum der Radiologie und Dermatologie, Klinikum der Johann-Wolfgang-Goethe-Universität, Theodor-Stern-Kai 7, D-6000 Frankfurt am Main 70

Nuclear Medicine in Clinical Oncology
Ed. by C. Winkler
© Springer-Verlag Berlin Heidelberg 1986

Table 1. Radiopharmaceuticals in nuclear lymphology and oncology (lymphatic neoplasias)

^{99m}Tc	(Mini)colloid [17, 20], Sb_2S_3 [55], rhecolloid [41 a], phytate, liposomes [55]
^{57}Co	Bleomycin [47]
^{67}Ga	Citrate [3, 4, 8, 18, 28, 30, 33–37, 42, 43, 45–48, 58, 61, 69, 71]
^{201}Tl	Cl [35, 36, 38, 51, 57, 63]
^{111}In	Monoclonal antibodies [47]
^{131}I	CEA and CA-19-9, radioimmuno-cocktail
^{58}Co ^{65}Zn	Hematoporphyrin [21]
^{11}C	Amino acids and other metabolites [39, 47]

Technique

For *scintigraphy of lymphokinetics* 55.5 – 74 MBq ^{99m}Tc-Sb_2b_3 (antimony-trisulfide colloid) are injected in several places around the tumor (<0.1 ml volume per injection site in 0.5 – 1.0 cm distance sub/intracutaneously modified according to [23]. A gamma camera with a large field of view interfaced to Informatek SIMIS 3 system (Sopha Medical) and a 140-keV general purpose collimator are used. Scans are taken between 2 and 4 h considering overlapping sites of the regions of interest and shielding the primary tumor with lead. For analogous gamma camera scans "preset cts" should amount to 10 000 (if injection site is outside the view of the gamma camera), 20 000 cts (injection site inside the view), 200 000 cts (inside without lead shield) [55].

In case of *lymphedema toe ergometry* is applied for better localization of lymph blocks and for quantitation of exercise-induced lymphonodular uptake of the lymphotropic radiopharmaceutical. For this procedure we propose the term "ergolymphoscintimetry." In swollen arms and legs, microcirculation may be studied using universal nuclear medicine techniques [44, 49, 53].

The technique of *^{67}Ga and ^{201}Tl tumor scintigraphy* has been described previously [33, 51 a].

Clinical Results

Our investigations include scintigraphy in malignant melanoma (MM). Lymph flow scintigraphy in tumors of the head and the neck has been presented elsewhere [2, 42, 54, 55].

Malignant Melanoma: Lymph Flow Scintigraphy

In 124 patients, 340 follow-up studies were performed. The following MM were revealed: superficial spreading (SSM), ($n = 65$); nodular (NM), ($n = 35$); lentiginous (LMM), ($n = 12$); acrolentiginous (ALM), ($n = 1$). All tumors were classified according to tumor thickness classes I– V (equivalent to <0.76 and >3.0 mm) as well as on the basis of the level of invasion [11, 68].

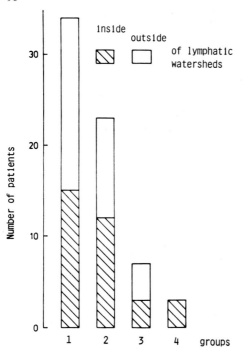

Fig. 1. Relation of lymph node groups to lymphatic watersheds

MM of the Trunk. Lymph nodes were localized scintigraphically in axillary, inguinal, parasternal, supraclavicular, and nuchal regions including 12 intransit LNs. None of the regions was predicted anatomically or clinically.

Axillary Type was visualized in 91% with the following subtypes: unilateral (50%) and bilateral (20%). These lymph flow types were occasionally combined with other flow pattern: parasternal and/or supraclavicular regions.

Lymphatic Watersheds (LWS). Attention must be paid to melanomas inside the "lymphatic watersheds" (LWS), which might involve multidirectional lymph flow pattern, i.e., lymphatic drainage to more than one LN-bearing area. LWS are defined as zones of anatomic variation about 2.5 cm to either side of the anterior and posterior midline as well as Sappey's line of the trunk. Figure 1 illustrates the number of regional LN (groups) with lymphatic drainage from a given primary lesion.

Among the 25 patients presenting with lymph flow to a single LN region, six had a primary lesion inside the LWS, thus sparing the patient an additional lymphadenectomy (which he might otherwise have undergone). On the other hand, in 50% of the primary tumors positioned outside the LWS, two [54] or three [55] regional lymph node drainage groups were identified. Importantly, in most of these cases, the lymph flow had crossed the LWS! These results clearly document that not only melanomas situated inside, but also those outside the LWS have an ambiguous lymphatic drainage. Although a peculiar alteration of the lymph flow pattern by the tumor cannot be excluded definitively, the anatomical thesis of "lymphatic watersheds" of the trunk should be revised [55].

MM of Upper Extremities. Twenty-two MMs presented with ipsilateral axillary lymph flow type.

MM of Lower Extremities. The lymph flow of all 13 tumors we scanned was drained by homolateral inguinal lymph nodes, which were clearly visualized in each patient, whereas the iliac and lumbar nodes presented with lower scintigraphic contrast. In tumors of the posterior lower legs, popliteal "intransit" lymph nodes were occasionally detected in addition to the regional inguinal nodes.

Malignant Melanoma: [201]*Tl Lymphnode Scintigraphy*

Eleven patients (four women, seven men) were scanned. All had previous surgery with complete removal of a malignant melanoma. Eight were suspected of having metastatic involvement of regional lymph nodes. Three were clinically free of recurrence or lymph node involvement. [201]Tl scan proved positive in seven patients by detecting focal accumulation in at least one tributary node. In one patient with a false-negative ^{201}Tl scan, the technique used was inadequate. All seven patients with positive ^{201}Tl scan had multiregional two-phase scintigraphy with early (20−30 min) and late (120 min p.i.) scans. For details, see [51 b].

Conclusions and Surgical Aspects

Increase in survival rate of high-risk melanoma patients after prophylactic dissection of regional LN is well documented. High-risk and low-risk melanoma patients were represented in our material in nearly identical proportions [44.2% vs 55.8%]. In 84% of the high-risk group, radical surgery was carried out after scintigraphy of lymphokinetics (SLK); 31% of our patients had histologically verified metastases.

Thus, preoperative decision making and, possibly, the recurrence rate of metastases may be improved by systematic application of SLK. Proper timing is decisive in the management of cutaneous MM. Since wide excision of the primary lesion induces a considerable manipulation of lymphatic drainage with subsequent interruption of lymph vessels and opening of collaterals, SLK should be performed immediately after clinical diagnosis of MM or − at the latest − after a simple excisional biopsy. Today, it is unquestionable that SLK need not necessarily identify metastases, but the procedure is capable of revealing those drainage groups implying greatest risk for harboring occult metastases.

Table 2. Present and future indications of scintigraphy of lymphokinetics (besides melanoma)

- Tumors of head and neck [42]
- Breast carcinoma [14, 16, 19, 62]
- Prostatic carcinoma [52]
- Ascites-peritoneal blockade [13]
- Bronchial carcinomas [32]
- Detection of thoracic duct leakage in congenital chylothorax [27]

Clinical Indications

Besides MM, a wide spectrum of other indications was elaborated by other groups (Table 2).

Mammary Lymphoscintigraphy

Parasternal lymphoscintigraphy [64] provides important information in the preoperative stage of breast carcinomas. Prognostic implications were stressed by Ege et al. [19] on the basis of a study in 1072 patients. Parasternal involvement increases with the stage of the disease. Regardless of the site of the primary tumor, parasternal lymphatics represent decisive risk factors. Nearly $\frac{1}{5}$ of the patients without axillary involvement have abnormal parasternal lymph nodes. From a surgeons's perspective [16], internal mammary lymphoscintigraphy was confirmed to serve as a key investigative tool in assessing the extent of the disease. The nuclear medicine procedure seems to be superior to computed tomography [14]. The correlation with histological findings is good; crossing of metastases from one breast to the other was shown [16, 19].

Scintigraphy of Lymphatic Malignancies

^{67}Gallium

Subsequent to our first multicenter report [33], many studies were published, including the Munich and NIH reports [4, 34].

General Sensitivity

The sensitivity of ^{67}Ga scintigraphy was categorized [37].

High. (90% − 100%) for malignant lymphoma, Hodgkin's, and non-Hodgkin's disease, Burkitt lymphoma, bronchial carcinoma, hepatoma, lymph node, and thoracic metastases of malignant melanoma (Fig. 4).

Low. (<50%) for melanoma, gastrointestinal tumors, brain tumors and metastases, thyroid carcinoma (exception, anaplastic), genitourinary carcinoma (exception, testicular, embryonic), breast carcinoma, neuroblastoma.

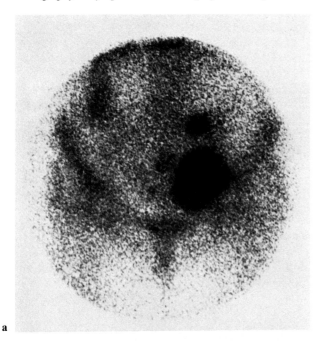

a

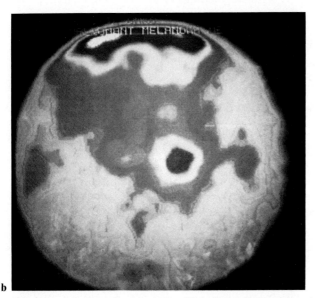

b

Fig. 2a, b. Scintigraphic detection of inguinal and iliacal lymph node metastases of a 27 year old female suffering from superficial spreading melanoma of the left lower leg after previous surgery one year ago. **a** [67]Ga analogous-scintigram showing at least 4 focal accumulations. **b** ^{201}Tl-computer-image, similar visualisation

Sensitivity Previously and Now

The overall detection rate of ^{67}Ga scintigraphy in lymphomas was originally reported to be 78%, increasing to 86% in endothoracic lesions [35, 58, see also 4, 18, 30, 69]. Considerable improvement of these data was achieved by using multipeak large-field gamma cameras with triple spectroscopy, applying nuclear tomography, and injecting higher amounts of ^{67}Ga − 5−10 mCi (i.e., up to 370 MBq) [3, 43]. ^{67}Ga uptake is higher in rapidly growing and non-differentiated tumors. It may vary, however, from site to site, even for histologically comparable or identical tumor classes, possibly due to differences in biological properties. Greater tumor uptake seems to be a sign of bad prognosis (see review and literature in [47]).

Tumor Size

Lesions under 1 cm in diameter are usually not visualized at all, while lesions around 2−3 cm are visualized in only 25% of cases. The best detectable size seems to range between 2 and 5 cm, whereas larger tumors escape detection, probably on account of central necrosis.

Hodgkin's Lymphoma

Histology is a major determinant of scintigraphic detectability: histiocytic types were described as being more often detectable (67%−74%) than mixed cell types (46%) [4].

Mediastinal involvement was ascertained by several authors with a sensitivity of up to 96% and an overall accuracy of 97% when ultrasound and ^{67}Ga scintigraphy were combined [9, 69]. CT is said to be incapable of differentiating enlarged but normal nodes from those arising from other causes [7]. Radiology often gives no answer as to whether a lesion has been adequately treated, especially when there is interfering radiation fibrosis.

Burkitt's Lymphoma

Another indication, in which the diagnosis, complete remission, or relapse are precisely decided by means of ^{67}Ga scintigraphy [61] is Burkitt's lymphoma.

Diagnosis, Staging, and Therapy Control

^{67}Ga is too expensive to be used as a screening tool. We have made use of this radiopharmaceutical preferentially for years for detecting occult (additional) lesions, when the diagnosis is already established clinically, or if there is a possibility of recurrent disease. In extended scars of the tumor region, ^{67}Ga scintigraphy was found to be superior to ultrasound and CT [43]. Again, this approach might change should prospective multicenter studies prove the high sensitivity of emission computerized tomography and if ECT becomes available in more oncology centers. In patients with limited diffuse stage I lymphomas who usually undergo local radiotherapy, the contribution of ^{67}Ga scintigraphy might increase the rate of identification of the site and extent of nodu-

Table 3. Nuclear medicine procedures in malignant lymphomas

Basic

- Tumor scintigraphy with ^{67}Ga, eventually supplemented by ^{201}Tl
- Bone scan (whole body), eventually supplemented by bone-marrow scan including liver spleen

Supplementary

- Brain scans
- Metastasis, cytostatic encephalopathy
- Parathyroid scans
- Lung perfusion scans (tumor microemboli, interstitial cytostatic pneumonia)
- Radionuclide ventriculography (EF for cardiotoxicity)
- Cardiac hot spot imaging (radiation necrosis of heart muscle)
- Hepatobiliary sequential scintigraphy (gallbladder obstruction by nodes)
- Hepatic (catheter), perfusion scintigraphy (control of catheter position in local chemotherapy)
- Renal clearance (^{123}I-hippuran, ^{99m}Tc-DTPA) (nephrotoxicity of cytostatics, obstructive uropathy)
- Double radionuclide/double compound scintigraphy (^{99m}Tc-Sb$_2$S$_3$/^{67}Ga) for metastasis' detection

---

lar lesions. Besides chest radiography, bone marrow examinations and CT nuclear medicine, investigations should be integrated as listed in Table 3. ^{67}Ga may also be employed in fevers of unknown origin, although ^{111}In leukocytes seem to be more sensitive in visualizing an abscess.

The role of ^{67}Ga for staging is limited to cervico- and thoraco-lymphonodular neoplasia. The existence and the extent of lesions prior to biopsy in unenlarged and impalpable lesions is a further domain of tumor scintigraphy. A staging laparotomy, however, is generally recommended regardless of the outcome of scintigraphy. On the other hand, both laparotomy and lymphangiography are avoidable, if ^{67}Ga indicates lesions in bone, abdominal region, or other organ involvement, proving stage IV [7, 35, 36, 50].

Concerning therapy control, our initial assumption is now generally accepted [31, 47]: The greatest clinical utility of ^{67}Ga is to assess the activity of the tumor under treatment. Therapy control, however, is effective only as far as the persistence of focal lesions after therapy is considered, i.e., as a sign of inadequate treatment. Negative ^{67}Ga scans are not definitive. Nevertheless, pre- and postoperative as well as pre- and posttherapy scans should be performed in any case.

Pediatric Oncology

Little attention has been paid to tumor scintigraphy in children [6, 18, 28, 48], although their sensitivity to ^{67}Ga scintigraphy is similar (87%) to that of adults [6]. The specificity is reportedly 100%. Occasionally, tumor scintigraphy is superior to chest radiography in revealing mediastinal involvement. ^{67}Ga uptake in the region of the thymus should not be mistaken as being tumor dependent. In contrast to the situation in adults, even abdominal lesions are more easily detected.

²⁰¹Thallium

This radionuclide has both myocardial and tumor-seeking properties. A universal spectrum of tumors is visualized [35, 36, 51 a, b, 57, 63]. Thyroid carcinoma belongs to the malignancies for which ²⁰¹Tl is eminently suitable [51, 57, 63]. By applying computer-assisted functional scintigraphy, kinetic differences of ²⁰¹Tl may be quantified to allow for separation of malignant and nonmalignant adenomas (Fig. 3): Regional lymphomas that do not lend themselves to staging by means of palpation, ultrasound, and CT are recognized as malignant if the functional patterns of the thyroid tumor and the suspicious regional lymphoma are identical or similar. In our 22 patients, ²⁰¹Tl-tumor scintigram was positive in 91%, and we were able to identify all regional malignant lymphomas [51 a]; difficulties arise shortly after thyroidectomy, where inflammatory salivary glands may be mistaken as evidence of malignant metastatic involvement of a node because after complete removal of the tumor there is no comparative kinetic reference.

Prospects

An outlook on present problems to be solved and future diagnostic and therapeutic prospects of nuclear lymphology must take into account the following aspects.

Problems of Lymph-Flow Scintigraphy

Illig [41] stressed the necessity of clarifying several questions: Does the lymphokinetic scintigram completely and reliably visualize all directions of lymph

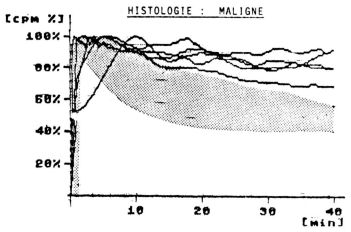

Fig. 3. Results of ²⁰¹Tl functional scintigraphy in thyroid carcinomas: comparison of tumor kinetics. Normal range spotted area in patients without thyroid carcinoma

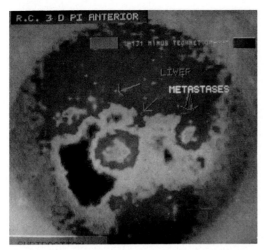

Fig. 4. Immunoscintigram in a 21-year-old female patient showing liver and extrahepatic lymph node metastases (confirmed by surgery) of a colonic carcinoma using a double tracer subtraction technique. J-131 labelled F (ab′)$_2$ fragments of monoclonal antibodies (Anti CA-19-9 anti-CEA) and Tc-99m colloid. Consider portal lymph node metastases (*bottom*)

flow or only the main pathways, as we assume? Is the present technique still appropriate? Are there influences due to previous diagnostic excision or subsequent to metastatic obstruction of lymph vessels?

New Radiopharmaceuticals

Among the newer radiopharmaceuticals (Table 1), labeled monoclonal antibodies seem to be most important for visualizing abdominal lymph nodes originating from colorectal carcinomas (Fig. 4) and lymph node metastases from breast carcinoma.

New Techniques

The combination of radioimmunoscintigraphy and emission computerized tomography seems to favor an optimal approach to tumor detection. Double radionuclide-double compound scintigraphy using peritumoral-interstitial injection of ^{99m}Tc complexes and ^{67}Ga holds promise for improved visualization of metastatic involvement of lymph nodes, but presently, experience with this approach is limited [41 a, 42, 55].

Ergolymphoscintimetry was recognized as an imaging procedure for analyzing lymphokinetics and detecting latent functional disturbances of lymph transport. Our preliminary unpublished data may be taken as evidence of the differential diagnosis between primary and secondary lymph edema making it possible to localize lymph blocks prior to vascular surgery.

The expense of positron emission tomography [39] means that it has no chance in this country.

Therapy

Intralymphatic administration of radiopharmaceuticals for therapeutic purposes includes several approaches: irradiating microspheres such as ^{90}Y, ^{46}Sc, ^{131}I-etiodol and -lipiodol, and ^{198}Au [5, 12, 65, 73].

Recently palladium-109 (^{109}Pd) was successfully coupled to a monoclonal antibody that reacts with a high molecular weight antigen associated with melanoma, thus showing its potential for tumor therapy [22].

References

1. Abramson DI, Dobrin PB (1984) Blood vessels and lymphatics in organ system. Academic Press, New York
2. Altmeyer P, Munz D, Steinhoff W, Hör G, Holzmann H (1981) Szintigraphische Identifizierung der Lymphdrainage maligner Rumpfmelanome. Akt Derm 7:127
3. Anderson KC, Leonard RCG, Canellos GP (1983) High dose gallium imaging in lymphoma. Am J Med 75:327
4. Andrews GA, Hübner KF, Greenlaw RH (1978) Ga-67 citrate imaging in malignant lymphoma: Final report of cooperative group. J Nucl Med 19:1013
5. Ariel IM, Resnick MI (1964) The intralymphatic administration of radioactive isotopes and cancer chemotherapeutic drugs. Surgery 55:355
6. Bekerman C, Port RB, Pang E (1978) Scintigraphic evaluation of childhood malignancies by ^{67}Ga-citrate. Radiology 127:719
7. Bekerman C, Hoffer PB, Bitran JD (1985) The role of gallium-67 in the clinical evaluation of cancer. Semin Nucl Med 15:72
8. Botsch H (1983) Galliumszintigraphie (Diagnostik bei entzündlichen Erkrankungen und Tumoren). Springer, Berlin Heidelberg New York Tokyo
9. Brascho DJ, Durant JR, Green LE (1977) The accuracy of retroperitoneal ultrasonography in Hodgkin's disease and non-Hodgkin's lymphoma. Radiology 125:485
10. Breit A, Czempiel H, Koernig-Kron K (1969) Die Lymphszintigraphie in der Tumortherapie (Erfahrung an über 800 Tumorpatienten). Strahlentherapie 138:74
11. Breslow A (1975) Tumor thickness, level of invasion, and node dissection in stage I cutaneous melanoma. Ann Surg 182:572
12. Chiappa S, Uslenghi C, Bonadonna G, Musumeci R (1970) Endolymphatic radiotherapy in malignant lymphomas – long-term results. Lymphology 1:13
13. Coates G, Bush RS, Aspin N (1973) A study of ascites using lymphoscintigraphy with ^{99m}Tc sulfur colloid. Radiology 107:577
14. Collier BD, Palmer DW, Wilson JF et al. (1983) Internal mammary lymphoscintigraphy in patients with breast cancer. Radiology 147:845
15. Deckart H, Lüning M, Gebert G, Henze E (1971) Möglichkeiten und Grenzen der abdominellen Lymphszintigraphie im Vergleich zur Lymphographie in der Beurteilung maligner Lymphoblastosen. Dtsch Gesundheitswes 9:391
16. Dionne L, Friede J, Blais R (1983) Internal mammary lymphoscintigraphy in breast carcinoma – a surgeon's perspective. Semin Nucl Med 13:35
17. Duson GL, Thrall H, Stevenson JS, Pinsky SM (1983) ^{99m}Tc minicolloid for radionuclide lymphography. Radiology 109:387
18. Edeling CJ (1983) Ga-67 in pediatric oncology. Clin Nucl Med 8:205
19. Ege GN (1977) Internal mammary lymphoscintigraphy in breast carcinoma: a study of 1072 patients. Int J Radiat Oncol Biol Phys 2:755
20. Fairbanks VF, Tauxe WN, Kiely JM, Miller WE (1972) Scintigraphic visualization of abdominal lymph nodes with ^{99m}Tc pertechnetate-labeled sulfur colloid. J Nucl Med 13:185

21. Fawwaz RA, Winchell HS, Frye F, Hemphill W, Lawrence JH (1969) Localization of [58]Co and [65]Zn − hematoporphyrin complexes in canine lymph nodes. J Nucl Med 10:581
22. Fawwaz RA, Wang TST, Srivastava SC et al. (1984) Potential of palladium-109-labeled antimelanoma monoclonal antibody for tumor therapy. J Nucl Med 25:796
23. Fee HJ, Robinson DS, Sample WF et al. (1978) The determination of lymph shed by colloidal gold scanning in patients with malignant melanoma: a preliminary study. Surgery 84:626
24. Fernholz HJ (1967) Lymphoszintigraphie im Kopf-Hals-Bereich. ROFO 4:106
25. Földi M, Casley-Smith JR (1983) Lymphangiology. Schattauer, Stuttgart, p 723
26. Frühling J (1981) Lymph and lymphatic pathophysiology. Radiopharmacol 2:223
27. Gates GF, Dore EK, Kanchanapoom V (1972) Thoracic duct leakage in neonatal chylothorax visualized by [198]Au lymphangiography. Radiology 105:619
28. Handmaker H, Ömara RE (1977) Gallium imaging in pediatrics. J Nucl Med 18:1057
29. Hay JB, Hobbs BB (1977) The flow of blood to lymph nodes and its relation to lymphocyte traffic and the immune response. J Exp Med 145:31
30. Henkin RE, Polycyn RE, Quinn JL (1974) Scanning treated Hodgkin's disease with ^{67}Ga citrate. Radiology 110:151
31. Herman TS, Jones SE (1978) Systematic restaging in patients with Hodgkin's disease − a southwest oncology group study. Cancer 42:1976
32. Höfer R, Benzer H (1967) Die indirekte Lymphographie der Lungen. In: Fellinger K, Höfer R (eds) Radioaktive Isotope in Klinik und Forschung. Urban und Schwarzenberg, München p 410
33. Hör G, Glaubitt D, Grebe SF, Hampe J, Haubold U et al. (1972) Tumorszintigraphie mit [67]Ga. In: Pabst HW, Hör G (eds) Nuklearmedizin − Klinische Leistungsfähigkeit und technische Entwicklung. Schattauer, Stuttgart, p 318
34. Hör G, Kempken K, Kriegel H, Langhammer H et al. (1974) Munich report on [67]Ga: a review of our experiences in nuclear biology, experimental and clinical nuclear medicine after four years use. Proc. Ist. World Congr. Nucl. Med. Berl., Tokyo 1974 (book of abstr.)
35. Hör G, Maul FD, Standke R, Munz D (1981) Scintigraphy in oncology. In: IAEA (ed) Medical radionuclide imaging 1980, Vienna, p 487
36. Hör G (1985) Nuklearmedizinisch-onkologische Einführung. In: Holzmann H, Altmeyer P, Hör G, Hahn K (eds) Dermatologie und Nuklearmedizin. Springer, Berlin Heidelberg New York Tokyo, p 113
37. Hoffer P (1980) Status of gallium-67 in tumor detection. J Nucl Med 21:394
38. Holzmann H, Altmeyer P, Hör G, Hahn K (eds) (1985) Dermatologie und Nuklearmedizin. Springer, Berlin Heidelberg New York Tokyo
39. Hübner KF, King P, Gibbs WD, Partain CL, Washburn LC et al. (1981) Clinical investigations with carbon-11-labelled amino acids using positron emission computerized tomography in patients with neoplastic diseases. Medical radionuclide imaging 1980. IAEA, Vienna, p 515
40. Hultborn KA, Jonsson L (1955) The use of calloidal [198]Au for the detection of lymph nodes in radical excision of the breast. Acta Radiol 43:132
41. Illig L: Lokale Lymphoszintigraphie in der Diagnostik der malignen Melanome der Haut. In: Holzmann H, Altmeyer P, Hör G, Hahn K (eds) Dermatologie und Nuklearmedizin. Springer, Berlin Heidelberg New York Tokyo
41a. Ito Y, Otsuka N, Nagai K, Muranaka A et al. (1982) Lymphoscintigraphy by subcutaneous injection of ^{67}Ga-citrate. Eur J Nucl Med 7:260
42. Jung H, Munz DL, Hör G, Frenkel G (1983) Lymphabflußuntersuchungen mit ^{99m}Tc-Antimontrisulfid-Kolloid und ^{67}Ga-Zitrat bei Malignomen im Gesichtsschädel- und Mundhöhlenbereich. Dtsch Z Mund-Kiefer-Gesichts-Chir 7:445
43. Kaplan WD, Anderson KC, Leonard RCF et al. (1983) High dose gallium in the evaluation of lymphoma (Abstr.). J Nucl Med 24:50
44. Kappert A (1985) Lehrbuch und Atlas der Angiologie. Erkrankungen der Arterien, Venen, Kapillaren und Lymphgefäße. Huber, Bern
45. Langhammer H, Hör G, Pabst HW (1970) Zur diagnostischen Diskrepanz von abdominaler Lymphknotenszintigraphie und röntgenologischer Lymphographie. Rontgenblätter 23:261

46. Langhammer H, Büll U, Kucharczyk D, Hör G, Frey KW, Pabst HW (1974) Zur Treffsicherheit der abdominalen Lymphknotenszintigraphie in der Tumordiagnostik. Med Welt 25:358
47. Larson SM, Carrasquillo JA (1984) Nuclear oncology 1984. Semin Nucl Med 14:268
48. Lepanto PB, Rosenstock J, Littman P (1976) Gallium-67 scans in children with solid tumors. Am J Rontgenol 126:179
49. Lofferer O, Mostbeck A: Nuclear medicine techniques in the diagnosis and differential diagnosis of swollen arms and legs. In: (25)
50. Mansfield CM, Park CH (1985) Contribution of radionuclide imaging to radiation oncology. Semin Nucl Med 15:28
51a. Maul FD, Wenisch HJC, Schumm P-M, Usadel KH, Bittner G et al. (1984) Zur szintigraphischen Differenzierung maligner und benigner Schilddrüsentumoren mit ^{201}Tl. In: Verhandlungen der Deutschen Gesellschaft für innere Medizin, vol 90. Bergmann, München, p 1026
51b. Maul FD, Altmeyer P, Bittner G, Wanner U et al. (1985) Die Thallium-201-Szintigraphie in der Diagnostik des metastasierenden malignen Melanoms. In: [38] p. 198
52. Menon M, Menon S, Strauss HW, Catalona WJ (1977) Demonstration of the existence of canine prostatic lymphatics by radioisotope techniques. J Urol 118:274
53. Mostbeck A, Partsch H, Kahn P (1985) Quantitative Isotopenlymphographie. In: Holzmann H, Altmeyer P, Hör G, Hahn K (eds) Dermatologie und Nuklearmedizin. Springer, Berlin Heidelberg New York Tokyo, p 426
54. Munz DL, Altmeyer P, Holzmann H, Encke A, Hör G (1982) Der Stellenwert der Lymphoszintigraphie in der Behandlung maligner Melanome der Haut. Dtsch Med Wochenschr 107:86
55. Munz DL (1983) Experimentelle und klinische Untersuchungen über die regionäre Lymphdrainage der Haut mit ^{99m}Tc markiertem Antimontrisulfid-kolloid − Bedeutung für das maligne Hautmelanom. Habilitationsschrift, Universität Frankfurt
56. Munz DL, Kötter R, Kornemann I, Brandhorst I, Hör G (1984) Bone marrow scanning versus bone scanning in the early diagnosis of neoplastic involvement of the skeletal system: A comparative parallel study. In: Schmidt HAE, Adam WE (eds) Nuklearmedizin. Schattauer, Stuttgart, p 664
57. Ochi H, Sawa H, Fukada T et al. (1982) Thallium-201-Chloride thyroid scintigraphy to evaluate benign and/or malignant nodules. Cancer 50:236
58. Pabst HW, Langhammer H (1980) Klinische Bedeutung des szintigraphischen Geschwulstnachweises mit tumoraffinen Testsubstanzen. Fortschr Med 98:653
59. Peters PE (1970) Zur Funktion der Lymphknotenbarriere des Menschen − Untersuchung mit ^{51}Cr-markierten Erythrozyten. ROFO 113:1
60. Potchen EJ, Welch MJ (1968) Radioisotopic assessment of extravascular albumin as an index of lymph transport. Lymphology 1:58
61. Richman SD, Appelbaum F, Levenson SM (1975) ^{67}Ga radionuclide imaging in Burkitt's lymphoma. Radiology 117:639
62. Rosenblum I, Stadler A, Wiznitzer T, Baron J (1982) Radionuclide mammalymphography in the preoperative investigation of suspected breast cancer. In: Schmidt HAE, Rösler H (eds) Nuklearmedizin. Schattauer, Stuttgart, p 830
63. Savioli M, Mango L, Spagnoli F, Cavallaro A (1983) ^{201}Tl scintigraphy of lymph node metastases in thyroid carcinoma: A case report. Tumor Diagn 3:138
64. Schenk P (1966) Szintigraphische Darstellung des parasternalen Lymphsystems. Strahlentherapie 130:4
65. Seitzman DM, Wright R, Halaby FA, Freeman JH (1963) Radioactive lymph angiography as a therapeutic adjunct. Am J Rontgenol 89:140
66. Sherman AJ, Ter-Pogossian M, Tocus EC (1953) Lymph node concentration of radioactive colloidal gold following interstitial injection. Cancer 6:1238
67. Siegl H, Wascher H (1967) Die Szintigraphie der zervikalen Lymphbahnen. Monatsschr Ohrenheilk Laryngol Rhinol 101:409
68. Sugarbaker EV, McBride CM (1976) Melanoma of the trunk: the results of surgical excision and anatomic guidelines for predicting nodal metastasis. Surgery 80:22
68a. Thompson CH, Stacker SA, Salehi N et al. (1984) Immunoscintigraphy for detection of lymph node metastases from breast cancer. Lancet II:1245

69. Turner DA, Fordham EW, Ali A (1978) Gallium-67 imaging in the management of Hodgkin's disease and other malignant lymphomas. Semin Nucl Med 8:205
70. Walker LA (1950) Localization of radioactive colloids in lymph nodes. J Lab Clin Med 36:440
71. Winkler C (1985) Nuklearmedizinische Tumordiagnostik. In: Hundeshagen H (ed) Nuklearmedizin, Part 3, Diagnostik II, Handbuch der medizinischen Radiologie. Springer, Berlin Heidelberg New York Tokyo, p 407
72. Zum Winkel K, Becker J, Jahns E, Scheurlen H, Herzfeld U (1967) Indikationsstellung und Dosimetrie bei der endolymphatischen Therapie mit J^{131}-Lipiodol. Strahlentherapie 133:4
73. Zum Winkel K (1972) Lymphologie mit Radionukliden. Hoffmann, Berlin
74. Zum Winkel K, Herbst H (1974) Möglichkeiten und Grenzen der Lymphszintigraphie. Dtsch Ärztebl 10:69

Bone Scintigraphy in Primary Malignant Bone Tumor

H. Creutzig[1]

Bone scintigraphy reflects the intensity of metabolic activity in the bone and therefore is a functional and not a morphological image. The sensitivity in detecting metastatic tumors of the skeleton has been proven to be much higher than X-ray techniques in many, but not in all, entities of primaries, while the specificity of conventional static imaging is very low. In secondaries, an increase in specificity by dynamic imaging is limited, the important differentiation between primary bone tumor and atypical osteomyelitis is impossible [1]. We will discuss the usefulness and limitations of dynamic bone scintigraphy in the diagnosis and follow-up of primary malignant tumors of the skeleton.

Malignant bone neoplasms are rare. Their estimated incidence is less than one case per 100 000 per year; they make up less than 1% of solid cancers. This incidence, however, is age-related; peak is 8% of cancers in the group of 15–19 years. In this peak group 60% are osteosarcomas and 30% Ewing's sarcomas, while in the aged group the most common tumor will be the chondrosarcoma.

There are no specific clinical signs: persistent local pain, especially in the young and around knee or shoulder, will be suspicious of malignancy. Only nonossifying fibroma and solitary enchondroma can be diagnosed by typical X-ray findings. In all other cases with an abnormal X-ray, open biopsy with histological examination is recommended as the only unequivocal test to exclude the diagnosis of malignancy.

The prognosis of malignant bone tumors depends on the grade and the stage of the tumor and the effectiveness of treatment. Any staging system must incorporate the significant prognostic factors, stratify the stages, and provide guidelines for adjunctive therapies.

The WHO system will not fullfil this and therefore should be only of historical interest as should our classification of uptake pattern in primary bone tumors [2]. The system used today is proposed by the Musculoskeletal Tumor Society and adopted by the American Joint Committee for Cancer Staging. It is based on three factors: (i) grading (G_{0-2}), (ii) extension of the primary tumor (T_{0-2}), and (iii) presence of metastases ($M_{0,1}$) [4].

Inactive benign lesions (G_0, T_0, M_0) are latent, static, and self-healing. Radiographic characteristics are lesions that are well-marginated by a mature shell of cortical-like reactive bone (Lodwick I a). In dynamic scintigraphy there is neither a hyperperfusion nor an increase in the early or late static scans (Table 1).

---

1 Abt. Nuklearmedizin, Hufelandstr. 55, D-4300 Essen

Nuclear Medicine in Clinical Oncology
Ed. by C. Winkler
© Springer-Verlag Berlin Heidelberg 1986

Table 1. Pattern of dynamic scintigraphy in primary bone tumors

	Benign inactive	Benign active	Benign aggressive low-grade sarcomas	High-grade sarcomas
Perfusion	N	+	+ +	+ − + + +
Early uptake	N	+ +	+ + − + + +	+ + +
Late uptake	N	+	+ +	+ + − + + +
Size (X-ray)	0	equal	larger	much larger

Active, progressing benign lesions (G_0, T_0, M_0) are mildly symptomatic and occasionally associated with pathological fractures. They grow steadily, but remain encapsulated. Radiographic characteristics are irregular marginated defects; expansion, bulging, and deformation of overlying reactive bone or cortex is frequently observed (Lodwick I b). In dynamic scintigraphy there is a distinct hyperperfusion and an increase in the static images corresponding closely to the radiographic defects.

Aggressive, invasive benign lesions (G_0, $T_{1,2}$, $M_{0,1}$) are symptomatic and grow rapidly, often associated with a pathological fracture. They penetrate the capsule and the natural barriers and may appear inflammatory. Despite the really benign cytologic characteristics, distant, usually pulmonary, metastases may occur. Radiographic characteristics are a ragged permeative interface with adjacent bone, cortical destruction, endosteal buttresses and periosteal Codman's triangles (Lodwick I c). In dynamic scintigraphy there is a marked hyperperfusion, a high uptake in the early and late static images, both beyond the radiographic limits.

The behavior of G_0 benign lesions is often better predicted by the combination of radiographic staging and clinical features or the findings of dynamic scintigraphy than by histology. Therefore, in all patients with radiographic signs of Lodwick I b or I c a dynamic scan should precede any surgery.

Low-grade sarcomas (G_1, $T_{1,2}$, M_0) present as a slow-growing, painless mass with an indolent, but steady, growth rate. They are not inhibited by the natural barriers and often produce extraosseous extension and neovascular bundle involvement. Radiographic characteristics are a generous reactive rim of cancellous bone admixed with defects of extracapsular and/or soft tissue extension (Lodwick II). Scintigraphic signs are the same as in aggressive benign lesions.

High-grade sarcomas usually appear as destructive symptomatic masses. Radiographic characteristics are no, or a poorly marginated, border between the lesion and the surrounding bone, patchy cortical destruction, early soft tissue extension, obliteration of periostal reaction, and ill-defined intramedullary extension (Lodwick III). In dynamic scintigraphy there is an extreme hyperperfusion, and a maximal uptake in both the early and the late scan, wide beyond the radiographic signs.

Low-grade sarcomas are parosteal or enosteal osteosarcoma, giant cell tumor, hemangioendothelioma; high-grade sarcomas the "classic" osteosarcoma, postradiation and Paget's sarcoma, chondrosarcoma, and giant cell sarcoma.

The clinical usefulness of radionuclide imaging in differentiation of malignant bone tumors is discussed controversely. McLean and Murray concluded from their experiences with 52 primary bone sarcomas that osteosarcoma, Ewing's sarcoma, and chondrosarcoma tend to be associated with a characteristic pattern permitting a particular diagnosis to be suggested [9], while Siuda et al. [11] could not make a clear distinction between benign and malignant tumors by ratio measuring and three-phase scintigraphy. Biopsy remains the only unequivocal diagnostic test [3]. In pulmonary metastases there might be an intensive uptake of Tc-99m-MDP, but the diagnostic test of choice is CT scanning [12]. Bone scanning is, however, the most sensitive test for detecting bone metastases and must therefore precede any other more invasive diagnosis and any treatment [6].

The dynamic bone scan may be helpful in the differentiation of benign lesions (G_0) into static, active, or aggressive (Table 1). In sarcomas it is less helpful for initial classification, but is more sensitive than X-ray or CT in detecting skip lesions and skeletal metastases [5, 7]. In the early follow-up during chemotherapy, dynamic scintigraphy may predict the later outcome of this therapy [7]. Therefore, bone scintigraphy should not only be done before, but also during treatment.

Dynamic scintigraphy

The technique of dynamic scintigraphy differs only little from the classic three-phase bone scintigraphy. For intra- and interindividual comparison, sequential computerized scintigraphy and exact standardisation of acquisition parameters is necessary. The best approach for this comparison has been proposed by Knop et al. [8]: they measure regional Tc-99m-MDP clearances for up to one hour after i.v. injection of the radiopharmaceutical over the tumor, normal bone, and soft tissue regions. One hour later, the uptake over the tumor region and the corresponding contralateral region is quantified by a static computerized scan. This technique is rather time consuming.

For less-equipped departments the COSS nuclear study group has proposed a minimal program: a computerized dynamic scintigraphy for 10 min, calculation of slope ratios or uptake ratios from a short dynamic study, and a late static image (Table 2). Analog images might be impressive, but the addition of

Table 2. Quantitative three-phase scintigraphy in primary bone tumor (COSS 85)

Tumor/contralateral region ratio
1.   10– 20 s after bolus injection of Tc-99m-MDP
2.   30– 40 s
3.   60– 70 s
4.   5–   6 min
5. 120–121 min

Documentation of activity, region size, count rate, etc.

---

quantitative data is necessary for predicting of treatment response. The study is repeated every second week during chemotherapy.

In good responders a normalization of tumor blood flow and a decrease in regional clearance by ⅔, or a decrease of uptake ratios in both the early and late static scan of more than 70%, is seen within 6 weeks of treatment start [8, 10]. In nonresponders there is a further increase in some or all parameters. In partial response a mixed pattern may occur: while there is a normalization in tumor perfusion, there are little changes in late uptake ratios. Only in good responders will an en-bloc resection of the tumor be useful. Two case reports will illustrate these findings:

Case report 1: The 15-year-old girl has been referred to bone scintigraphy to confirm an inflammatory process in the right knee. A painful swelling has been treated by her surgeon without any X-ray diagnosis. The late static image is shown in Fig. 1: it is diagnostic for a benign aggressive or a malignant bone tumor, in combination with age and symptoms of the patient for a classic osteosarcoma. The pelvic scan (Fig. 2) shows a skip lesion at the region of the trochanter minor, it is a $G_2T_2M_1$ tumor. While the tumor is confirmed by X-ray, both CT and angiography are negative for the skip lesion. The patient is treated preoperatively with chemotherapy following the COSS protocol [13, 8].

Time-activity curves over the tumor and the contralateral side show a response of perfusion, but no normalization (Fig. 3). Histologically, a near total avitality is seen in the posttreatment biopsy (regression grade III after Salzer), and an amputation is done.

Another 3 months later (Fig. 4) the skip lesion seems to be unchanged in the late scan and is not detectable by CT. The study is repeated another 4 months later after a pleural metastasis has been removed surgically: the perfusion is normal, but both the early and the late scan show an maximal uptake in the skip lesion (Fig. 5). CT is now also positive and maximal-dose chemotherapy is started. Another 3 weeks later multiple skeletal metastases are seen on the late pelvic scan (Fig. 6). The patient died one month later.

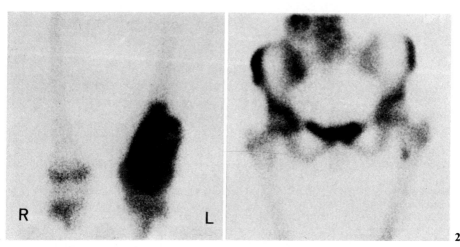

Fig. 1. Late static scan from ventral in a 15 year old girl – intensive uptake beyond the limits of radiographic signs – diagnostic for malignant or benign agressive bone tumor (010369-12. 1. 84)

Fig. 2. Pelvic scan in the same patient with a faint uptake in the trochanter minor region left. "Skip lesion"

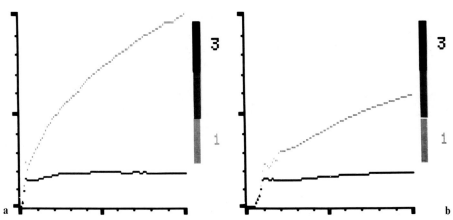

Fig. 3. Time-activity curve for ten minutes over tumor (gray) and contralateral knee (black) **a** before and **b** after six months of treatment. There is an 45% decrease in early (10 min) uptake

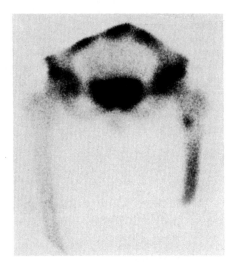

Fig. 4. Scan in the same patient three months after amputation. The uptake in the skip lesion is unchanged

Case report 2: This 17-year-old girl was referred for scintigraphy after a plain X-ray was done because of a sport accident 2 days before. The radiological diagnosis of osteosarcoma was confirmed by scintigraphy. During treatment the late uptake decreased, and the time-activity curves normalized. The good response was confirmed by a total avitalization of tumor mass in the posttreatment biopsy and a normal postsurgical follow-up.

Valid data of the late prognosis in scintigraphically good responders are not available. From short-term experience (1–2 a) dynamic scintigraphy will best predict the outcome. Therefore, this technique should be used not only in prospective protocols, but in every patient with primary malignant bone tumor before and after initial treatment. As in the diagnosis of acute osteomyelitis [1],

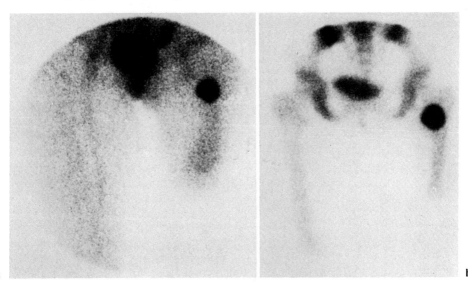

a   b

Fig. 5a, b. The same patient another three months later. The perfusion is normal, but there is an intensive uptake both in the early (**a**) and the late scan (**b**)

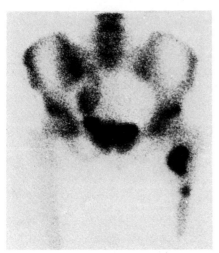

Fig. 6. Multiple skeletal metastases another three weeks later and prefinal

there seems to be no difference in the usefulness of dynamic Tc-99m-MDP scintigraphy and quantitative gallium-67 imaging [14].

In summary, bone scintigraphy may indicate a malignant or benign bone tumor, is highly sensitive in detecting both skip and distant bone metastases, and must therefore be done in the initial diagnostic procedure after an X-ray suggests a bone tumor. Moreover, dynamic bone scintigraphy will predict treatment response; at least in prospective studies it is done during initial treatment every second week. In the "routine" follow-up it should be repeated before any biopsy.

References

1. Creutzig H (1984) Nuklearmedizinische Diagnostik der Osteomyelitis. Nuklearmediziner 7:133
2. Creutzig H, Bornemann H, Schwarzrock R (1978) Szintigraphie bei primären Knochentumoren und tumor-like lesions. Nuklearmediziner 1:31
3. Eilber FR, Caulkins E (1984) Bone tumors – clinical and radiological investigation. In: Enneking WF (ed) Current concepts of diagnosis and treatment of bone and soft tissue tumors. Springer, Berlin Heidelberg New York Tokyo
4. Enneking WF (1984) Staging of musculoskeletal neoplasm. In: Enneking WF (ed) Current concepts of diagnosis and treatment of bone and soft tissue tumors. Springer, Berlin Heidelberg New York Tokyo
5. Fischer M, Wasyleweski AH, Ritter J (1985) Die Wertigkeit der Knochenszintigraphie bei malignen Knochentumoren. In: Hahn K (ed) Pädiatrische Nuklearmedizin, vol 3. Kirchheim, Mainz
6. Kloiber R (1984) Scintigraphy of bone tumors. In: Enneking WF (ed) Current concepts of diagnosis and treatment of bone and soft tissue tumors. Springer, Berlin Heidelberg New York Tokyo
7. Knop J, Montz R (1983) Bone scintigraphy in patients with osteogenic sarcoma – Cooperative osteogenic sarcoma study group COSS 80. J Cancer Res Clin Oncol 106 [Suppl]:49
8. Knop J, Stritze P, Montz R (1985) Knochenszintigraphie zur Erfolgsbeurteilung einer Chemotherapie beim Osteosarkom. Nuklearmedizin 24:75
9. McLean RG, Murray ICP (1984) Scintigraphic pattern in certain primary malignant bone tumors. Clin Radiol 35:379
10. Müller St, Schober O, Creutzig H (1985) Analyse der ersten Phase im Knochenszintigramm. In: Feine U (ed) 2. Tübinger Knochensymposium
11. Siuda S, Büll U, Pottmeyer A (1984) Szintigraphische Beurteilung von primären Knochentumoren. Nuklearmediziner 7:89
12. Vanel D, Henry-Amar M, Lumbroso J (1984) Pulmonary evaluation of patients with osteosarcoma. Am J Roentgenol 143:519
13. Winkler K, Beron G, Kotz R (1984) Neoadjuvant chemotherapy for osteogenic sarcoma: results of a cooperative German/Austrian study (COSS-80). J Clin Oncol 5:33
14. Yeh SD, Rosen G, Caparros B (1984) Semiquantitative Gallium scintigraphy in patients with osteogenic sarcoma. Clin Nucl Med 9:175

Scintigraphic Detection of Bone Metastases

E. K. J. PAUWELS[1], H. E. SCHÜTTE, J. W. ARNDT, and A. VAN LANGEVELDE

Following the introduction of suitable radiotracers for skeletal imaging, the detection of malignant bone disease became one of the important fields of interest in nuclear medicine. In many nuclear medicine departments bone scans may account for more than half of all imaging procedures. In oncology many applications of bone scintigraphy have been mentioned, and it is recognized that the bone scan is no longer solely used for the mapping of bone metastases, but among other applications also for therapy monitoring and the localization of sites for biopsy or further diagnostic imaging. It should be emphasized that in an era of limited funds for health care it is important to understand how useful bone scanning is. It is the purpose of this chapter to explore the indications for bone scintigraphy in the evaluation of patients with osseous metastases. In addition to this survey the cost-effectiveness of bone scanning in relation to its diagnostic yield and the proper choice of bone seeking radiopharmaceuticals for the detection of skeletal metastases will be discussed.

Choice of Radiopharmaceutical

After the introduction of Tc-99m polyphosphate [1] it was found that other Tc-99m labeled bone-seeking agents revealed higher uptake in bone. Continuing research for more efficacious radiopharmaceuticals for bone imaging has brought us to the use of Tc-99m labeled pyrophosphate (PPi), ethylene hydroxy diphosphonate (EHDP), and methylene hydroxy diphosphonate (MDP) within a relatively short period in the mid-1970s. Of these compounds Tc-99m MDP is still widely used. Fogelman [2], however, has pointed out that the detection rate of bone metastases was not improved with the introduction of MDP and it was suggested that neither EHDP nor MDP is superior to the other in cinical practice. Investigations on other diphosphonates have also been performed [3, 4], but these compounds were found to be not very useful, as they displayed a lower bone affinity than MDP for both normal and abnormal osseous tissue. Improvements in the scintigraphic image quality and the lesion detection rate were reported with the use of the recently developed bone agents Tc-99m hydroxy methylene diphosphonate (HDP) and Tc-99m-dicarboxy propane

---

1 Department of Diagnostic Radiology, Division of Nuclear Medicine, University Hospital, Rijnsburgerweg 10, NL-2333 AA Leiden

Nuclear Medicine in Clinical Oncology
Ed. by C. Winkler
© Springer-Verlag Berlin Heidelberg 1986

diphosphonate (DPD). A few studies with cross-over clinical comparison of these agents were published [5-7], and it was concluded that these newer agents do not possess relevant clinical advantages over the traditionally used MDP as to the visualization of bone metastases. In order to compare the image quality and lesion detectability of Tc-99m HDP and Tc-99m MDP, Van Duzee et al. [8] demonstrated that there were small but significant improvements in scintigraphic parameters at 2 h after injection with the use of Tc-99m HDP. In addition to these findings it was shown that Tc-99m HDP images obtained at 2 h after injection are of high cosmetic and diagnostic quality as compared with 3-h bone scans [9] and that all lesions visualized at 3 h are also clearly visible at 2 h. In an unpublished recent study using commercially available HDP, we have compared bone scans obtained with this Tc-99m labeled HDP preparation and Tc-99m labeled MDP at 2 h after injection in 10 patients suffering from bone metastases and various malignancies.

Visual reading of MDP and HDP scintigrams revealed the same number and locations of bone metastases.

Semiquantitative image evaluation included the rating of radiopharmaceutical concentration in normal bone and soft tissue, the lesion definition on the scan and the overall image quality ("cosmetics") of the scintigram.

In this evaluation, the images, with no signs of identification as to imaging agent and patient name, were placed on a view box. Visual grading occurred on a four-point scale. In this double-blind comparative study we found a statistically significant ($P<0.0001$) superiority of the HDP image over MDP with respect to normal bone visualization at 2 h after injection and the overall image quality ("cosmetics") ($P<0.001$) (Dr. Heideman, Dept. Medical Statistics, University of Leiden). Also the other parameters pointed to better imaging characteristics for HDP than for MDP, although these differences were not statistically significant.

From this recent investigation and from other studies we believe that there is sufficient evidence that HDP is the best agent for scintigraphic imaging of the skeleton and the detection of bone metastases. At present, the use of HDP will result in the best possible bone scan in the majority of patients even at 2 h after injection. It is our experience that incidentally patients may benefit from the use of Tc-99m MDP or Tc-99m DPD as these agents may give slightly better images in selected cases.

The search for new bone-seeking agents is a continuing one. It needs to be emphasized that tracers showing high uptake in normal bone do not necessarily display bone lesions to a desirable degree. The ideal combination remains the high uptake in normal bone and the bone lesion with low uptake in soft tissue. Some recent data have become available as to the use of a new agent which displays a high bone lesion to normal bone ratio: dimethyl amino diphosphonate (DMAD). Studies by Rosenthall [10] and Smith [11] have demonstrated that lesions barely or not visible with MDP were disclosed with MDAD. Unfortunately, the normal bone to soft tissue ratio was very low for this agent, and this poor visualization of the normal skeleton does not make DMAD the preferred agent. The introduction of this new bone-scanning agent may, however, show the way to a new class of imaging agents.

Yield of Bone Scanning for the Detection of Bone Metastases

Skeletal scintigraphy for the detection of osseous metastases may lead to a false-negative result in 3%−5% of the cases. This may be caused by obesity of the patient or may be due to little reactive bone turnover, which occurs in fast-growing or indolent metastases. False negative results may lead to delay in treatment, increase patient suffering and may ultimately result in increased health care cost.

False positive scintigraphic findings include benign lesions which are wrongly reported as malignant. In this respect it should be realized that bone scintigraphy cannot differentiate between benign and malignant disease as bone-seeking agents accumulate in both types of lesions. Only under certain conditions the skeletal abnormalities may be positively interpreted as malignant and the interpreter of the bone scan should be aware of this. False positive results may have serious consequences and may have considerable disadvantages for the treatment of the patient. Ultimately, such results will also increase health costs.

Once the site of osseous pathology has been assessed using scintigraphy, roentgenologic examination should follow. The importance of radiography may be illustrated by our findings in 138 patients suffering from malignant disease. In 65 cases we noticed osseous abnormalities. Roentgenological evaluation revealed malignant secondary lesions in 55 patients. In the other 10 patients scintigraphic lesions were attributed to fractures or osteoporotic collapse of vertebrae [12].

Although it is impossible to differentiate between malignant and benign bone lesions with scintigraphy, the following characteristics of the abnormal bone scan may be of assistance in the interpretation.

Pattern of Scintigraphic Abnormalities

The bone scintigram in Paget's disease is very often characteristic of this disorder, so that the diagnosis is unequivocal. There is a characteristic, sharply defined area of homogeneously high uptake of radioactivity in the affected bone, although an area of even higher uptake within one lesion is unequivocal. In long bones, the area of high activity is always bordered by the articular surface on one side and by normal bone on the other side [13]. Augmented deposition of the radiopharmaceutical that occurs solely in the joints is very seldom due to malignant disease, but rather to arthrosis or arthritis.

Hematogenic Metastases

Some malignant diseases show an arterial or venous pattern of metastatic disease. Peripheral bone lesions are more likely to be malignant in a patient with lung carcinoma than in a patient with breast carcinoma. In the latter case, bone metastases preferentially occur in the axial skeleton. If, in the case of breast carcinoma, only peripheral skeletal lesions are observed, these abnormalities may be attributed to fracture or osteomyelitis rather than to bone metastases.

Solitary or Multiple Bone Lesions

Multiple lesions scattered over the whole skeleton, preferentially in the ribs and spine, are often due to metastases. Fractures in ribs, on the other hand, are characterized by a linear row of hot spots. Solitary lesions are difficult to interpret and roentgenologic evaluation should be carried out in all cases. In case of doubt, a few months later a repeat scan may display the proliferative nature of the disease in case of malignancy.

Bone Pain and the Results of the Bone Scans

Bone pain as an indicator for the presence or absence of skeletal metastases is not very reliable. Front et al. [14] demonstrated that only about 30% of individual bone metastases in breast carcinoma were painful, and it was concluded that scintigraphy is not only indicated in patients with bone pain. In addition to this, the question arises of whether a parameter as subjective as pain is useful in all cases. In some cases very painful bone lesions may conceal other bone metastases which are less painful.

Schütte [15] demonstrated that 60% of painful abnormalities disclosed by bone scintigraphy in patients suffering from malignancy were due to bone metastases. On the other hand, in 70 patients with bone pain, who were not known to have a malignancy, only 1 out of 30 abnormal bone scans appeared to be due to bone metastases, whereas all other lesions were caused by degenerative and benign disease, as demonstrated by radiography. Finn et al. [16] performed bone scintigraphy in patients with breast carcinoma, prostate carcinoma, and gynecologic tumors who were clinically suspected of having bone metastases. It was found that metastases were demonstrated respectively in 40%, 30%, and 7% of the cases. The authors described bone scintigraphy as a technique "to answer identifiable questions that have a reasonable probability of being answered."

In the past decade many facts and figures have become apparent on the usefulness of bone scintigraphy in various malignant disorders. In what follows pertinent data on the yields and value of bone scans will be presented on the basis of a literature review.

Scintigraphic Detection of Specific Metastases

Breast Carcinoma

Early reports [17] on the yield of bone scanning in patients with breast carcinoma gave high numbers for the presence of bone metastases, but these findings are no longer justified. At present, the yield of bone scintigraphy amounts to about 2% in stages I and II and about 30% in stage III [18].

At the early stages of breast carcinoma, skeletal scintigraphy has been advocated if clinical or biochemical signs of metastatic disease are present. In view of the low diagnostic yield in asymptomatic patients, baseline scintigraphy, as an aid in interpreting follow-up bone scans, is not recommended for the same reason. The high yield at later clinical stages of breast carcinoma makes skeletal scintigraphy useful both for diagnostic work-up and follow-up.

Prostate Carcinoma

Osteoblastic metastases may be clinically occult. However, with larger tumor sizes the probability of presence of bone metastases increases [19]. Diagnostic yields in relation to tumor stages have been reported to be: T1, 7%; T2, 19%; T3, 39%; and T4, 65%. Strikingly, alkaline and acid phosphatase serum concentration and bone pain are not good indicators for the presence or absence of bone metastases. For this reason bone scanning should be performed at both the early and later stages of prostate cancer.

Lung Carcinoma

Frequently occurring lytic metastases usually cause bone pain. In a study by Hooper [20], bone scintigraphy revealed metastases in 35.7% of the cases with clinical symptoms and in less than 4% of the patients without bone pain. Considering this low yield in the absence of bone pain, it is advocated that bone scanning be performed only when clinical symptoms are present. In oat cell and adenocarcinoma, asymptomatic and osteoblastic lesions may be present, and bone scintigraphy may be indicated for the staging of the patient.

Gynecologic, Bladder, and Gastrointestinal Tumors

The yield of bone scanning is reported to be very low in all stages [21] and it is advisable to perform this examination only in cases in which the presence of metastases is clinically suspected.

Multiple Myeloma

In this disease, little reactive bone formation is present, and this may be the reason why a false-negative rate of about 25% has been reported [22]. Frank et al. [23] have noted that increased tracer accumulation is often due to fractures, based on myeloma. As a general rule, roentgenologic evaluation of the skeleton is advised, although false-negative results have been reported in 15% of the cases.

Kidney Carcinoma

Bone metastases are often lytic and better demonstrable with radiography. As the majority of lesions are symptomatic, radiography should be the method of choice in later clinical stages of renal cell carcinoma [24]. A recent report by Rosen and Murphy [25] showed that about 8% of patients in early clinical stages of renal cell carcinoma had bone metastases demonstrated by scintigraphy. On the basis of this number, it remains questionable whether to perform bone scanning in the early stages of kidney carcinoma.

Cost-Effectiveness of Routine Bone Scanning

Many authors have indicated the usefulness of serial bone scanning on a routine basis in patients suffering from malignancies [26]. This repeated bone scintigraphy would allow the early recognition of high-risk patients and the early installment of therapy with decreasing costs of health care. Taking the high sensitivity of the bone scan into account, this looks like a valid argument for performing the examination routinely. However, under these conditions only the conversion of a normal to abnormal bone scan has diagnostic value. In order to assess the value of serial bone scintigraphy one has to know the incidence of this conversion. Not many data are available as to this incidence. In a literature survey, McNeil [27] has indicated that about 8% − 20% of patients with early staged breast carcinoma convert from normal to abnormal bone scan results within about 2 years of surgical treatment. These data are deduced from patient groups that were under treatment in the past decade and it can be expected that the incidence of bone metastases will be lower with earlier surgical treatment, radiotherapy, and adjuvant chemotherapy which is common now. Given the overall cost of a bone scan of US$ 200, an estimated incidence of conversion of 10% over 4 years, and serial bone scanning each half year over a period of 4 years, it would cost US$ 160 000 to detect osseous metastases in 10 patients, which amounts of US$ 16 000 per patient. The significance of these numbers is even clearer if a diagnostic yield of 2% to 5% is assumed.

On the basis of these numbers, routine serial bone scanning is difficult to justify, especially if one realizes that many of these cases will be symptomatic as far as bone pain and rises in phosphatase levels are concerned. In these selected symptomatic patients, radiographs of the involved skeletal areas may rapidly determine the nature of the lesion and only at that stage whole-body skeletal scintigraphy is necessary to determine the extent of the disease. Thus, it is believed that whole-body bone scanning may generally be desired in patients showing the clinical signs of disseminated skeletal disease. In addition to this, bone scintigraphy may be performed in individual cases on occasions in which it is necessary to ascertain the absence of bone metastases or to evaluate treatment. In these cases financial considerations are different, as the cost of the individual bone scan is low in terms of total cost of patient care.

References

1. Subramanian G, McAfee JG, Blair RJ et al. (1972) A potential radiopharmaceutical for skeletal imaging. J Nucl Med 13:947−950

2. Fogelman I, Citrin DL, McKillop JH et al. (1979) A clinical comparison of Tc-99m HEDP and Tc-99m MDP in the detection of bone metastases: concise communication. J Nucl Med 20:98–101

3. Wang TST, Fawwaz RA, Johnson LJ et al. (1980) Bone-seeking properties of Tc-99m carbonyl diphosphonic acid, dihydroxy-methylene diphosphonic acid and monohydroxy-methylene phosphonic acid: concise communication. J Nucl Med 21:767–770

4. Unterspann S (1976) Experimental examinations on the suitability of organo-aminomethane-bisphosphonic acid for bone scintigraphy by means of Tc-99m in animals. Eur J Nucl Med 1:151–154

5. Pauwels EKJ, Blom J, Camps JAJ et al. (1983) A comparison between the diagnostic efficacy of Tc-99m MDP, Tc-99m DPD and Tc-99m HDP for the detection of bone metastases. Eur J Nucl Med 8:118–122

6. Vorne M, Vähätalo S, Lantto T (1983) A clinical comparison of Tc-99m-DPD and two Tc-99m MDP agents. Eur J Nucl Med 8:395–397

7. Schroth HJ, Hausinger F, Garth H et al. (1984) Comparison of the kinetics of methylene-diphosphonate (MDP) and dicarboxypropan-diphosphonic acid (DPD), two radio-diagnostics for bone scintigraphy. Eur J Nucl Med 9:529–532

8. Van Duzee BF, Schaefer JA, Ball JD et al. (1984) Relative lesion detection ability of Tc-99m HMDP and Tc-99m MDP: concise communication. J Nucl Med 25:166–169

9. Pauwels EKJ, Blom J, Aarts JCNM (1984) A comparison between whole body scans made at two hours and three hours after intravenous injection of Tc-99m HDP as to image quality and lesion detectability. Clin Nucl Med 9:75–78

10. Rosenthall L, Stern J, Arzoumanian A (1982) A clinical comparison of MDP and DMAD. Clin Nucl Med 7:403–406

11. Smith ML, Martin W, McKillop JH et al. (1984) Improved lesion detection with dimethyl-amino-diphosphonate: a report of two cases. Eur J Nucl Med 9:519–520

12. Schütte HE, Park WM (1983) The diagnostic value of bone scintigraphy in patients with low back pain. Skeletal Radiol 10:1–4

13. Vellenga CJLR, Pauwels EKJ, Bijvoet OLM et al. (1984) Untreated Paget disease of bone studied by scintigraphy. Radiology 153:799–805

14. Front D, Schneck SD, Frankel A et al. (1979) Bone metastases and bone pain in breast cancer. JAMA 242:1747–1748

15. Schütte HE (1979) The influence of bone pain on the results of bone scans. Cancer 44:2039–2041

16. Finn SD, Larson EB, Rudd TR et al. (1982) Clinical use of radionuclide bone imaging in a university medical center. JAMA 248:439–442

17. Roberts JG, Gravelle IH, Baum M et al. (1976) Evaluation of radiography and isotopic scintigraphy for detecting skeletal metastases in breast cancer. Lancet 1:237–239

18. Pauwels EKJ, Heslinga JM, Zwaveling A (1982) Value of pre-treatment and follow-up skeletal scintigraphy in operable breast cancer. Clin Oncol 8:25–32

19. Biersack HJ, Wegner G, Distelmaier W et al. (1980) Ossäre Metastasierung des Prostatakarzinoms in Abhängigkeit von Tumorgröße und Geschwulstdifferenzierung. Nuklearmedizin 19:29–32

20. Hooper RG, Beechler CR, Johnson MC (1978) Radioisotope scanning in initial staging of bronchogenic carcinoma. Am Rev Respir Dis 118:279–286

21. Harbert JC, Rocha L, Smith FP et al. (1982) The efficacy of radionuclide bone scans in the evaluation of gynecologic cancers. Cancer 49:1040–1042

22. Woolfenden JM, Pitt MJ, Durie BGM et al. (1980) Comparison of bone scintigraphy and radiography in multiple myeloma. Radiology 134:723–728

23. Frank JW, LeBesque S, Buchanan RB (1982) The value of bone imaging in multiple myeloma. Eur J Nucl Med 7:502–505

24. Clyne CAC, Frank JW, Jenkins JD et al. (1983) The place of the Tc-99m-polyphosphonate bone scan in renal carcinoma. Br J Urol 55:174–175

25. Rosen PR, Murphy KG (1984) Bone scintigraphy in the initial staging of patients with renal cell carcinoma. J Nucl Med 25:289–291

26. McNeil BJ, Pace PD, Gray EB et al. (1978) Pre-operative and follow-up bone scans in patients with primary carcinoma of the breast. Surg Gynecol Obstet 147:745–748

27. McNeil BJ (1984) Value of bone scanning in neoplastic disease. Semin Nucl Med 14:277–286

Metaiodobenzylguanidine in the Diagnosis of Neuroblastomas

U. Feine[1]

The neuroblastoma is the second most common childhood malignant tumor. The diagnosis of most abdominal or mediastinal tumors is done as a rule with X-ray, CT, or ultrasound, yet the type can normally only be determined by taking a tissue sample. In an early examination, a third of the children older than 1 year show the disseminated form with distant metastases and often a diffuse bone/bone marrow infestation.

The tumor consists of embryonic cells from the sympathetic nerve cell row. In 1957 the high catecholamine production of these tumors, which is similar to that of the pheochromocytoma, was discovered and analyzed by means of the 24-h urine excretion.

In 1983/84 Kimmig [4] and our nuclear medicine pediatrics group [2] in Tübingen at the same time showed that ^{131}I-MIBG was actively absorbed and stored in the neuroblastoma. Metaiodobenzylguanidine (MIBG) labeled with ^{131}I has been used since 1981 by the working group of Beyerwaltes [1] in Ann Arbor for the clinical diagnosis of pheochromocytoma [5, 7].

MIBG is inserted into the level of the noradrenaline in a way similar to that of the sympathetic blocker, guanethidine, and is actively stored in the sympathetic nerve cells.

In 1984 at the Nuclear Medicine Congress in Helsinki [3] we introduced the results of a multicenter study at 6 different pediatric/nuclear medicine clinics with a total of 60 examinations of children with neuroblastoma. This study showed that the sensitivity of ^{131}I-MIBG in the diagnosis of neuroblastoma was very high and that high specificity was present as well.

Tables 1 – 4 reflect these results.

Table 1 shows the number of diagnostic cases and the therapies reported to us as of August 1984 by each of the clinics participating in the study.

Table 2 shows that, with one exception, all neuroblastoma children with raised catecholamine levels in the 24-h urine sample evidenced a clear absorption of ^{131}I-MIBG. The one negative case was examined with ^{123}I after 6 h but not after 24 h, and a late scintigraph was not made, so that the storage in the tumor did not come out clearly on the last day. (See below also our results with ^{123}I- MIBG.)

---

1 Nuclearmedizinische Abteilung, Medizinisches Strahleninstitut der Universität, Röntgenweg 11, D-7400 Tübingen

Nuclear Medicine in Clinical Oncology
Ed. by C. Winkler
© Springer-Verlag Berlin Heidelberg 1986

Table 1. Diagnostic and therapeutic attempts with ^{131}I-MIBG in neuroblastoma

	Cases (n)	Diagnostic (n)	Therapeutic (n)
Copenhagen	14	22	1
Tübingen	11	21	5
Heidelberg	7	7	0
Münster	7	7	0
Mainz	6	6	2
Düsseldorf	2	2	0
Total	47	65	8

Table 2. Results of diagnostic scintiscans in neuroblastoma with ^{131}I-MIBG in relationship to the excretion of catecholamines: Highly or medium elevated catecholamine levels (vanillinmandelic acid and homovanillic acid) in 24 h urine

Correct positive scan	39/40
False negative scan	1/40

Table 3. Results of diagnostic scintiscans in neuroblastomas with ^{131}I-MIBG in relationship to the excretion of catecholamines: Normal or borderline elevated catecholamine levels in the 24 h urine

Correct negative scans in cases without suspicion of relapse or metastatic lesion	10/10
Correct positive scans in cases with beginning relapse or metastatic lesion	8/10
False negative scan in a case with possible generalisation	1/10
Negative scan in a catecholamine negative primary tumor	1/10

Table 3 shows that all patients in the tumor-free stage were really negative, and at boderline values of catecholamine level 80% could be recognized as tumor positive. This result indicates the high value of MIBG diagnosis for the early recognition of the recurrence of tumors. Table 4 gives the sensitivity of all investigated cases of neuroblastoma, and also those where catecholamine was negative, as around 90%. The sensitivity of the catecholamine positive tumor cases is 96%.

The specificity was 100% when it is taken into consideration that other neurogenic tumors like the pheochromocytoma can be also positive.

Table 4. Results of diagnostic scintiscans in children with suspected neuroblastomas

---

A. 5 neuroblastomas without determination of the catecholamine levels
    1/5 positive scan
    4/5 negative scans

B. 5 suspected neuroblastomas. Final diagnosis:
    2 Non-Hodgkin lymphomas
    1 Rhabdomyosarcoma
    1 Liposarcoma
    1 Malignant neuroectodermal tumor

All tumors   Sensitivity 90%
Catecholamine-positive tumors   Sensitivity 96%
                                    Specificity 100%

Since attaining these results of the multicenter study we have conducted another 35 examinations of neuroblastoma children, in part with ^{131}I, but also with ^{123}I-MIBG.

The results can be summarized as follows:

1. The sensitivity of the primary neuroblastoma determination, before cytostatic treatment, continues to be very high for tumors with raised catecholamine secretions. To date, we have observed only one histologically verified neuroblastoma located in the neck region which was positive for ^{123}I-MIBG despite the absence of catecholamine secretion (Fig. 1).
2. After cytostatic treatment and external irradiation the absorption of MIBG in the tumor may be significantly lower. We observed two later tumors that were histologically strongly dedifferentiated. These tumors would not absorb

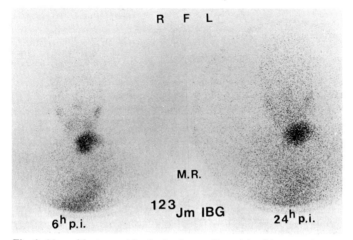

Fig. 1. Neuroblastoma, histologically confirmed by biopsy, without elevated catecholamine levels, in the neck region of a 4-year-old boy with good uptake of ^{123}I-MIBG. Blockade of the thyroid gland with iodine

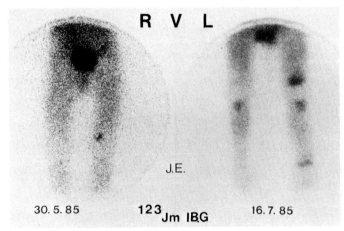

Fig. 2. Three-year-old boy, stage IV in remission after therapy. Beginning bone marrow infiltration at the left distal femur. After 6 weeks increased infiltration. Scan 24 h after 2.5 mCi ^{123}I-MIBG

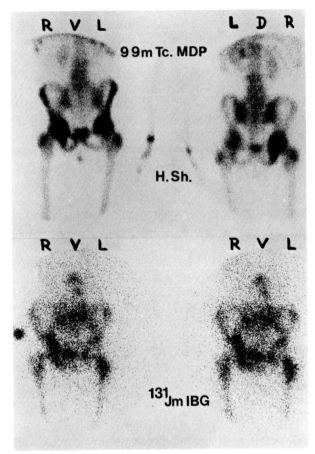

Fig. 3. Eight-year-old girl with neuroblastoma stage IV in remission after therapy, pain in region of the right pelvis without X-rays signs. Bone scan with local increased uptake in the ischium right side. MIBG scan: diffuse bone marrow uptake in the whole pelvis

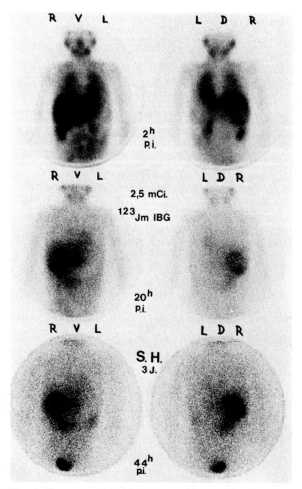

Fig. 4. Three-year-old girl with neuroblastoma behind the liver. Scintigraphy 2−44 h after injection of 2.5 mCi ^{123}I-MIBG. The tumor can be differentiated from the liver 20 h after injection, and after 44 h there is MIBG storage only in the tumor

any more MIBG, nor did they have significantly raised levels of catecholamine.

3. Although the tumor diagnosis of the neuroblastoma can normally be accomplished with other examination techniques, such as ultrasound, CT, and X-ray, MIBG storage can confirm the specific diagnosis of a neuroblastoma and allows a better recognition of the spreading of the tumor.

4. MIBG is especially well suited to the early discovery of a reoccuring tumor and diffuse bone marrow metastases where the catecholamine level has not yet significantly increased. We were able to demonstrate this in numerous cases where the radiodiagnoses of the bone marrow were negative and the catecholamine levels were borderline (Figs. 2 and 3).

5. Comparative investigations between [131]I- and ^{123}I-MIBG indicate that both isotopes can be used in the diagnosis if exposures are made after 24 h when using [123]I. These later pictures are indispensable, since tumors occasionally will not stand out against the background radiation during the first 24 h and can thus be overlooked. The comparison of five children who were treated with [131]I- and ^{123}I-MIBG did not give any false-negative findings. On the other hand, the soft radiation of the ^{123}I with 160 keV gives a clearly better resolution and presentation of details with the gamma camera than the harder 364 keV radiation of ^{131}I, especially of dispersed tumor localisations. In one case this resulted in a more certain diagnosis than could have been achieved with [131]I (Fig. 4).

6. Finally, the ^{131}I-MIBG diagnostic with quantitative evaluation is indispensable to the preparation and indication setting of a ^{131}I-MIBG therapy. It is also essential to the control of the course of therapy and calculation of dosages. Whole-body scintigrams from dorsal and ventral views with quantitative analyses can be a big advantage here.

Comments on the methodology:

^{131}I-MIBG was given intravenously in doses of 0.5 – 1 mCi (16 – 37 MBq) with the highest possible specific activity (20 – 30 mCi per mg MIBG).

Whole-body scans given 24 – 96 h after the i.v. injection to detect peripheral bone marrow centers will produce a certain tumor diagnosis.

^{123}I-MIBG was administered in doses of 2 – 5 mCi (75 – 200 MBq); local scans and whole body scans were necessary after 6 h, 20 – 24 h and 40 h. Especially important are the pictures after 24 h and later, since, as already discussed, many tumors can only later be differentiated from the background radiation.

The thyroid gland was carefully blocked with iodide tablets.

In conclusion, it can be said that [131]I- and ^{123}I-MIBG have an important role to play today in the diagnosis of neuroblastomas. The following indications are now given:

1. Suspicion of neuroblastoma because of a histologically unknown tumor and/ or increased catecholamine secretion
2. Staging of a known neuroblastoma
3. Control of progress and early recognition of relapses and detection of the diffuse bone marrow metastases
4. Therapy planning and therapy control

References

1. Beyerwaltes WH (1981) New horizons for therapeutic nuclear medicine in 1981. J Nucl Med 22:549 – 554
2. Feine U, Treuner J, Niethammer D, Borchelt G, Dopfer R, Eibach E, Grünbach S, Kaiser W, Klingebiel T, Meinke J, Müller-Schauenburg W (1984) Erste Untersuchungen zur szintigraphischen Darstellung von Neuroblastomen mit 131-J-metajodbenzylguanidin. Nuc Compact 15:23 – 26

3. Feine U et al. (1984) Scintigraphic imaging of neuroblastoma with 131 MIBG and first attempts of its therapeutic use. 22nd Int Annual Meeting Soc. Nuclear Medicine Europa, Helsinki, 1984. In: Nuklearmedizin. Schattauer, Stuttgart

4. Kimmig B, Brandeis WE, Eisenhut M, Bubeck B, Herrmann HJ, zum Winkel K (1983) Szintigraphische Darstellung eines Neuroblastoms. Nuc Compact 14:320 – 326

5. Sisson JC, Shapiro B, Beierwaltes WH et al. (1984) Radiopharmaceutical treatment of malignant pheochromocytoma. J Nucl Med 24:197 – 206

6. Treuner J, Feine U, Niethammer D, Müller-Schauenburg W, Meinke J, Eibach E, Dopfer R, Klingebiel T, Grünbach S (1984) Scintigraphic imaging of neuroblastoma with ^{131}I-m iodobenzylguanidine. Lancet I:333 – 334

7. Wieland et al. (1980) Radiolabeled adrenergic neuro-blocking agent: adrenomedullary imaging with 131 I iodobenzylguanidine. J Nucl Med 21:349

Scintigraphic Imaging of Pheochromocytomas by Means of Metaiodobenzylguanidine (MIBG)

B. Shapiro[1], J. C. Sisson, O. Geatti, P. Eyre, M. Lynn, and W. H. Beierwaltes

Introduction

Pheochromocytomas and functioning paragangliomas (extra-adrenal pheochromocytomas) remain a significant clinical problem [1, 2], and, while unusual, are by no means rare tumors [2, 3]. The clinical manifestations are protean [1, 2], but the introduction of sensitive and specific assays for plasma catecholamines, urinary catecholamines, and catecholamine metabolites have made the biochemical diagnosis of pheochromocytoma easier [4–6]. Successful therapy hinges on the accurate location of all tumor deposits to permit their extirpation [1, 2, 7].

The preoperative location of the site(s) of lesions responsible for the hypercatecholaminemia remains a challenge despite the introduction of CT [8–10] and high-resolution ultrasound [11, 12] which have replaced intravenous urography with nephrotomography as noninvasive techniques. Venography with venous sampling may provide a functional means of locating pheochromocytomas, but is invasive and cumbersome [9, 13]. Arteriography is likewise invasive. If the feeding vessels of the tumor can be opacified, the lesion may be delineated. However, in the case of extra-adrenal lesions, these vessels cannot always be identified [14, 15]. All procedures involving the administration of intravascular contrast may lead to allergic reactions or provoke pheochromocytoma crisis [14].

The introduction of the radiopharmaceutical, ^{131}I metaiodobenzylguanidine (^{131}I MIBG) has led to a safe, noninvasive, and sensitive technique for the location of pheochromocytomas [16]. This technique has been shown to be efficacious in the location of benign, sporadic intra-adrenal [16, 17], benign, sporadic extra-adrenal abdominal [16, 17], and extra-abdominal [17, 18] and malignant [17, 19] lesions. The technique is especially helpful in the case of suspected postoperative recurrence [19, 20]. Familial lesions including multiple endocrine neoplasia types 2a and 2b (MEN 2a and 2b) may be located at an early stage of evolution from adrenal medullary hyperplasia to pheochromocytoma [21]. Other familial pheochromocytomas associated with neurofibromatosis [22], von Hippel-Lindau disease [17], or not associated with any obvious syndrome [23] may be detected.

1 Division of Nuclear Medicine, Department of Internal Medicine, University of Michigan, Ann Arbor, MI 48 109, USA

Nuclear Medicine in Clinical Oncology
Ed. by C. Winkler
© Springer-Verlag Berlin Heidelberg 1986

Radiolabeling of MIBG with ^{123}I offers a radiopharmaceutical with considerable advantages over ^{131}I-MIBG, namely, lower radiation dosimetry, high photon flux, shorter half-life, better photon detection and greater sensitivity. Preliminary experience has shown that ^{123}I-MIBG provides better lesion delineation and the localization of smaller lesions than can be revealed by ^{131}I MIBG [24].

The initial impression of total specificity of ^{131}I MIBG uptake for pheochromocytoma must now be tempered by the observation that this radiopharmaceutical is taken up by neuroblastomas [25], carcinoid tumors [26], medullary carcinoma of the thyroid [27], and a variety of other neuroendocrine tumors [17, 28]. The radiopharmaceutical is perhaps better characterized as a neuroendocrine tumor-seeking agent than a pheochromocytoma-seeking agent.

This paper summarizes the overall experience with radioiodinated MIBG scintigraphy at the University of Michigan.

Materials and Methods

Patient Population

A total of 540 patients were studied at the University of Michigan Medical Center for known or suspected pheochromocytoma between June 1980 and April 1985. Multiple studies were obtained in a total of 65 patients (in some cases more than two studies were obtained), the total number of studies being 719. These included cases studied before and after curative surgery, at serial intervals to monitor the evolution of MEN 2a and 2b syndromes and the progression of malignant disease.

Biochemistry

Plasma catecholamine concentrations were determined using radioenzymatic assay [29] on plasma samples obtained from an indwelling venous cannula (in place for 30 min) in the fasting, supine state. Urinary catecholamine and catecholamine metabolite excretion rates were determined on 12-h, overnight urine collections using the technique of Van Euler and Lishajko [30].

[131]I MIBG Scintigraphy

[131]I MIBG with a specific activity of at least 1.8 mCi/mg was prepared using the technique of Wieland et al. [31] and was administered by slow intravenous injection over $20-30$ s. The dose was 0.5 mCi/1.7 m^2 body surface area to a maximum of 0.5 mCi [16, 17]. The thyroidal uptake of free ^{131}I was diminished by the administration of iodides. Multiple overlapping images of the head, neck, chest, abdomen, and pelvis were obtained using a large field-of-view gamma camera equipped with a high-energy, parallel hole collimator and in-

terfaced to a dedicated minicomputer. A symmetrical 30% window at the 365 keV photopeak was used [16, 17]. Images containing 100 000 counts (or 20-min acquisition time) were displayed in analog and digitized form on film. A small number [32] of the earlier studies were performed with images containing 50 000 counts and were displayed on Polaroid [17]. A small number of studies were performed initially in which sequences of imaging other than the now standardized images at 1, 2, and 3 days were obtained: day 1 only (3 studies), day 2 only (43 studies), day 3 only (2 studies) at 1 and 2 days (88 studies), at 1 and 3 days (5 studies), and at 2 and 3 days (44 studies) [17]. All further experience was obtained with images at 1, 2, and 3 days (534 studies).

Anatomical orientation for the ^{131}I MIBG scintigrams was provided by surface markers and in selected cases by scintigraphy of other organs: the kidneys by ^{99m}Tc DTPA, liver and spleen by ^{99m}Tc sulfur colloid, skeleton by ^{99m}Tc MDP, myocardium with ^{201}Tl, and cardiac blood pool with ^{99m}Tc-labeled red blood cells [17, 18, 32]. By obtaining the ^{131}I MIBG and orientation scintigrams without moving the patient, it was possible to superimpose abnormal foci of ^{131}I MIBG uptake on the orientation scintigram using the computer-stored data [17, 18, 32].

[123]I MIBG Scintigraphy

A small number of patients (19) and volunteers (5) were studied using ^{123}I MIBG in a dose of up to 10 mCi administered by slow intravenous injection (specific activity, 6.5−11.7 mCi/mg). Multiple overlapping images of the head, neck, thorax, abdomen, and pelvis were obtained 2−4 h, 17−20 h, and 40−48 h after injection. In some patients simultaneous ^{131}I and ^{123}I MIBG studies were performed [24, 33]. The instrumentation was as described above for ^{131}I MIBG scintigraphy using a 20% window at the 159 keV photopeak [33].

Single photon emission tomography (SPECT) was performed in eight cases using a General Electric 400 T tomographic Anger camera and Star computer. Acquisition was performed using a low-energy, all-purpose collimator and 20% window at the 159 keV photopeak. Sixty-four projections were obtained over 360° at 15−20 s per projection. Uniformity correction was applied during acquisition and a filtered back projection algorithm was used to generate 1-pixel thick transaxial, sagittal, and coronal sections. A dynamic rotating display of the 64 projections was also examined [33].

Correlation of ^{131}I and ^{123}I MIBG Scintigraphy with Biochemical Studies, Other Medical Imaging Techniques and Final Outcome

The biochemistry obtained prior to referral to the University of Michigan was "abnormal" in almost all instances, but had been obtained with a wide variety of assays of variable sensitivity and specificity and under a range of clinical conditions, pharmacological interventions, and states of salt loading; thus, the results of plasma and urinary catecholamines obtained under carefully controlled circumstances at this institution were given primary importance.

Review of all available medical imaging studies (or when this was not possible the reports of such studies) was undertaken. This included various combinations of intravenous urography, CT, ultrasound, angiography, venography with venous sampling, bone scans, and skeletal radiographs.

Follow-up CT, NMR, and venous sampling (some of them directed by the preceding ^{131}I MIBG scintigraphy) were also reviewed where these were performed.

Finally the results of surgical explorations and tumor resection were examined. All patients have been subjected to follow-up for up to as long as 4½ years.

Scintigraphy (^{131}I MIBG) was classified as true-positive, true-negative, false-positive, and false-negative using previously described rigid criteria [17]. In the case of ^{123}I MIBG scintigraphy, similar criteria were used, but the fact that the normal adrenal medullae were readily visualized was taken into account [24, 33].

Results

No side effects were observed as a consequence of ^{123}I or ^{131}I MIBG administration.

The results of the initial ^{131}I MIBG scintigraphy performed in each case are recorded in Table 1. This excludes the multiple imaging such as that performed to evaluate the evolution of MEN 2a and 2b and malignant pheochromocytomas.

In 19 cases initial scans were repeated for confirmation of the presence of a lesion and the second scan was congruent with the first in each instance. Serial studies were performed at 3 to 18-month intervals in 32 patients with malignant pheochromocytoma and showed variable patterns of tumor extension (varying from no change to rapid progression) in untreated cases and variable patterns of tumor extension or regression in patients treated with a variety of interventions (including teleradiotherapy, chemotherapy, and ^{131}I MIBG therapy [34, 35]). The details of these findings, however, lie outside the scope of this discussion.

The overall prevalance, sensitivity, specificity, positive predictive accuracy, and negative predictive accuracy are presented in Table 2.

The results of ^{123}I MIBG scintigraphy in 5 normal controls and 19 patients with pheochromocytoma are presented in Table 3.

Discussion

The results obtained show that the earlier experience has been confirmed and ^{131}I MIBG scintigraphy is a safe, noninvasive, and sensitive technique for the location of pheochromocytomas of all types [16 – 23]. These impressions have

Table 1. Diagnostic scintigraphy for suspected pheochromocytoma with ^{131}I MIBG

	Total	True-positive	True-negative	False-positive	False-negative
Sporadic intraadrenal pheochromocytoma	34	30	0	0	4
Sporadic abdominal extra-adrenal	8	6	0	0	2
Sporadic thoracic extra-adrenal	9 (1 malignant)	9	0	0	0
Sporadic cervical extra-adrenal	4 (2 malignant)[a]	1	0	0	3
Unknown sites	4	0	0	0	4
MEN 2	37 (3 malignant)	22	13	0	2
Neurofibromatosis	18 (1 malignant)	6	12	0	0
Von Hippel-Lindau	2 (1 malignant)	2	0	0	0
Simple familial	3 (2 malignant)	3	0	0	0
Sporadic malignant	67	61	0	0	6
"False-positives"	3[b]	0	0	3	0
Pheochromocytoma excluded[c]	252	0	252	0	0
Pheochromocytoma probably excluded[d]	99	0	99	0	0
Totals	540	140	376	3	21

[a] Two cases of nonfunctioning paragangliomas (also appear in Table 4)
[b] One case each of retroperitoneal neuroendocrine tumor and metastatic choriocarcinoma (also appear in Table 4); one case of probable dilated renal pelvis
[c] Entirely normal biochemistry and radiology
[d] Minimal elevations of catecholamines, but normal radiology

been supported by the observations of other independent workers. The results of the present series, the previous University of Michigan experience, and that of larger series in the USA, France, and Germany are presented in Table 4.

We would recommend that where available, ^{131}I MIBG scintigraphy be the initial localizing procedure of choice to screen the entire body for pheochromocytoma deposits in a sensitive and noninvasive manner. CT, venography with sampling, and/or arteriography may be used to better define the anatomical relations of abnormal foci of ^{131}I MIBG uptake [17, 40, 41]. In those cases where ^{131}I MIBG scintigraphy is negative and suspicion of pheochromocytoma remains high, the latter procedures may yet disclose the location of the lesions [17, 40, 41].

[123]I MIBG scintigraphy provides a far greater useful photon flux and permits the better delineation of lesions and the detection of smaller lesions than does ^{131}I MIBG [24, 33, 42]. It also permits the performance of single photon emission computed tomography (SPECT) and rotating display images which may

Table 2. Summary of overall results of ^{131}I MIBG scintigraphy at the University of Michigan (June 1980 to March 1985)

Number	Sensitivity	Specificity	Negative predictive accuracy	Positive predictive accuracy	Prevalence
540	87%	99%	95%	98%	30%

Table 3. Results of ^{123}I MIBG scintigraphy (modified from [33])

	Positive[a, b]	Negative
Primary pheochromocytomas	4[c]	0 (Bilateral adrenal, 2 pararenal, left atrial)
Recurrent pheochromocytoma	2	0 (Abdominal extra-adrenal, left atrial)
Malignant pheochromocytoma	9[d]	0
No pheochromocytoma	0	4[b] (Three status postsuccessful pheoresection, one essential hypertension)
Normal volunteers	0	5[b]

[a] In every instance all lesions seen with ^{131}I MIBG were more clearly delineated; SPECT in 7 cases revealed diagnostic information not available from planar images

[b] The adrenal medullae were visualized in 9 of 15 patients still possessing adrenal glands. Five of the remaining patients had multiple abdominal tumor deposits that were difficult to differentiate from adrenal medullae; the adrenal medullae of all normal volunteers were visualized

[c] One pararenal lesion was not visualized by ^{131}I MIBG scintigraphy, but clearly visualized by ^{123}I MIBG scintigraphy

[d] In 5 cases ^{123}I MIBG demonstrated additional lesions not visualized by ^{131}I MIBG

Table 4. Summary of overall results at University of Michigan and comparison with other series

	Reference	Number	Sensitivity	Specificity	Negative PDA	Positive PDA	Prevalence
Michigan (Present series)	–	540	87	99	95	98	30
Michigan (Previous summary)	[17]	421[a]	87	99	95	97	30
Southampton	[39]	46	88	95	88	95	52
Mayo Clinic	[37]	42	79	96	85	94	45
Tours	[38]	27	89	94	94	89	33
Combined German experience	[36]	191	88	94	94	98	34

[a] Based on number of scans

PDA, predictive accuracy

further improve its efficacy [33]. This agent may be that of choice if problems with expense and supply can be solved. The fact that the normal adrenal medullae are regularly visualized means that quantitation of ^{123}I MIBG may be required to distinguish normal from hyperplastic or tumorous adrenal medullae [43].

The initial impression of absolute specificity of MIBG uptake for pheochromocytoma must be modified in light of uptake of this tracer by a variety of neuroendocrine tumors [25 – 28] (see also Appendix). The efficacy of ^{131}I MIBG scintigraphy for neuroblastoma appears to have been established [25, 44], but its role in the location of other lesions is under investigation.

Appendix: Scintigraphic imaging of lesions other than pheochromocytomas

	True-positive	True-negative	False-positive	False-negative
Neuroblastoma	14	2	0	2
Carcinoid tumors	2	0	0	9
Medullary carcinoma of the thyroid (MCT)[a]	1	0	0	16
Oat-cell tumors	0	0	0	1
Insulinoma	0	0	0	1
Other tumors[b]	2	0	0	0
Nonfunctioning paragangliomas	2	0	0	0
Chemodectomas (carotid body tumors)[c]	2	0	0	3

[a] Sporadic MCT and MCT associated with MEN 2a and 2b
[b] One retroperitoneal neuroendocrine tumor, one metastatic choriocarcinoma
[c] Catecholamine, secreting and nonsecreting

References

1. Freier DT, Eckhauser FE, Harrison TS (1980) Pheochromocytoma: a persistently problematic and still potentially lethal disease. Arch Surg 115:388 – 391
2. Manger WM, Gifford RW (1982) Hypertension secondary to pheochromocytoma. Bull NY Acad Med 58:139 – 158
3. St. John Sutton MG, Sheps SG, Lie JT (1981) Prevalence of clinically unsuspected pheochromocytoma. Review of a 50-year autopsy series. Mayo Clin Proc 56:354 – 360
4. Bravo EL, Tarazi RC, Gifford RW, Stewart BH (1979) Circulating and urinary catecholamines in pheochromocytoma: diagnostic and pathophysiologic implications. New Engl J Med 301:682 – 686
5. Freier DT, Harrison TS (1973) Rigorous biochemical criteria for the diagnosis of pheochromocytoma. J Surg Res 14:177 – 180
6. Bravo EL, Tarazi RC, Fouad FM, Vindt DG, Gifford RW (1981) Clonidine-suppression: a useful aid in the diagnosis of pheochromocytoma. New Engl J Med 305:623 – 626
7. Van Heerden JA, Sheps SG, Hamberger B (1982) Pheochromocytoma: current status and changing trends. Surgery 91:367 – 373
8. Stewart BH, Bravo EL, Haaga J, Meaney TF, Tarazi R (1978) Localization of pheochromocytoma by computed tomography. New Engl J Med 299:460 – 461

9. Dunnick NR, Doppman JL, Gill JR, Strott CA, Keiser HR, Brennan MF (1982) Localization of functional adrenal tumors by computed tomography and venous sampling. Radiology 142:429−433

10. Adams JE, Johnson RJ, Rickards D, Isherwood I (1983) Computed tomography in adrenal disease. Clin Radiol 34:39−49

11. Yeh H-C (1980) Sonography of the adrenal glands, normal glands and small masses. AJR 135:1167−1177

12. Bowerman RA, Silver TM, Jaffe MJ, Stuck KJ, Hinerman DL (1981) Sonography of adrenal pheochromocytomas. AJR 137:1227−1231

13. Jones DH, Allison CA, Hamilton CA, Reid JL (1979) Selective venous sampling in the diagnosis and localization of pheochromocytoma. Clin Endocrinol 10:179−186

14. Rossi P, Young IS, Panke WF (1968) Techniques, usefulness and hazards of arteriography of pheochromocytoma: review of 99 cases. JAMA 205:547−553

15. Kinkhabwala MN, Conradi H (1972) Angiography of extra-adrenal pheochromocytoma. J Urol 108:666−668

16. Sisson JC, Frager MS, Valk TW, Gross MD, Swanson DP, Wieland DM, Tobes MC, Beierwaltes WH, Thompson NW (1981) Scintigraphic localization of pheochromocytoma. New Engl J Med 305:12−17

17. Shapiro B, Copp JE, Sisson JC, Eyre PL, Wallis J, Beierwaltes WH (1985) 131-I-meta-iodobenzylguanidine for the locating of suspected phcochromocytoma: experience in 400 cases (441 studies). J Nucl Med

18. Shapiro B, Sisson JC, Kalff V, Glowniak JV, Satterlee WG, Glazer GW, Francis IR, Bowers R, Thompson NW, Orringer M, Gross MD, Beierwaltes NJ (1984) The location of middle mediastinal pheochromocytomas. J Thorac Cardiovasc Surg 87:814−820

19. Shapiro B, Sisson JC, Lloyd R, Nakajo M, Satterlee WG, Beierwaltes WH (1984) Malignant pheochromocytoma: clinical, biochemical and scintigraphic characterization. Clin Endocrinol 20:189−203

20. Kalff V, Sisson JC, Beierwaltes WH (1982) Adrenal gland identification: pre-operative assessment. Surgery 91:374−376

21. Valk TW, Frager MS, Gross MD, Sisson JC, Wieland DM, Swanson DP, Mangner TJ, Beierwaltes WH (1981) Spectrum of pheochromocytoma in multiple endocrine neoplasia. A scintigraphic portrayal using ^{131}I-meta-iodobenzylguanidine. Ann Intern Med 94:762

22. Kalff V, Shapiro B, Lloyd R, Sisson JC, Holland K, Nakajo M, Beierwaltes WH (1982) The spectrum of pheochromocytoma in hypertensive patients with neurofibromatosis. Arch Intern Med 142:2092−2098

23. Glowniak JV, Shapiro B, Sisson JC, Thompson NW, Coran AG, Lloyd RV, Kelsch RC, Beierwaltes WH (1985) Familial extra-adrenal pheochromocytoma: a new syndrome. Arch Intern Med 145:257−261

24. Lynn MD, Shapiro B, Sisson JC, Swanson DP, Mangner TJ, Wieland DM, Meyers LJ, Beierwaltes WH (1984) Portrayal of pheochromocytoma and normal human adrenal medulla by 123-I-meta-iodobenzylguanidine (123-I-MIBG). J Nucl Med 25:436−440

25. Treuner J, Feine U, Niethammer D, Muller-Schaumburg W, Meinke J, Eibach E, Dopfer R, Klingebiel TH, Grumbach ST (1984) Scintigraphic imaging of neuroblastoma with ^{131}I-MIBG. Lancet 1:333−334

26. Fischer M, Kamanabroo D, Sanderkamp H, Proske T (1984) Scintigraphic imaging of carcinoid tumors with ^{131}I-MIBG. Lancet 2:165 (letter)

27. Endo K, Shiomi K, Kasagi K, Konishi J, Torizuka K, Nakao K, Tanimura H (1984) Imaging of medullary carcinoma of the thyroid with ^{131}I-MIBG. Lancet ii:233

28. Smit AJ, Van Essen LH, Hollema H, Muskiet FAJ, Piers OA (1984) ^{131}I-MIBG uptake in a non-secreting paraganglioma. J Nucl Med 25:984−986

29. Peuler JD, Johnson GA (1971) Simultaneous single isotope radioenzymatic assay of plasma norepinephrine, epinephrine and dopamine. Life Sci 21:625−636

30. Von Euler US, Lishajko F (1959) The estimation of catecholamines in urine. Acta Physiol Scand 45:122−132

31. Wieland DM, Wu J-I, Brown LE, Mangner TJ, Swanson DP, Beierwaltes WH (1980) Radiolabeled adrenergic neuron-blocking agents: adrenomedullary imaging with [131I]iodobenzylguanidine. J Nucl Med 21:349−353

32. McEwan AJ, Shapiro B, Sisson JC, Beierwaltes WH, Ackery DM (1985) Radi-oiodobenzylguanidine for the scintigraphic location and therapy of adrenergic tumors. Semin Nucl Med 15:132−153
33. Lynn MD, Shapiro B, Sisson JC, Beierwaltes WH, Meyers LJ, Ackerman R, Mangner TJ (1985) Improved visualization of pheochromocytomas and normal adrenal medullae with ^{123}I-MIBG scintigraphy. Radiology (in press)
34. Sisson JC, Shapiro B, Beierwaltes WH (1984) Radiopharmaceutical treatment of malignant pheochromocytoma. J Nucl Med 25:198−206
35. Sisson JC, Shapiro B, Glowniak JV, Beierwaltes WH, Mangner TJ, Wieland DM, Carey JC, Petry NA, Copp JE, Eyre PL (1984) ^{131}I-MIBG treatment of malignant pheo-chromocytoma. J Nucl Med 25:p 72
36. Anonymous (1983) Clinical value of adrenomedullary scintigraphy with ^{131}I-MIBG. Nucl Compact 14:318 (Editorial)
37. Brown ML, Sheps SG, Sizemore G (1984) MIBG in the evaluation of suspected pheo-chromocytoma: Mayo Clinic experience. J Nucl Med 25:p 94 (Abstract)
38. Baulieu JL, Guilloteau C, Canbom C, Viel C, Baulieu F, Itti R, Pourcelot L, Besnard JC (1984) MIBG scintigraphy: A one-year experience. J Nucl Med 25:p 111 (Abstract)
39. Ackery DM, Tippett P, Condon D et al. (1984) New approach to the localization of phaeo-chromocytoma: Imaging with ^{131}I-MIBG. Br Med J 288:1587−1591
40. Francis IR, Glazer GM, Shapiro B et al. (1983) Complementary roles of CT scanning and 131-I-MIBG scintigraphy in the diagnosis of pheochromocytoma. Am J Roentgenol 141:719−725
41. Shapiro B, Copp JE, Eyre P et al. (1984) A new and efficient approach to the diagnosis and location of pheochromocytomas. Clin Res 32:300A (Abstract)
42. Horne T, Hawkins LA, Britton KE, Granowska M, Bouloux P, Besser GM (1984) Imaging of pheochromocytoma and adrenal medulla with 123-I-meta-iodobenzylguanidine. Nucl Med Commun 5:763−768
43. Hawkins LA, Britton KE, Shapiro B (1980) Selenium 75 seleno-methyl-cholesterol: a new agent for quantitative functional scintigraphy of the adrenals: physical aspects. Br J Radiol 53:883−889
44. Munkner T (1985) ^{131}I-metaiodobenzylguanidine scintigraphy of neuroblastomas. Semin Nucl Med 15:154−160

Nuclear Medicine in the Diagnosis of Skin Tumors

H. J. BIERSACK[1]

Nuclear medicine offers a variety of diagnostic tools for the evaluation of skin tumors which include the radioactive phosphorus (^{32}P) uptake test, tumor imaging with ^{67}Ga, ^{201}Tl, and immunoscintigraphy with radiolabeled antibodies. These procedures and their results are briefly described in this paper.

The ^{32}P Uptake Test

Increased uptake of the β-emitter ^{32}P-orthophosphate in neoplasms has been described as early as 1940 [10]. Later, the metabolic pathways of radioactive phosphorus were investigated in detail revealing the combination of phosphorus with tissue components like nucleoproteins and phospholipids [23]. The synthesis of these substances was shown to be accelerated in malignancies when compared to normal cells, with the exception of bone, intestine, and liver [13]. In view of the possibility of using ^{32}P for tumor diagnosis, the increased uptake of radiophosphorus in inflammatory processes may interfere occasionally with a differential diagnosis [2]. In most cases, however, it is possible to identify inflammations, so that the ^{32}P uptake test has proved to be useful for tumor detection in clinical practice since 1942. Positive results have been obtained in breast cancer [11, 12, 16], testicular tumors [19], thyroid cancer [20], and eye tumors [3, 6, 21, 22]. Since 1952 ^{32}P has also been used for the evaluation of skin tumors [1, 2, 4]. Whereas Geiger counters were initially used as detectors, for the past 15 years these have been replaced by semiconductor counting systems for determining radiophosphorus uptake.

Methods

The Clinical Counting System (Technical Associates) has been used in our institute for the ^{32}P uptake test in patients with skin tumors. The system is equipped with a so-called eye probe, 5 mm in diameter. A dose of $3-4$ µCi ^{32}P/kg body weight are injected intravenously. With regard to the radiation load, the bone marrow has to be taken into account as critical organ; $30-40$ mrad/µCi ^{32}P must be recond with.

---

1 Institut für klinische und experimentelle Nuklearmedizin der Universität, D-5300 Bonn

Examinations are performed 24 and 48 h p.i. In view of the temperature-dependent sensitivity of the detector, a calibration for 37°C body temperature is necessary. To avoid temperature-related faults, standard controls before and after the clinical examination should be performed. Radioactive contamination of the detector is avoided by covering the lesion with a dustic film. The counting period is usually 2–3 min. In addition to the measurement over the tumor, another measurement must be performed in a reference area, which can be in the vicinity of the tumor or in an area at a contralateral extremity. The following formula is used to determine significant differences in count rates:

$$\frac{N_1 - N_2}{\sqrt{N_1 + N_2}} = t \qquad \begin{array}{l} N_1 = \text{count rate tumor} \\ N_2 = \text{count rate unaffected skin} \end{array}$$

A t value of ≥ 2 is regarded to be significant, representing a probability of at least 95% for a nonrandom difference.

Patients

A total of 35 patients with malignant tumors of the skin including basal cell epithelioma were investigated (Table 1), and additionally 10 patients with precancerous lesions. Eleven patients with benign lesions without signs of inflammation served as controls.

Results

The clinical results are summarized in Table 2. In all of the patients with malignant tumors or precancerous lesions an increased ^{32}P uptake was observed. In contrast, increased uptake was not established in any of the 11 cases with benign lesions. Although only a limited number of cases were studied, we are confident that the following conclusions may be safely drawn: 1. A clear distinction between malignant melanoma and benign naevus is possible, 2. cutaneous metastases of melanoma can be detected even in the presence of benign naevi, and 3. the test renders possible the detection of recurrences of previously treated skin tumors.

Table 1. Investigated patients

Malignant tumors	N	Precancerous lesions	N
Malignant melanoma	14	Bowen's disease	4
Reticulosarcoma	3	Actinic keratosis	3
Squamous cell carcinoma	4	Junctional naevus-	3
Cutaneous lymphoma	4	cell naevus	
Basal cell epithelioma	10		
Total	35	Total	10

Table 2. Results of the ^{32}P test

Diagnosis	Positive	Negative
Malignant melanoma	25	0
Basal cell epithelioma	10	0
Precancerous lesions	10	0
Benign lesions[a]	0	11

[a] No inflammation!

^{67}Ga Scintigraphy

Conventional gallium scans are considered to be of limited value in the detection of metastatic melanoma. In the early examinations of melanomas by means of gallium, a high specificity was described whereas the sensitivity was only 50% [17]. Jackson et al. [7] reported on a prospective trial of gallium scanning as multisystem surveillance for metastatic melanoma in 36 patients. In 69% of these cases the results were true-positive, and 6% were false-positive. Romolo and Fisher [18] studied the predictive value of preoperative conventional gallium scans in patients with deep stage I or clinical stage II melanoma. The gallium scan predicted the lymph node status with an efficiency of 50%, a sensitivity of 39%, and a specificity of 96%. Kirkwood et al. [8] described a new method of tomographic gallium scanning using high radioactivity doses (10 mCi) and a special detecting system − the so-called Anger tomographic multiplane scanner (Phocon).

In these studies, 114 scans were performed in 67 patients during a 3-year period. Sensitivity for proof of tumors located in superficial lymph nodes, in the abdomen, mediastinum, and osseous sites was 68% (lung or mediastinum), 90% (lymph nodes and soft tissue), and 100% (abdomen, bone). Overall sensitivity was 82%, and specificity was 99% in 570 organ system assessments. When a site was clinically occult but gallium-positive, the authors established that 6 out of 7 results were true positive in lymphatic sites, and in all of the mediastinal and abdominal sites. It must be stressed, however, that these excellent results of the Yale melanoma group [8] could only be achieved by using high doses of ^{67}Ga and a highly specialized tomographic scanner for gallium imaging.

^{201}Tl Imaging

Since 1976, ^{201}Tl has been used for the detection of a variety of different malignant tumors. Neoplastic tissue shows increasing concentration of radioactivity during a relatively long period, while in inflammatory lesions the concentration decreases relatively early following an initially high uptake [15]. For this test 2 mCi ^{201}Tl are injected intravenously. Measurements are performed after 2 min and 2 h following the injection of the test substance. Maul et al. [15] reported clinical results with 11 patients with melanoma, 7 of them having metastases. In all of the 7 cases, increased thallium uptake was detected, while 3 of 4 patients without spread were true-negative. Despite the low number of cases investigated it could probably be assumed that gallium can be substituted by thallium as test substance for skin tumors.

Radioimmunoscintigraphy

A whole series of cell surface antigens have hitherto been discovered in malignant melanomas. It has been possible to produce antibodies against some of these antigens which could be used for radioimmunoscintigraphy [5, 9, 20]. Although the data of antibody scintigraphy in melanoma patients are presented elsewhere in this book, the results using ^{99m}Tc-labeled $F(ab')_2$ fragments of a melanoma antibody (22,28S/SORIN) shall be summarized here briefly. For these studies, 6 to 8 mCi of ^{99m}Tc-labeled antibody fragments are administered intravenously. Scintigraphy is performed 1–6 h after injection. Background activity decreases fast due to renal excretion of fragments. Physiological uptake is observed in liver, spleen, and kidneys. High radioactivity uptake can be observed in the primary tumors as well as in distant metastases. Scheidhauer et al. (pers. communication) reported on a sensitivity of 73% in 30 patients. In some cases, both primary tumor and metastases were positive. There were, however, patients with "positive" primary tumor and "negative" metastases or vice versa. Thus, the relatively low detection rate might be due to different antigen patterns of primary tumors and metastases. It seems obvious that a "mixture" of different antibodies could probably improve the results.

References

1. Bauer FK, Steffen CG (1955) Radioactive phosphorus in the diagnosis of skin tumors. JAMA 158:563
2. Biersack HJ, Rodermund OE, Meurin G, Winkler C (1976) Radiophosphor (^{32}P)-Test bei Präkanzerosen und malignen Tumoren der Haut. Hautarzt 27:133
3. Biersack HJ, Schlieter F (1978) Der ^{32}P-Test in der ophthalmologischen Tumordiagnostik. 59. Jahrestagung der Deutschen Roentgengesellschaft, Bonn 1978, p 76 (Abstracts)
4. Cramer H, Pabst HW (1952) Tumordiagnostik mit radioaktiven Isotopen. Z Krebsforsch 58:163
5. Ghose T, Ferrone S, Jmai K, Norwell ST, Luner SJ, Martin RH (1981) Imaging of human melanoma xenografts in nude mice with a radiolabeled monoclonal antibody. JNCI 69:823
6. Hagler WS, Jarrett WH, Schnauss RH, LaRose JH, Palms JM, Wood RE (1972) Diagnosis of malignant melanoma of ciliary body or chorioid: Use of radioactive phosphorus uptake test. South Med J 65:49
7. Jackson FI, McPherson TA, Lentle BC (1977) Gallium-67 scintigraphy in multisystem malignant melanoma. Radiology 122:163
8. Kirkwood JM, Myers JE, Vlock DR, Neumann R, Ariyan S, Gottschalk A, Hoffer P (1982) Tomographic Gallium-67 citrate scanning: useful new surveillance for metastatic melanoma. Ann Intern Med 97:694
9. Larson SM, Brown IP, Wright PW, Carrasquillo JA, Hellström I, Hellström KE (1983) Imaging of melanoma with I-131 labeled monoclonal antibodies. J Nucl Med 24:123

10. Lawrence JJ (1940) Studies on neoplasms with the aid of radioactive phosphorus. J Clin Invest 19:267
11. Low-Beer BVA (1946) Surface measurements of radioactive phosphorus in breast tumors as possible diagnostic method. Science 104:399
12. Marinelli LD, Goldschmidt B (1942) Uptake of radioactive phosphorus by breast tumors. Radiology 39:454
13. Marshak A (1940) Uptake of radioactive phosphorus by nuclei of liver and tumors. Science 92:460
14. Matzku S, Tilgen W (1985) Experimentelle Grundlagen der Radioimmundiagnostik und -therapie humaner Melanome mit monoklonalen Antikörpern. In: Holzmann H, Altmeyer P, Hör G, Hahn K (eds) Dermatologie und Nuklearmedizin. Springer, Berlin Heidelberg New York Tokyo, p 137
15. Maul FD, Altmeyer P, Bittner G, Wanner U, Baum RP, Standke R, Wenisch HJC, Holzmann H, Hör G (1985) Die Thallium-201-Szintigraphie in der Diagnostik des metastasierenden malignen Melanoms. In: Holzmann H, Altmeyer P, Hör G, Hahn K (eds) Dermatologie und Nuklearmedizin. Springer, Berlin Heidelberg New York Tokyo, p 198
16. McCorkle HJ, Low-Beer BVA, Bell HG, Stone RS (1948) Clinical and laboratory studies on the uptake of radioactive phosphorus by lesions of the breast. Surgery 24:409
17. Milder MS, Frankle RS, Bulkley GB, Ketcham AS, Johnston GS (1973) Gallium-67 scintigraphy in malignant melanoma. Cancer 32:1350
18. Romolo JL, Fischer SG (1979) Gallium-67 scanning compared with physical examination in the preoperative staging of malignant melanoma. Cancer 44:468
19. Roswitt JB, Sorrentinó J, Yalow R (1950) The use of radioactive phosphorus in the diagnosis of testicular tumors. J Urol 63:724
20. Swedenburg RW, Tuttle WM, Corrigan KE (1955) Isotope techniques for mediastinal tumors. AMA Arch Surg 71:378
21. Terner JS, Leopold JH, Eisenberg IJ (1956) The radioactive phosphorus uptake test in ophthalmology. AMA Arch Ophthal 55:52
22. Thomas CI, Krohmer JS, Storaasli JP (1952) Detection of intraocular tumors with radioactive phosphorus. AMA Arch Ophthal 47:276
23. Tuttle WM, Erf LA, Lawrence JH (1941) Studies on neoplasms with the aid of radioactive phosphorus. J Clin Invest 20:577

IV. Radioimmunodetection

Principles of Radioimmunodetection of Tumors

S. von Kleist[1]

The technique which has become known as radioimmunodetection (RAID) is the outcome of a long, continuous development which has its roots in the last century, since as early as 1895 it was claimed for the first time that injected heterologous antibodies were taken to the tumour against which they had been prepared [1]. Yet it took another 50 years to actually demonstrate that such antibodies fixed onto the malignant cells. A prerequisite for this was to label the antibodies with the right radioisotope and to show that the coupling procedure did not destroy the ability of the immunoglobulins to combine with the antigen. It was Pressman and his group who resolved these problems and who in 1957 introduced the concept of injecting antitumour antibodies to localize tumours in experimental systems. He and his colleagues proved that the antibodies, when radiolabelled and injected intravenously, could be detected by external scanning procedures in the tissues that had served as antigen source for immunization [2, 3]. Although these experiments were completed in 1965, it still took 10 more years until the first clinical trials could be run. These were made possible among other things by the discovery in human carcinomas of what are known now as tumor-marker substances, such as alpha-fetoprotein (AFP) or carcinoembryonic antigen (CEA). Based on both systematic animal studies with xenotransplanted tumors and close collaboration between the two disciplines, nuclear medicine and immunology, the successful in vivo localization of primary tumors and metastases in patients developed rapidly, despite many initial setbacks an failures [4−6].

The RAID technique evidently has improved greatly due to the use of better reagents, for instance affinity-purified polyclonal or monoclonal antibodies, yet it is equally evident that it is not perfect, and many a problem has still to be resolved before it can be recommended for routine use.

In clinical oncology, radioimmunodetection appears to be possible and indicated for all patients in whom a tumor marker is either elevated or at least present in the serum and where the site of the marker production, in other words the tumor location, is not known. Since the sensitivity and specificity of the immunological tumor localization and the resolution of an immunoscintigram depends not only on the quality of the antibody but also on the radiolabel, the choice of the label is therefore of considerable importance. The first successful clinical images by external scanning were obtained in 1978 by

---

1 Institut für Immunbiologie der Albert-Ludwigs-Universität, Stefan-Meier-Straße 8, D-7800 Freiburg i. Br.

Nuclear Medicine in Clinical Oncology
Ed. by C. Winkler
© Springer-Verlag Berlin Heidelberg 1986

Goldenberg et al. [5], who used ^{131}I-labelled antibodies against CEA. Although radionuclides of this element have become the most commonly employed labels for monoclonal and polyclonal antibodies applied in immunoscintigraphy, they are far from being ideal for in vivo tumor imaging for the following reasons: Besides having a long half-life of 8 days, they have a high energy of emission, namely 364 keV, which is not very convenient for gamma scintigraphy, and they emit beta particles. Another considerable disadvantage is the fact that one usually observes a high uptake or greater concentration of the radionuclide in the thyroid, the liver, the spleen and the bladder, because the radiolabel is excreted through the urinary tract as iodide, and all these concentrations in the tissues may obscure secondary tumors, especially when they are located in the pelvic region.

According to several authors, the metallic radionuclide [111]Indium seems to offer some advantages over iodine [7−10], since its half-life is shorter, and so tumour imaging can be delayed until selective uptake by the neoplastic tissues has been achieved. Furthermore, the emitted energy is more suitable for detection by standard gamma cameras and there is no beta-particle emission. In addition, although the uptake ratio of nontumor to tumor tissues is approximately equal for both iodine and indium, namely 2.5:1, the fact that it seems to be less for indium in the rest of the body, notably the liver, makes the visualization of the malignancies with this label easier. This is especially true of secondaries in the pelvic region, since there is reduced urinary excretion. The main advantage, however, is that blood pool image subtraction no longer seems to be necessary, as blood clearance appears to be increased [7]. It thus seems that indium is a most suitable radionuclide for immunoscintigraphy, which can be reliably coupled to both monoclonal and polyclonal antibodies.

As pointed out above, the efficacy of the radioimmunodetection depends also on the quality of the antisera employed. Since to date we still have no truly tumor-specific antigen in human cancers and consequently no specific antitumor antibodies, we are left with almost the same difficulties that our pioneer predecessors faced 40 years ago. Therefore, and to compensate for the reagents' lack of tumour specificity, one will have to screen carefully the isotope-antibody conjugates, especially monoclonal antibodies, before injecting them into the patients. This is necessary to avoid damage inflicted by the antibody (either directly or via complement binding) on normal cells carrying the same epitopes as the envisaged tumour cells.

Let me take as an example of the problems one can encounter the most widely used target antigen for tumour imaging with monoclonal antibodies, CEA. For the screening, and to demonstrate the in vivo tumour specificity of anti-CEA monoclonal antibodies with a potential use in patients, animal models such as nude mice transplanted with human cancer xenografts are usually employed [11, 12]. It is often overlooked that such models have severe shortcomings inasmuch as such transplanted animals do not contain the homologous or any other normal tissues that could serve as specificity controls. An even more important deficiency is that the mice have no circulating human white blood cells, such as granulocytes or lymphocytes, which are most frequently carriers of cross-reacting antigens or CEA-related molecules.

We and others have shown that CEA contains at least eight different epitopes that can be distinguished by different monoclonal antibodies. Most of these determinants, however, are repeated on the widely distributed "nonspecific cross-reacting antigen" or NCA which, as we have shown, exists in three molecular species and is also present in circulating cells such as the already mentioned granulocytes [13–16]. Out of more than 30 CEA-reactive monoclonal antibodies from various laboratories that we have so far tested by immunoprecipitation, only five were truly CEA specific; all the others also recognized CEA-related, hence cross-reactive, antigens. What can happen if such antibodies are injected into patients is already summarized in the title of the paper recently published by Dillman et al. [17], namely, "a lack of radioimmunodetection and complications associated with (or caused by) the monoclonal anti-CEA-antibody cross-reacting with an antigen on circulating cells." The authors reported that in five of the six patients the injected anti-CEA-monoclonal antibody caused a 40%–90% decrease of their circulating granulocytes. Besides this, a systemic toxicity with fever, rigors and emesis was also observed.

What has been described here for an anti-CEA-monoclonal antibody is of course valid for monoclonal antibodies against other known tumor markers, too. It is therefore of utmost importance that the still very limited range of monoclonal antibodies, all of which so far react only preferentially and not specifically with tumors, be enlarged.

Since we have dealt above with the resolution and specificity of immunoscintigrams, we shall now discuss the sensitivity of the method which for the moment is still limited to tumors with a diameter of 1–2 cm. The lack of a greater sensitivity is partly due to an excessive background activity of the radiolabels, partly to other factors we shall mention later. To reduce the blood pool activity caused by radioiodinated antibodies, computer-assisted subtraction techniques, for instance by means of ^{99}Technetium-labelled normal immunoglobulin injections, were recommended and successfully employed [18, 19]. More recently, other techniques have been studied, which use a second antibody directed against the radiolabelled first (specific) antibody to optimize the clearance of radioactivity in the blood while maximizing the activity in the tumor. One new principle of reducing the presence of circulating labelled antibodies is to use liposome-entrapped secondary antibodies so as to complex and deliver to the liver the primary antibody which is not fixed onto the tumor. It was recently reported by the Charing Cross Hospital Group that the liposomally entrapped secondary antibody was indeed able to reduce blood levels of free iodine-labelled anti-CEA antibodies without reducing the amount of anti-CEA bound to the tumor [20]. Sharkey et al. used a similar approach when they administered a second antibody directed against radiolabelled primary anti-CEA antibodies 24 h after injection of the primary antibody. They found that the tumor/nontumor ratios were significantly improved 24 h thereafter [21].

Although these studies, which were conducted in animals, indicate that reducing background radioactivity by injection of second antibody may be useful for improving the radioimmunodetection of tumors, more studies are certainly needed before this new technology can be used in patients.

A further critical problem which has limited the radioimmunoimaging of human tumors smaller than 2 cm in diameter has been the low uptake of radio-labelled antibodies. Several factors that are hard to control can be made responsible for this, e.g. the low affinity of the antibody for the target antigen, the low concentration of the target antigen in the tumor in relation to the normal surrounding tissues and probably an antigen-antibody complex formation or fixation of the antibody on circulating cells and its elimination via the opsonized cells by the reticuloendothelial system [22].

In conclusion, I believe one can certainly say that radioactively labelled monoclonal or other antibodies directed against tumor-associated antigens can indeed detect malignant tumors in patients. The techniques employed, however, are not yet perfect, and more fundamental investigations are needed, especially to prevent any negative consequences of cross-reactions of the antibodies with normal cells with cytotoxic effects.

These studies are all the more necessary, since the same immunological approach initially developed for tumor localization is now also used for therapeutic purposes.

References

1. Héricourt J, Richet C (1895) Traitment d'un cas de sarcome par la sérothérapie. C R Seances Acad Sci 120:948
2. Pressman D, Day ED, Blau M (1957) The use of paired labeling in the determination of tumorlocalizing antibodies. Cancer Res 17:845
3. Korngold L, Pressman D (1954) The localization of antilymphosarcoma antibodies in the Murphy lymphosarcoma of the rat. Cancer Res 14:96
4. Goldenberg DM et al. (1974) Photoscan localization of GW-39 tumors in hamsters using radiolabelled anticarcinoembryonic antigen immunoglobulin. Cancer Res 34:1
5. Goldenberg DM et al. (1978) Use of radiolabelled antibodies to carcinoembryonic antigen for the detection and localization of diverse cancers by external photoscanning. N Engl J Med 298:1384
6. Berche C et al. (1982) Tomoscintigraphy for detecting of gastrointestinal and medullary thyroid cancer: First clinical results using radiolabelled monoclonal antibodies against carcinoembryonic antigen. Br Med J 285:285
7. Halpern SE et al. (1983) Stability, characterization and kinetics of 111-In labelled monoclonal antitumor antibodies in normal animals and nude mouse human tumor models. Cancer Res 43:5347
8. Rainsbury RM et al. (1983) Location of metastatic breast carcinoma by monoclonal antibody chelate labelled by Indium 111. Lancet ii:934−939
9. Epenetos AA et al. (1984) Tumour imaging using an improved method of DPTA-coupled monoclonal antibodies radiolabelled with metallic radionuclides. Lancet ii:169
10. Armitage NC et al. (1984) Indium-111, a superior radiolabel for the imaging of colorectal cancer using the antitumor monoclonal antibody 791 T/36. Lancet ii (in press)
11. Buchegger et al. (1983) Radiolabelled fragments of monoclonal antibodies against carcinoembryonic antigen for localization of human colon carcinoma grafted into nude mice. J Exp Med 158:413
12. Moshakis V et al. (1981) Localization of human tumor xenografts after i.v. administration of radiolabelled monoclonal antibodies. Br J Cancer 44:91
13. Imai K et al. (1984) Immunologic characterization and molecular profile of CEA detected by monoclonal antibodies. J Immunol 132:2992
14. Wagener C et al. (1984) Binding of five monoclonal anti-CEA antibodies with different epitope specificities to various carcinoma tissues. Int J Cancer 33:469

15. Koga Y et al. (1985) Further comparative studies on chemical properties of CEA in tumor tissues and closely related antigens in adult feces and meconium. Mol Immunol 22:67
16. Grunert F et al. (1985) Two CEA and three NCA species, although distinguishable by monoclonal antibodies, have nearly identical peptide patterns. Int J Cancer 36:357
17. Dillman RO et al. (1984) Lack of radioimmunodetection and complications associated with monoclonal anticarcinoembryonic antigen antibody cross-reactivity with an antigen on circulating cells. Cancer Res 44:2213
18. Deland FH et al. (1980) Imaging approach in radioimmunodetection. Cancer Res 40:3046
19. Goldenberg DM, Deland FH (1982) History and status of tumor imaging with radio-labelled antibodies. J Biol Response Mod 1:121
20. Barratt GM et al. (1983) Improved radioimmunodetection of tumors using liposome-entrapped antibody. Biochim Biophys Acta 762:154
21. Sharkey RM, Primus FJ, Goldenberg DM (1984) Improved radioimmunodetection of tumors by second antibody. Proc Am Assoc Cancer Res 25:252
22. Kaplan JH, Groves JN (1984) Characterization of antigen-antibody interactions relevant to the radioimmune imaging of tumors. Fed Proc 43:1510

Immunoscintigraphy of CEA-Producing Tumors with Special Emphasis on the Use of Mab Fragments and ECT

A. Bischof-Delaloye[1], B. Delaloye, F. Buchegger, V. von Fliedner, and J.-P. Mach

Introduction

The first reports that carcinoma could be detected in patients by external scanning following injection of purified I-131-labeled anti-CEA antibodies were made by Goldenberg et al. [1, 2]. They claimed that almost all the CEA-producing tumors could be detected by this method and that there were no false-positive results. However, our experience with highly purified goat anti-CEA antibodies [3] and the same blood pool subtraction technique used by Goldenberg was that only 42% of CEA-producing tumors (22 out of 53 tested) could be detected by this method [4]. Furthermore, we found that in several patients the labeled anti-CEA antibodies localized nonspecifically in the reticuloendothelium, particularly in the liver. Despite the use of the subtraction technique, it was difficult to differentiate this nonspecific uptake from the specific uptake in liver metastases. The discrepancy in the results obtained by the group of Goldenberg and our own is unlikely to be due to a difference in the quality of the anti-CEA antibodies used, since a direct measurement of the radioactivity in tumors resected after injection showed that our antibodies were capable of excellent tumor localization [4]. Furthermore, in a few patients scheduled for tumor resection, we injected simultaneously 1 mg goat anti-CEA antibodies labeled with 1 mCi I-131 and 1 mg control normal goat IgG labeled with 0.2 mCi I-125. With this paired labeled method adapted to the patient situation, we demonstrated that the antibody uptake was four times higher than that of control normal IgG [4].

These results were very encouraging in terms of specificity of tumor localization. However, the direct measurement of radioactivity in tumors also showed that only $0.05-0.2\%$ of the injected radioactivity was recovered in the resected tumors $3-8$ days after injection [4].

The obvious advantages of monoclonal antibodies (Mab) are their homogeneity and their specificity for the immunizing antigen. Another advantage of Mab is that they each react with a single antigenic determinant and thus should not be able to form large immune complexes with the antigen (provided the antigenic determinant is not repetitive).

1 Centre Hospitalier Universitaire Vaudois, Division autonome de médecine nucléaire, CH-1011 Lausanne

Nuclear Medicine in Clinical Oncology
Ed. by C. Winkler
© Springer-Verlag Berlin Heidelberg 1986

The first Mab used for immunoscintigraphy in patients was Mab 23 anti-CEA [5]. As early as 1981, the well-characterized Mab 23 was injected intravenously into 26 patients with large bowel carcinomas and two patients with pancreatic carcinomas. Each patient received 0.3 mg purified Mab labeled with $1-1.5$ mCi I-131.

The patients were studied by planar scintigraphy 24, 36, 48, and 72 h after injection. In 14 of the 28 patients (50%), a hot area corresponding to the tumor was detected $36-48$ h after injection. In six patients, the scans were doubtful, and in the remaining eight patients, they were entirely negative [5].

The results were slightly better than those obtained with polyclonal anti-CEA antibodies [4]. There was less background radioactivity in the liver, but the method could not yet be considered as clinically useful in comparison with the other modern methods of tumor diagnosis.

The introduction of emission computerized tomography (ECT) improved the detection especially of small lesions [5, 6], since its contrast is less volume dependent and the overlap of active structures can be eliminated to a great extent.

With this method, 15 out of 16 carcinoma tumor sites (10 colorectal carcinomas; 1 stomach, 1 pancreas, and 4 medullary thyroid carcinomas) could be detected.

The poor imaging qualities of I-131 and the fact that patients are exposed to high levels of radiation, however, detract from the advantages of this technique. I-123 could overcome these two major disadvantages of I-131 [7], but its 13.2-h period precludes scans later than 48 h.

In order to further improve this method, we produced a series of 26 new hybridoma-secreting anti-CEA antibodies and selected them first, in vitro, by criteria of high affinity for CEA [8] and low cross-reactivity with glycoproteins present on the surface of granulocytes, termed NCA-55 and NCA-95. Furthermore, $F(ab')_2$ and Fab fragments were prepared from three selected Mab and tested for their capacity to localize, in vivo, in human colon carcinoma heterotransplanted in nude mice [9]. Groups of $4-7$ mice were injected simultaneously with I-131-labeled Mab or fragments and with normal IgG or their corresponding fragments labeled with I-125. The mice were dissected $2-5$ days later.

The ratios of tumor antibody concentration to normal organ antibody concentration increased dramatically with the use of fragments. The ratios of tumor antibody concentration to normal organ antibody concentration (average of all normal organs) were 7 for intact Mab, 25 for $F(ab')_2$, and 85 for Fab. The specificity indices calculated by dividing the tumor-to-normal-organ ratios for antibody by the corresponding ratio for control IgG were 3.4 for intact Mab, 8.2 for $F(ab')_2$, and 19 for Fab [9].

The scanning results obtained with these experimental animals were in agreement with those obtained by direct measurement of radioactivity. With intact Mab, tumor grafts of $0.5-1$ g did not give contrasted positive scans until 3 days after injection, whereas fragments of Mab allowed the detection of smaller tumors at an earlier time. The best results were obtained with Fab fragments of Mab 35, which allowed the clear detection of a 0.1-g tumor graft 48 h after injection [9].

Patients and Method

Based on the above experimental results, we examined in a retrospective study 30 patients with colorectal carcinoma after injection of 1.5 mg $F(ab')_2$ (13 patients) and 1 mg Fab (17 patients) fragments of Mab 35 labeled with I-123 (2.3 – 8 mCi; mean, 3.95 mCi). The isotope was prepared from the I-127 (p, 5n) Xe-123 reaction and provided by the *Eidgenössisches Institut für Reaktorforschung* at Würenlingen, Switzerland.

All patients gave informed consent. For 2 days before and 3 days after injection, the thyroid was blocked with Lugol's solution. The evening before and 1 h prior to injection, the patient received an antihistaminic drug (Clemastine 2 mg) in order to prevent allergic reactions. In addition, 100 mg prednisolone was injected intravenously 1 h before the administration of the antibody. No intracutaneous testing was performed.

Anterior and posterior whole-body scans were performed simultaneously using a rotating dual-head scintillation camera with a whole-body attachment linked up with an array processor and a computer. Whole-body tracer distribution was studied 1, 6, 24, and 48 h after injection; the lower and upper abdomen were examined by ECT at 6 and 24 h in all patients and at 48 h in 11 patients. Additional regions were studied if other metastatic lesions were suspected either anamnestically or on the basis of the planar whole-body images.

Following the last antibody-ECT of the upper abdomen, another ECT of the liver was performed after injection of Tc-99^m sulfur colloid (3 – 4 mCi), with the patient remaining in the same position.

For all tomographic reconstructions, 30 views per camera head were stored with an angular increment of 6°; low-energy all-purpose collimators were used. Six hours after injection an average 70 000 counts per view were collected in about 30-s exposures, at 24 h 50 000 counts in 60-s exposures, and at 48 h some 30 000 counts in 120-s exposures. At 48 h, the patient had thus to be immobile for at least one hour per region. The camera was checked daily for center alignment, uniformity, and sensitivity of both heads. The slice thickness of the reconstructed sections was 12 mm.

Transverse, sagittal, and coronal sections were obtained for all regions examined. Figure 1 demonstrates the scintigraphic aspect of a carcinoma of the ascending colon on transverse, coronal and sagittal sections 6 h after injection.

Results

All primary tumors were visualized by this technique regardless of the level of circulating CEA or the type of fragment used. All but one could already be clearly distinguished on the 6-h scans.

Figure 2 shows the results obtained in a patient with carcinoma of the sigmoid. The transverse section on the left shows accumulation of activity in the iliac vessels and in the tumor which is situated anteriorly with respect to the right iliac vessels. On the coronal section, the location of the tumor in the right lower pelvis above the urinary bladder is confirmed. This unusual location of a

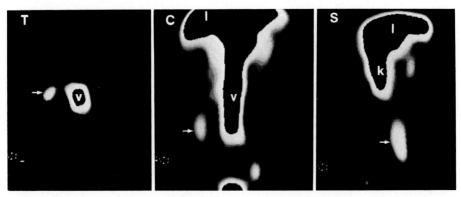

Fig. 1. Adenocarcinoma Dukes C of the ascending colon imaged 6 hours after injection of I-123-labeled anti-CEA Mab Fab. The tumor is well separated from big vessels (*V*), liver (*l*) and kidney (*k*) on the transverse (*T*), coronal (*C*), and sagittal (*S*) section

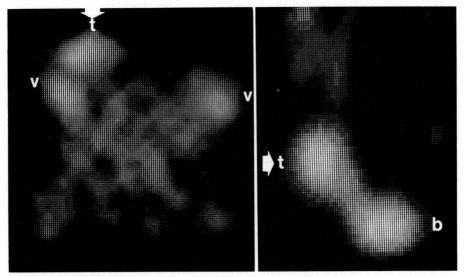

Fig. 2. Results obtained in a patient with carcinoma of the sigmoid. The transverse section on the left shows accumulation of activity in the iliac vessels (*v*) and in the tumor (*t*) which is situated anteriorly with respect to the right iliac vessels. On the coronal section the location of the tumor (*t*) in the right lower pelvis above the urinary bladder (*b*) is confirmed

sigmoid tumor was proved at laparotomy. All but one of the local recurrences were visualized by this technique. In one patient, the recurrent tumor could not be visualized with the radiolabeled Fab fragments of the antibody, but antibody uptake occurred in numerous bone metastases. These were previously unknown and only later confirmed by a conventional bone scan.

Two other patients presented with bone metastases which were all well visualized with both types of labeled Mab fragments, whereas no uptake could be detected in two small lung metastases in a patient under chemotherapy. As no increase in the size of these lung metastases could be observed during the 10 months following the examination, it might be suggested that there was no active tumor present at the time of the investigation with the radiolabeled antibody. In another patient, two recent lung metastases were clearly visualized.

It was possible to identify 12 patients with liver metastases. In 10 patients, uptake of the antibody could be detected, one of which was previously unknown and confirmed at surgery. Liver metastases remained undetected in two patients; one had liver cirrhosis, and the other had undergone repeated partial hepatectomy, the recent metastasis being located at the hepatectomy section.

Discussion and Conclusion

The poor signal-to-noise ratio observed after injection of the labeled antibody remains one of the major problems in immunoscintigraphy. Circulating antibody and nonspecific tracer uptake may mask the tumor uptake, which has been shown to be nonuniform and rather low even with specific antibodies. Several attempts have been made to improve the tumor definition and localization on the scans. With I-131, the first radiolabel used, it became possible to perform late scans after the decrease of circulating activity. The poor counting statistics of these images, however, made the detection of small tumors difficult. Different subtraction techniques were used in order to separate target from nontarget activity. These techniques, however, are not free from artefacts [10], which are mainly due to the different photon energies of the radionuclides used and to the differences in the in vivo distribution of pertechnetate, serum albumin, or red cells in comparison with antibodies.

F (ab')$_2$ and Fab fragments of Mab give higher tumor-to-background ratios than the intact antibody by reduced binding to reticuloendothelium and faster urinary excretion [8, 9]. But even when renal excretion is prevented, there remains an inverse relationship between size and tumor uptake of the intact Mab and its fragments [11]. The tumor-to-background ratios and the specificity indices of the anti-CEA Mab fragments used in the present study have been shown to be higher for F (ab')$_2$ fragments compared with the intact antibody in nude mice bearing human colon carcinoma. For Fab fragments these ratios even increased [9]. Thus, both types of antibody fragments could reasonably be used with the I-123 label.

The major advantage of using tomoscintigraphy and I-123-labeled Mab fragments is the high quality of the images: it therefore becomes possible to distinguish tumor accumulation of radioactivity from physiologic organ concentration and circulating radioactivity without the artefacts inherent in subtraction techniques. We are aware that our optimistic results in terms of sensitivity have to be confirmed in a prospective study.

In any case, we think that small fragments of Mab with high affinity for a relatively abundant tumor marker such as CEA represent the best tracer for diagnostic purposes. Because of their higher tumor-to-background ratio, Fab fragments seem to be preferable to F (ab')$_2$ fragments for the visualization of small tumors and liver metastases.

References

1. Goldenberg DM, Deland F, Kim E et al. (1978) Use of radiolabeled antibodies to carcinoembryonic antigen for the detection and localization of diverse cancers by external photoscanning. N Engl J Med 298:1384–1388
2. Goldenberg DM, Kim E, Bennett SJ et al. (1983) Carcinoembryonic antigen radioimmunodetection in the evaluation of colorectal cancer and in the detection of occult neoplasms. Gastroenterology 84:524–532
3. Mach JP, Carrel S, Merenda C et al. (1974) In vivo localization of radiolabeled antibodies to carcinoembryonic antigen in human colon carcinoma grafted into nude mice. Nature 248:704–706
4. Mach JP, Carrel S, Forni M et al. (1980) Tumor localization of radiolabeled antibodies against carcinoembryonic antigen in patients with carcinoma. N Engl J Med 303:5–10
5. Mach JP, Buchegger F, Forni M et al. (1981) Use of radiolabelled monoclonal anti-CEA antibodies for the detection of human carcinomas by external photoscanning tomoscintigraphy. Immunol Today 2:239–249
6. Berche C, Mach JP, Lumbroso JD et al. (1982) Tomoscintigraphy for detecting gastrointestinal and medullary thyroid cancers: first clinical results using radiolabelled monoclonal antibodies against carcinoembryonic antigen. Br Med J 285:1447–1451
7. Epenetos AA, Mather S, Granowska M et al. (1982) Targeting of iodine-123-labelled tumour-associated monoclonal antibodies to ovarian, breast and gastrointestinal tumours. Lancet 8306:999–1005
8. Haskell CM, Buchegger F, Schreyer M et al. (1983) Monoclonal antibodies to carcinoembryonic antigen: ionic strength as a factor in the selection of antibodies for immunoscintigraphy. Cancer Res 43:3857–3864
9. Buchegger F, Haskell CM, Schreyer M et al. (1983) Radiolabeled fragments of monoclonal anti-CEA antibodies for localization of human colon carcinoma grafted into nude mice. J Exp Med 158:413–427
10. Ott J, Grey LJ, Zivanovic MA et al. (1983) The limitations of the dual radionuclide subtraction technique for the external detection of tumours by radioiodine-labelled antibodies. Br J Radiol 56:101–108
11. Halpern SE, Buchegger F, Schreyer M et al. (1984) Effect of size of radiolabeled antibody and fragments on tumor uptake and distribution in nephrectomized mice. J Nucl Med 25:112

Beta-hCG and Related Germ Cell Tumor Antigens in Radioimmunodetection

H. N. Wellman[1], L. Lin, R. Rowland, and G. Sledge

Beta-human chorionic gonadotropin (Beta-hCG) has figured prominently in one of the most important developments in modern day oncology. Currently, beta-hCG and alpha-fetoprotein (AFP) are probably the best two examples of tumor markers. These glycoproteins, which can be employed as on-codevelopmental antigens for the production of monoclonal antibodies used to detect tumors, have been involved in benchmark studies in tumor physiology and biochemistry. They are mostly associated with germ cell tumors (GCT), of which testicular carcinomas are by far the most important, representing the commonest tumors in men between ages of 15 and 35. Carcinoma affecting such a large population at the prime of their lives takes on particular importance. The astounding improvement in cure and survival rates recorded by Einhorn et al., working at Indiana University, is a basis for the success story in working with this tumor [11]. With a chemotherapeutic regimen of cis-platinum, vincristine, and bleomycin (PVB), a cure rate of only 10% in the 1960s has improved to 95% – 99% for stage I or II and 60% – 70% for stage IV in individuals with nonseminomatous germ cell tumors (NSGCT). Since on-codevelopmental antigens have played an important role in the diagnosis and management of these tumors, discussion of these tumor-associated antigens is inextricable from some discussion of the diagnosis and management of the tumors themselves.

Because it is the first solid tumor to show such a high cure rate, testicular tumor thus represents a landmark tumor in adult oncology. In order to appreciate the potential of and need for radioimmunodetection (RAID) in these disease processes, the recent changes in the diagnosis and management of GCT, principally testicular carcinoma, must be understood.

Some degree of confusion exists with regard to the pathologic classification of testicular GCT. There is general agreement that two major groups exist, namely, the seminomatous and the nonseminomatous. For a number of years, seminoma has not been as much of a diagnostic and management problem – with there being general agreement that the primary management be radiation therapy – since it is a responsive tumor. The real problem has been with non-seminomatous tumors, not only in their diagnosis and management, but also in their classification. In the British scheme, all NSGCT are classified as terato-

---

1 Indiana University, Department of Radiology, Division of Nuclear Medicine, 926 West Michigan Street, Indiana University Medical Center, Indianapolis, IN 46223, USA

Nuclear Medicine in Clinical Oncology
Ed. by C. Winkler
© Springer-Verlag Berlin Heidelberg 1986

carcinomas, whereas in the American system, teratoma is the term reserved for a tumor having more than one germ layer of tissue, other tumors being classified as embryonal carcinomas of the testis [32]. The recent dramatic improvement in cure and survival has primarily been with NSGCT, which comprise about 60% of testicular carcinomas, while seminomas comprise 40%. More recently, better pathologic definition of these tumors has been accomplished with electron microscopy. With regard to tumor markers, the nonseminomatous GCT are much more frequently found to have beta-hCG and AFP; only occasionally is a seminoma associated with these tumor markers.

The whole management of NSCGT has changed dramatically within the past 5–10 years. Diagnostically, not only has the availability of serum markers been of import, but also a marked improvement in the detection of metastatic disease has been achieved through X-ray, CT, and ultrasound techniques. Burney and Klatte of our institution have reported on the excellent results obtainable with these modalities [5]. Accuracy rates of 87% for computed tomography (CT) and 83% for ultrasound (US) in detecting metastatic spread of disease in the abdomen and chest were reported. There are drawbacks to both procedures, ultrasound being very operator dependent and greatly affected by abdominal and bowel gas. CT has the drawback of not being helpful in examining very thin individuals who lack contrasting fat tissue. As the investigators indicate, thin people should go to ultrasound and fat people to CT to obtain the best results with these modalities. More recently, MRI studies in our institution have been of little additional help compared with CT and US. Other investigators have reported lesser accuracies, and all groups are unanimous in their view that the problem cases are patients with borderline enlarged lymph nodes [31, 38]. A significant number of patients are false-positive. This is one area where more specific tests, such as RAID would be helpful in improving diagnostic accuracy and staging.

The success with the PVB regimen used at Indiana has led to a considerable modification of the surgical management of most patients with NSGCTs. Donohue and Rowland of our institution recently reported that there has now been an actual reversal of surgical management, with the emphasis in most patients placed on the utilization of cytoreductive chemotherapy (SRC) after initial orchiectomy [8, 9, 33], reserving staging laparotomies for stage I and II NSGCT. Thus, there is the need for RAID in those patients who might be falsenegative according to results of the other diagnostic and imaging techniques and yet are strongly suspected of having disseminated disease on the basis of persistently elevated tumor markers.

The key role played by hCG and AFP in the management of the GCT logically led to optimism that these agents might be utilized for RAID [23]. There are both alpha and beta subunits of hCG. The alpha subunit has glycoproteins that closely resemble TSH, LH, and FSH and thus lacks specificity. The beta subunit, on the other hand, does not have these cross-reactivities and is more specific as an oncodevelopmental antigen. The beta subunit is seen in about 50% of patients with NSGCT and has occasionally been found in patients with lung, liver, breast, stomach, or pancreas carcinomas as well. AFP in oncodevelopmental glycoprotein appears to function somewhat like albumin in the fetus. It, too, is elevated in something approaching 50% of patients with NSGCT, but is also found in many other diseases. There is no consistency as to whether a given patient with NSGCT will have both of these on-codevelopmental antigens present, but on average, 84% of patients will have elevated levels of one or the other or both of these glycoproteins. There are now very sensitive radioimmunoassays based on monoclonal antibodies to these "shed" (or more likely secreted) antigens. The presence of a rise and fall over the course of treatment of a patient with these tumor markers has played a significant role.

With such a high level in patients with NSGCT, there was a logical basis for exploring the use of these markers in the RAID of disseminated testicular tumors. Seminoma, by the way, is very seldom associated with an elevation of hCG. More recently, it has become apparent that these are just the first two of many testicular GCT-associated antigens that might be present. Also, hCG is known to be primarily associated with the syncytiotrophoblastic component of GCT and AFP with yolk sac elements. Other recently reported on-codevelopmental antigens are the placental alkaline phosphotase (PLAP), stage-specific embryonic antigen (SSEA-1), 5F9.3 antigen, K4, K21 and P12 antigens, and SP-1 − the pregnancy-specific beta glycoprotein. Antibodies, especially monoclonal antibodies, to these oncodevelopmental antigens including fractionated antibodies, have been reported, mostly in animals, but some in patient clinical series.

Prominent among the groups working in this area has been that of Goldenberg, DeLand and Kim, working mainly at the University of Kentucky. They have also collaborated with Javadpour at the National Institutes of Health. As early as 1981, this group reported their initial results in five patients with testicular GCT studied with RAID using iodine-131 labeled hCG or AFP [17]. At that initial stage, hCG already appeared to be more specific than AFP. Although in using either labeled antibody, it was found that tissue background was very high and had to be corrected for by the simultaneous injection of technetium-labeled blood pool and extracellular fluid space tracers with subtraction imaging. The authors concluded, however, that even though there were elevated serum levels of the two markers, it did not hinder the successful tumor localization for RAID. The choice of which labeled tracer to use was based upon the oncodevelopmental glycoprotein predominating in an individual patient serum. The authors had to utilize what they then described as elaborate computer processing to make possible visualization of the monoclonal antibody localization. Goldenberg further updated the data from this group, reporting on studies in 25 patients with labeled hCG RAID [14]. In this group were 10 patients with testicular cancer, all of whom had positive findings correlating with other imaging and surgical procedures for presence of tumor. More recently, DeLand reported on a total of 60 patient studies with polyclonal antibodies to hCG [16]. Successful studies were reported in 25 of these patients. A detection rate of 100% was reported in the patients with GCT. In this group of patients, four with testicular cancer were found to have sites with the hCG RAID techniques when other detection methods were negative. The investigators also noted that the plasma levels of hCG had no relationship to the detection of tumors in vivo. In the same report, results for 21 patients out of a group of 51 studied with either polyclonal or monoclonal antibodies to AFP were reported. Results, again with AFP, were not as good as with hCG, with an overall true-positive detection rate of 74% and a false-positive rate of 6%. The best results were obtained in patients with embryonal carcinoma of the testes. Also, hepatocellular and ovarian carcinoma yielded good results. However, results with seminoma and lung cancer were poor. Besides the problems of the high levels of background with the secreted or shed antigens, with monoclonal antibodies there may be a difference in the epitopes expressed between the primary and metastatic tumor, reducing the possibility of specific targeting. Thus, there is still some question as to whether some mixture of antibodies should be used. Availability of specific cellular antigens should contribute to the selection of monoclonal antibodies that will provide the highest ratio of antigen-antibody reaction in vivo, as well as the opportunity of engineering mixtures of monoclonal antibodies for improved tumor sequestration (one might call these oligoclonal antibody techniques). The authors conclude from the data that there is still promise in utilizing tumor-associated antibodies, although their investigation with labeling radionuclides for cancer detection and therapy is still a highly developmental technique and requires much continued evaluation. They also speculate that the availability of single photon emission computed tomography (SPECT) techniques will improve immunodetection utilizing labeled antibodies.

Investigators working in Japan reported on the utilization of iodine-131-labeled AFP in clinical studies [34, 39]. They had performed basic investigations in animals injected with labeled AFP from human testicular tumor, with successful localization of the labeled antibodies with RAID. However, in clinical cases, despite the use of an Anger-type tomographic apparatus for imaging, these authors had to conclude that they saw no specific tumor localization. This, in part, was due to the very high background and to the fact that no subtraction techniques were utilized, as reported by other groups above. The authors conclude that this may have been in part due to the chemotherapy that the patients had already received with *cis*-diamminodichloroplatinum.

Very recently, Wahl et al., from the University of Michigan reported on the utilization of the 5F9.3 monoclonal antibody [36], an antibody raised against testicular GCT. This has some cross-reactivity with teratocarcinomas. It has been successfully labeled with iodine-131 and a case report of the successful localization of metastatic choriocarcinoma in a 29-year-old woman has been made. The patient had undergone extensive surgical and radiation therapy and had received 45 courses of chemotherapy over a 4-year period. In follow-up, she was found to have a rising hCG level, but no macroscopic evidence of disease or evidence on CT scans as to the site of the disease. Specific localization of 5F9.3 monoclonal antibody in the left chest and midabdomen revealed sites of metastatic choriocarcinoma, later confirmed with tissue diagnosis. Very important in this report is the apparent specificity of 5F9.3 monoclonal antibody, to the extent that the antigen does not appear to be secreted or shed and, indeed, may then be a legitimate surface antigen and thus not require techniques of background subtraction employed by DeLand et al. These findings are very encouraging. Aspirates from the tumor analyzed for radioactivity showed a tenfold background-to-target ratio of the uptake of the activity. The preliminary findings with this particular monoclonal antibody offer promise for patients who have rising hCGs, while no other obvious foci of metastatic disease are evident from clinical investigations or other imaging techniques.

Another group of promising GCT-related oncodevelopmental antigens are the stage-specific embryonic antigens, specifically SSEA-1. Ballou et al., recently reported on the use of a monoclonal antibody to SSEA-1 [4]. This oncodevelopmental antigen was derived from human teratocarcinoma. Interestingly, these authors compared a whole antibody and its divalent antigen-binding peptic fragment [F(ab')2 μ], which was prepared using the techniques reported by Lin of our group, labeled, and utilized in animals [24]. These techniques show the possibility for improving the localization of monoclonal antibody, and it is our intent to use similar techniques in the future. The Fab fragment was shown to have a shorter half-life in serum and an improved lesion-to-background ratio, although uptake in the tumor was not as high as the whole antibody. Nonetheless, the authors conclude that, despite a lesser uptake, the improvement in reduction of background obviates the need for dual tracer technique for subtraction of background-enhanced tumor detection. There is promise that, by maximizing the affinity, specificity, and use of appropriate fragments, tumor localization with labeled monoclonal antibodies for RAID can be greatly enhanced.

Rettig et al., very recently reported on high molecular weight glycoproteins of human teratocarcinoma defined by monoclonal antibodies to their carbohydrate determinants [30]. The K4, K21, and P12 antibodies that react to specific carbohydrate sequences present in high molecular weight glycoproteins were identified. These are thought to be specific surface antigens to this testicular teratocarcinoma line and, if so, may lead to progress in isolating a more specific group of surface antigens for better specificity and affinity for future RAID studies. Their preliminary immunocytochemical studies on human teratocarcinomas indicate that the expression of K4, K21, and P12 distinguishes different histological types within tumors. Especially the highly restricted distribution of K21, which is undetectable in normal adult tissue, makes this antigen a potential target for immunological imaging in tumors and immunotherapy of human teratocarcinoma.

Another promising potential oncodevelopmental antigen is found in the isoenzymes of placental alkaline phosphatase (PLAP). This is the old so-called Regan enzyme. A number of authors are now reporting on monoclonal antibodies to these PLAP antigens [2, 3, 12, 18, 23, 26, 29]. Some authors report that all GCT, including seminomas and malignant teratomas, have been identified as having PLAP as a surface antigen. Very few other tumors have been found to have this particular oncodevelopmental antigen. In our own experience, utilizing tissue from the large group of testicular carcinoma patients studied here at Indiana University, we have prepared monoclonal antibodies with the similar consistent finding of most of the GCT expressing the PLAP oncodevelopmental antigen. However, we are presently in the process of developing monoclonal antibodies to this particular antigen for future exploration of its use as a labeled specific monoclonal antibody to GCT for RAID.

Likewise, in this group of patients with testicular carcinoma, we had previously studied the specificity and affinity of 21 different antibodies to beta hCG by screening using histochemical staining techniques. Unfortunately, the background staining was found to be so excessive, presumably because of the secretion or shedding of the antigen, that it was not deemed prudent to go on with developing a radiolabeled antibody for use in the human subjects. Such activities would have just duplicated those reported already by other groups, and it is clear that antibodies with greater affinity and specificity must be developed if RAID is to become a successful complementary imaging technique to the already very useful CT and US techniques. Especially in light of the deficiencies of CT and US, only an antibody with high specificity and affinity would help identify questionable metastatic sites as well as reveal those not evident on the other studies. Furthermore, with the incredible success in the treatment of GCT now, the need for RAID studies will be limited to a relatively small proportion of this disease group.

We have been employing a murine monoclonal IGG-1 antilactoferrin antibody and lactoferrin-conjugated affinity column to boost the effectiveness of various methods for radionuclide labeling and possible proteolytic fragmentation of antibody molecules. The possibility of producing carbohydrate-free antibody molecules using the tunicamycin-containing culture medium is also being evaluated. Carboydrate-free antibodies may prevent recognition by the reticuloendothelial system, decreasing background radioactivity and scint-images and facilitating detection of smaller foci of involved nodes.

In summary, beta-hCG and AFP as oncodevelopmental antigens, have played an extremely important role, so to speak, as a generic model for identifying a group of antigens with an affinity and specificity, making possible successful RAID. The pioneering efforts of the investigators working with these agents has certainly demonstrated the feasibility of employment of this imaging technique. The results with these particular oncodevelopmental antigens in GCT have not been ideal. The realization that a secreted or shed antigen may result in poor target-to-nontarget ratio requiring elaborate techniques for imaging subtraction could only be realized by painstaking research. The need for more specific, probably cell surface, antigens as a means of making monoclonal antibodies with higher specificity and affinity is clear, and there already are good possibilities for the identification of such antigens. It will require long, painstaking research to develop the optimal monoclonal antibody or mixture of antibodies, or so-called oligoclonal antibodies to best cover the possibilities for any given tumor. Our group, along with others, will be exploring these other potential oncodevelopmental antigenic glycoproteins for the purpose of developing more specific antibodies for RAID. Other proposals include the utilization of unique administration routes, particularly administration through the lymphatic pathways by localized injections. This would not be unlike the ingenious technique reported by Kaplan et al., on iliopelvic radionuclide lymphoscintigraphy in patients with testicular cancer [20]. Weinstein et al. have also reported on the utilization of lymphatic administration of monoclonal antibodies for improved diagnosis and therapy of tumor metastases [37]. The more widespread availability now of newer generations of single photon emission computed tomography (SPECT) apparatus, as discussed by DeLand, will also improve the contrast enhancement necessary for RAID. All in all, we are probably only in the very early phases of employing RAID in the diagnosis and management of GCT as well as the whole field of oncology. The fact that in an extremely complicated area, such as the antioncodevelopmental glycoprotein monoclonal antibodies, there has been even a limited degree of initial success is very encouraging.

References

1. Abramson CS, Kersey JH, LeBien TW (1981) A monoclonal antibody (Ba-1) reactive with cells of human B lymphocyte lineage. J Immunol 126:83–88
2. Beckstead JH (1983) Alkaline phosphatase histochemistry in human germ cell neoplasms. Am J Surg Pathol 7:341–349
3. Benham FJ, Andrews PW, Knowles BB, Bronson DL, Harris H (1981) Alkaline phosphatase isozymes as possible markers of differentiation in human testicular teratocarcinoma cell lines. Dev Biol 88:279–287
4. Ballou B, Reiland J, Levine G, Knowles B, Hakala TR (1985) Tumor location using F(ab')2μ from a monoclonal IgM antibody: pharmacokinetics. J Nucl Med 26:283–292
5. Burney BT, Klatte EC (1980) Abdominal ultrasound and computed tomography in testicular cancer. In: Einhorn LH (ed) Testicular tumors: management and treatment Masson, New York, pp 83–115
6. DeLand FH, Goldenberg DM (1985) Diagnosis and treatment of neoplasms with radionuclide-labeled antibodies. Semin Nucl Med 15(1):2–11
7. DeLand FH, Kim EE, Simmons G, Goldenberg DM (1980) Imaging approach in radioimmunodetection. Cancer Res 40:3046–3049
8. Donohue JP (1980) Surgical management of testis cancer. In: Einhorn LH (ed) Testicular tumors: management and treatment. Masson, New York, pp 29–46
9. Donohue JP, Rowland RG (1984) The role of surgery in advanced testicular cancer. Cancer 54:2716–2721
10. Eckelman WC, Paik CH, Reba RC (1980) Radiolabeling of antibodies. Cancer Res 40:3036–3042
11. Einhorn LH, Williams SD (1980) The management of disseminated testicular cancer. In: Einhorn LH (ed) Testicular tumors: management and treatment. Masson, New York, pp 117 149
12. Epenetos AA, Travers P, Gatter KC, Oliver RDT, Mason DY, Bodmer WF (1984) An immunohistological study of testicular germ cell tumours using two different monoclonal antibodies against placental alkaline phosphatase. Br J Cancer 49:11–15
13. Gaylis FD, Fraley EE, Bronson DL (1984) In vitro models of human testicular germ-cell tumors. World J Urol 2:2–5
14. Goldenberg DM, Kim EE, DeLand FH (1981) Human chorionic gonadotropin radioantibodies in the radioimmunodetection of cancer and for disclosure of occult metastases. Proc Natl Acad Sci USA 78:7754–7758
15. Halsall AK, Fairweather DS, Bradwell AR et al. (1981) Localization of malignant germ-cell tumors by external scanning after injection of radiolabelled anti-alpha-fetoprotein antibody. Br Med J 283:942–944
16. Harris H (1980) Multilocus enzyme systems and the evolution of gene expression: the alkaline phosphatases as a model example. Harvey Lect 76:95–124
17. Javadpour N, Kim EE, DeLand FH, Salyer JR, Shah U, Goldenberg DM (1981) The role of radioimmunodetection in the management of testicular cancer. JAMA 246:45–49

18. Jemmerson R, Fishman WH (1982) Convenient selection of monoclonal antibodies to isoenzymes of placental alkaline phosphatase using the catalytic activity of the antigen in enzyme-antigen immunoassay. Anal Biochem 124:286−292

19. Jeppsson A, Wahren B, Stigbrand T, Edsmyr F, Andersson L (1983) A clinical evaluation of serum placental alkaline phosphatase in seminoma patients. Br J Urol 55:73−78

20. Kaplan WD, Garnick MB, Richie JP (1983) Iliopelvic radionuclide lymphoscintigraphy in patients with testicular cancer. Radiology 147:231−235

21. Kim EE, DeLand FH, Nelson MO, Bennett S, Simmons G, Alpert E, Goldenberg DM (1980) Radioimmunodetection of cancer with radiolabeled antibodies to alpha-feto-protein. Cancer Res 40:3008−3012

22. Lange PH, McIntire KR, Waldmann TA (1980) Tumor markers in testicular tumor: current status and future prospects. In: Einhorn LH (ed) Testicular tumors: management and treatment. Masson, New York, pp 69−81

23. Lange PH, Millan JL, Stigbrand T, Vessella RL, Ruoslahti E, Fishman WH (1982) Placental alkaline phosphatase as a tumor marker for seminoma. Cancer Res 42:3244−3247

24. Lin LC, Putnam FW (1978) Cold pepsin digestion: a novel method to produce the F fragments from human immunoglobulin M. Proc Natl Acad Sci USA 75:2649−2653

25. Millan JL, Stigbrand T (1981) "Sandwich" enzyme immunoassay for placental alkaline phosphatase. Clin Chem 27:2014−2018

26. Millan JL, Stigbrand T, Ruoslahti, Fishman WH (1982) Characterization and use of an allotype-specific monoclonal antibody to placental alkaline phosphatase in the study of cancer-related phosphatase polymorphism. Cancer Res 42:2444−2449

27. Moldofsky PJ, Sears HF, Mulhern CB, Hammond ND, Powe J, Gatenby RA, Steplewski Z, Koprowski H (1984) Detection of metastatic tumor in normal-sized retroperitoneal lymph nodes by monoclonal-antibody imaging. Eng J Med 311:106−107

28. Narayan P, Carroll PG, DeWolf WC (1984) Teratocarcinoma: basic research and its clinical relevance. World J Urol 2:6−11

29. Paiva J, Damjanov I, Lange PH, Harris H (1983) Immunohistochemical localization of placental-like alkaline phosphatase in testis and germ-cell tumors using monoclonal antibodies. Am J Pathol 111:156−165

30. Rettig WJ, Cordon-Cardo C, Ng JSC, Oettgen HF, Old LJ, Lloyd KO (1985) High-molecular-weight glycoproteins of human teratocarcinoma defined by monoclonal antibodies to carbohydrate determinants. Cancer Res 45:815−821

31. Richie JP, Garnick MB, Finberg H (1982) Computerized tomography: how accurate for abdominal staging of testis tumors? J Urol 127:715−717

32. Roth LM, Gillespie JJ (1980) Pathology and ultrastructure of germinal neoplasms of the testis. In: Einhorn LH (ed) Testicular tumors: management and treatment. Masson, New York, pp 1 29

33. Rowland RG (1984) Surgical management of post-chemotherapy residual testis tumor. In: Ratliff TL, Catalona WJ (eds) Urologic oncology. Nijhoff, Boston, pp 256−274

34. Sakahara H, Endo K, Nakashima T, Ohta H, Torizuka K, Okada K, Yoshida O, Hirai H (1984) Experimental studies on the tumor imaging using antibodies to human alpha-feto-protein: fluctuations in the iodine-labeled antibody activities. Kaku-Igaku 21:805−813

35. Sidi AA, Chiou R-K, Lange PH (1984) Recent reflections on tumor markers. World J Urol 2:18−25

36. Wahl RL, Jackson G, Laino L, Kroenberg S, Khazaeli MB, LoBuglio AF, Patillo RA, Beierwaltes WH (1985) Monoclonal antibody radioimmunodetection of occult chorio-carcinoma: case report. Presented at Central Chapter Society of Nuclear Medicine, Chicago, Illinois, March 1985 (abstract)

37. Weinstein JN, Parker RJ, Keenan AM, Dower SK, Morse III HC, Sieber SM (1982) Monoclonal antibodies in the lymphatics: toward the diagnosis and therapy of tumor metastases. Science 218:1334−1337

38. Williams RD, Feinberg SB, Knight LC, Fraley EE (1980) Abdominal staging of testicular tumors using ultrasonography and computed tomography. J Urol 123:872−875

39. Yanagisawa M, Miki M, Hirai H (1981) Clinical evaluation of tumor positive imaging with I-125 (or-131)-labeled anti-human AFP specific antibody for AFP producing tumor line (JTG-1) and clinical cases. Nippon-Hinyokika-Gakkai-Zasshi 72:1559−1568

Radioimmunodetection with Monoclonal Antibodies Against Prostatic Acid Phosphatase

S. E. Halpern[1] and R. O. Dillman

Carcinoma of the prostate is one of the most common tumors. In the USA, it accounts for approx. 18% of all cancers of males and 24,000 deaths annually. The initial treatment a patient receives is highly dependent on the stage of the tumor at the time of its initial recognition. Therapy chosen in view of known distant metastases is also dictated to some extent by their distribution. It would be valuable, therefore, to have a diagnostic agent that could specifically indicate the presence and extent of metastases at both the early and late stages of prostate carcinoma. Currently, we are limited to the measurement of serum acid phosphatase levels, which, while useful when elevated, are not highly sensitive; computerized tomography (CT) which cannot specifically indicate metastases or radionuclide bone scanning, while useful, is also nonspecific. The invention of monoclonal antibodies (MoAb) [1] provides the potential for both specificity and sensitivity in diagnostic testing. This report describes our effort to develop a radiolabeled MoAb against prostatic acid phosphatase (PAP) and use it for the radioimmunodetection (RAID) of prostatic cancer.

Materials and Methods

Monoclonal antitumor antibodies were formed against PAP by the Hybritech Corporation using the standard hybridoma technique. The antibody was derived by immunizing mice with human seminal fluid which is known to have a high PAP concentration, then screening with radiolabeled PAP. The resulting hybridoma was grown in the peritoneal cavity of nude mice and the MoAb produced was further refined by ammonium sulfate precipitation and diethyl-aminoethanol (DEAE) column chromatography. This MoAb has been designated PAY-276. It is an IgGIK and has an affinity for the antigen of greater than 10^9 mol/l. It is greater than 80% immunoreactive. This MoAb is thought to recognize only the PAP unique to benign or malignant prostate tissue.

The MoAb was labeled with ^{111}In using the method of Krejcarek and Tucker [2], as modified by our group. This technique produces high labeling efficiency (80%−95%) with specific activities of 5 µCi/mcg or greater without significant

---

1 Veterans Administration, Medical Center, 3350 La Jolla Village Drive, San Diego, CA 92161, USA

Nuclear Medicine in Clinical Oncology
Ed. by C. Winkler
© Springer-Verlag Berlin Heidelberg 1986

damage to the MoAb from the labeling process. The latter is assessed using in vitro studies which indicate the same immunoreactivity as the stock material and in vivo distribution studies in Balb/C mice that indicate a distribution typical of other IgG MoAbs. The following is a brief description of the labeling process.

Diethylenetriaminepentaacetic acid (DTPA) is reacted with five equivalents of triethylamine and the reaction product is lyophilized. The lyophilized salt is then dissolved in dry acetonitrile. This is necessary because water will inhibit the subsequent reactions. The preparation is then reacted with isobutylchloroformate forming the carboxycarbonic anhydride of DTPA. The anhydride in turn is reacted with amine groups on the MoAb resulting in the conjugation of the antibody, i.e., the chelating side chain is attached to the protein. Since the anyhdride also reacts with water in the environment, a large amount of free DTPA is formed. This must be removed before radiolabeling occurs or the efficiency of the ^{111}In chelation will be low. Separation of the MoAb-DTPA complex from the free DTPA is accomplished by passing it through a Sephadex G-75 column. The void volume is pooled (it contains the MoAb) and labeled with ^{111}In by reacting the ^{111}In as the citrate with buffering at pH 4.0. Thirty minutes are necessary for this portion of the reaction. In all of the studies to be described 1 mg of the side chain conjugated MoAb was used for labeling, having been mixed with equal molar amounts of human serum albumin prior to the reaction. To rid the preparation of unreacted ^{111}In, a scavenging agent is added to the reaction vial. This results in the unlabeled ^{111}In being immediately sequestered and rapidly eliminated in the urine. After the first 24 h nearly all of the ^{111}In that is not protein bound has been eliminated from the body by the kidney.

Seven patients with metastatic prostate carcinoma were studied. Three of them received a 1-mg dose, one received 2.5 mg, two received 5 mg, and one received 20 mg of the antibody. In all cases only 1 mg of the side-chain labeled antibody was used, the rest of the preparation being made up of unchelated PAY-276. Five mCi of ^{111}In was reacted in all cases. The radiopharmaceutical was administered intravenously over a period of 2 h following which imaging was accomplished at the end of infusion, then at 4, 24, 48, 72, and occasionally 144 h postinjection. Blood was drawn at multiple time points and used to follow complete blood counts, serum chemistries, and disappearance of the radiolabeled MoAb from the vascular compartment. Urine was collected through 24 h in all patients.

Results

There were no acute or chronic untoward effects from the administration of the radiopharmaceutical. One patient died approximately 2 weeks following administration of the radiopharmaceutical; however, death was due to his malignancy. The serum chemistries were normal in all of the patients except for the one patient who died, and these values were abnormal before administration as well as following the MoAbs.

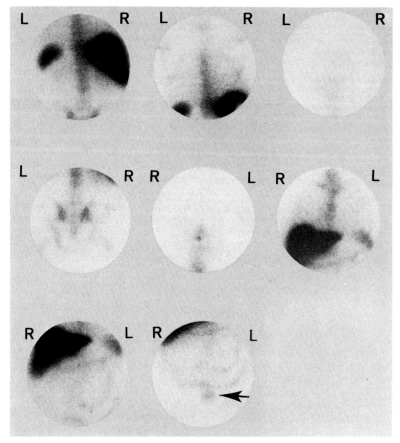

Fig. 1. These scans, which were performed 72 h following the administration of ¹¹¹In-PAY-276, clearly indicate the prostate gland (*arrow*), yet bony metastases present in the patient were not detected

The blood disappearance curves indicated that in the majority of the patients there was a rapid disappearance of the radiopharmaceutical from the blood. Unlike other MoAb systems that we have studied [3] this did not necessarily appear to be correlated with the antibody dose administered. Approximately 30% – 70% of the radiopharmaceutical remained in the blood at 6 h while only 10% – 25% remained in the blood at 24 h. By 72 h 1% – 5% was all that remained.

The scans indicate that a large amount of the radiopharmaceutical is removed by the liver within the first few hours of its administration (Fig. 1). The spleen and bone marrow are also frequently imaged. The patient in Fig. 1 had widely metastatic bone metastases from his tumor. These were not detected by imaging, however, the unresected prostate is seen in this case and in most other cases in which the prostate had not been surgically excised. Figures 2 and 3

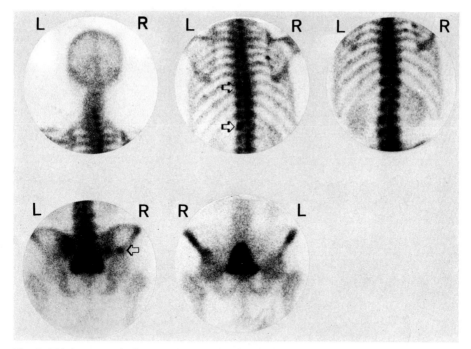

Fig. 2. This bone scan indicates at least three sites of metastatic disease (*arrows*)

demonstrate uptake in sites of bony metastases by diphosphonate bone scanning and radioimmunodetection, respectively. The bone scan was performed approx. 3 months prior to the MoAb study. A large lesion is seen in the L5 vertebra on the antibody study which is not present on the bone scan. One of the thoracic vetebral lesions is imaged by the antibody study, but not the other areas indicated by the bone scan.

At least one lesion was detected in five of the seven patients in this study. Conversely, only 11 of 52 lesions indicated on bone scans were detected (21%).

Discussion

The results of this work indicate that successful radioimmunoimaging is dependent on a host of variables. PAY-276, for example, has high immunoreactivity, can be stably labeled with a radionuclide that has outstanding imaging characteristics, is used in a system where antigen is known to exist on the tumor, is nontoxic, and yet is capable of detecting less than 25% of the bony lesions.

Multiple factors are probably responsible for this. First there is the rapid and large accumulation of radiopharmaceutical by the liver and the swift egress of the ^{111}In-PAY-276 from the vascular compartment. These events deny the metastatic lesions an adequate chance to acquire the antibody. When we com-

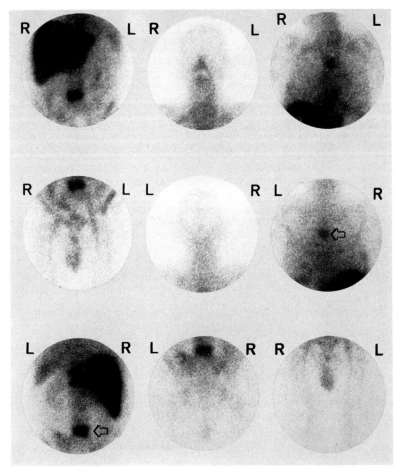

Fig. 3. ^{111}In-PAY-276 study in the patient whose bone scan appears in Fig. 2. Note the dramatic areas of increased uptake (*arrows*). Further note that one of the previous sites indicated on the bone scan does not take up the ^{111}In radiopharmaceutical

pared the blood disappearance curve of PAY-276 with that of another IgG ^{111}In antiprostate MoAb, we found PAY-276 to be removed from the vascular compartment faster than the other MoAb. Our work in the melanoma system [3] indicates that a short duration of circulation decreases the chance of detecting lesions. In the case of PAY-276 this could be one reason for the poor tumor detection.

The cause of the high liver uptake is not known, however certain possibilities exist. One of these is intravascular immune complex formation. Small amounts of PAP that is specific for PAY-276 do circulate in the serum and should form immune complexes. The search for PAP:[111]In-PAY-276 immune complexes has been difficult, however, because these complexes are too small to be easily separated from uncomplexed ^{111}In-PAY-276 via high pressure liquid chromatography (HPLC) technique. An indirect method established in our laboratory suggests that they may well have been formed.

In this technique we removed blood from patients 24 h postadministration of ^{111}In-PAY-276 and administered it to Balb/C mice. Control mice received only the radiolabeled antibody. The livers of the mice that received the serum doubled the uptake of ^{111}In observed in controls. Our interpretations of these data are based on our studies in another circulating antigen system. We had previously shown that circulating carcinoembryonic antigen (CEA) produced in nude mice bearing CEA-producing human tumors will result in high liver uptake of the ^{111}In anti-CEA preparation [4]. The greater the circulating CEA levels, the greater the amount of radiopharmaceutical that went to the liver. Thus, immune complexes formed with IgG anti-CEA monoclonal antibodies were removed by the liver of the mouse in the manner observed following the administration of ^{111}In-PAY-276-laden patient serum from subjects with prostate cancer. Interestingly enough, CEA:^{111}In anti-CEA immune complexes formed in the human were not removed by the human liver as they were in the mouse. In this case, the immune complexes circulated for a long time in the vascular compartment. To add to the confusion, if patients developed circulating antimouse antibodies and immune complexes formed with ^{111}In anti-CEA, they were rapidly removed by the human liver. Thus, while we know that complexes with circulating antigen form in the human following administration of ^{111}In-PAY-276, they may or may not be related to the marked liver uptake. Obviously more work needs to be done in this area.

It is entirely possible that the liver uptake of this MoAb could be the result of unique characteristics of the MoAb such as the configuration or array of the carbohydrate groups in the molecule. Indeed, each MoAb system that we have studied to date has shown distribution characteristics in the human somewhat unique unto itself. Yet another reason (speculations) for the poor tumor detection could have something to do with the blood flow to the bony metastases. Tumors with very high blood flow (provided antigen is present) become inviting targets for radioimmunoimaging detection. The blood flow to prostatic cancer metastatic to bone may not be very great.

Finally, work in nephrectomized mice (unpublished data of the authors) suggests that removal of the Fc portion of the molecule may result in a reduction of the amount of protein sequestered by the liver. This further suggests that the offending entity may be the carbohydrate groups on the molecule. If this is the case with PAY-276, its F (ab')$_2$ may yet prove a good MoAb for radioimmunodetection. It must be remembered, however, that data derived in the nude mouse model may not always be a valid method for indicating that a derived immunoreactive molecule will be useful clinically.

In summary, we have studied seven patients with ^{111}In antiprostatic acid phosphatase MoAb with mediocre results. The difficulty in radioimmunoimaging with this particular antibody was secondary to rapid removal of the radiopharmaceutical from the blood and its sequestration by the liver. The possibility that the antibody might be a useful entity following the removal of the Fc portion of the molecule is discussed in theoretical terms.

References

1. Köhler G, Milstein C (1975) Continuous cultures of fuse cells secreting antibody of pre-defined specificity. Nature 256:495–497
2. Krejcarek GE, Tucker KL (1977) Covalent attachment of chelating groups to macromolecules. Biochem Biophys Res Commun 71:581–585
3. Halpern SE, Dillman RO, Witztum KF, Hagan PO, Dillman JB, Sobol R, Frinke J, Bartholomew R, David G, Carlo D (1985) Radioimmunodetection in melanoma employing ^{111}In-P96.5 monoclonal antibodies: a preliminary report. Radiology 155:493–499
4. Hagan PO, Halpern SE, Chen A, Krishnan L, Frincke J, Bartholomew RM, David GS, Carlo D (in press) In vivo kinetics of radiolabeled monoclonal anti-CEA antibodies in animal models. J Nucl Med

Immunoscintigraphy of Ovarian Cancer by Means of HMFG2 Monoclonal Antibody

M. Granowska[1], C. C. Nimmon, and K. E. Britton

Human milk fat globule 2 (HMFG2) antibody is a monoclonal antibody, class IgG_1, against the HMFG protein, which is a large glycoprotein (300 KD). It is present on the epithelial surface membrane lining of the duct of the breast, the crypts of the colon, and the inside lining of ovarian follicles [1, 2].

With malignant changes in these tissues, architectural disruption occurs, the epithelial surface lining becomes exposed to blood and the antigen is present in increased density. HMFG2 thus is against a tumour-associated antigen and not specific for ovarian cancer. Its presence and site of uptake may be demonstrated in histological tissue sections by immunoperoxidase staining. The hybridoma producing HMFG2 was derived from the fusion of the mouse myeloma cell line NSI with the spleen cells of a mouse which had received an initial injection of delipidated HMFG protein followed by a boost with cultured normal milk epithelial cells [3]. It is provided by the Imperial Cancer Research Fund Laboratories, London.

Labelling of HMFG2

^{123}I iodine is produced by the Atomic Energy Research Establishment, Harwell, using a high energy cyclotron so that the product ^{123}I is free of ^{124}I and contains less than 0.05% ^{125}I. It is available throughout Europe on a Wednesday morning. It is dissolved in sodium hydroxide, dispensed into sterile vials and may be dried. Iodogen (Tetrachlorodiphenylglycoluril, Pierce Chemicals) is dissolved in dichlormethane to make an iodogen solution and evaporated to dryness at 20 °C in sterile propylene tubes. The iodogen reagent thus coats the inside of these tubes which are used for the labelling procedure. To this tube 10 mCi (400 MBq) ^{123}I, 0.1−0.2 ml 0.1 M citrate buffer pH 6, 400 µg IgG_1 monoclonal antibody (2 mg/ml in 0.1 M citrate/tris buffer pH 7.4) and 10 µl potassium iodide (6×10^{-5} M in water) are added and mixed together by gentle shaking for 10 min. To remove free ^{123}I, the mixture is decanted onto a Sephadex G50 filtration column in a 20-ml syringe which has been pre-washed with 1% serum albumin in phosphate buffered saline. After a 5-ml void volume, the eluate is collected, activity assayed and passed through a micropore filter into sterile

---

1 St. Bartholomew's Hospital, Dept. of Nuclear Medicine, West Smithfield, London EC1A, 7BE, UK

Nuclear Medicine in Clinical Oncology
Ed. by C. Winkler
© Springer-Verlag Berlin Heidelberg 1986

vials. Chromatographic quality control is undertaken and the reagent used if there has been over 70% labelling efficiency. Using the iodogen technique in this way, over 95% of the immunoreactivity of HMFG2 is shown to be preserved using the ELISA technique and by direct radioimmunoassay.

[111]In Indium 6 mCi (240 MBq) is used to label HMFG2 conjugated using the bicyclic bisanhydride of diethylene triamine penta acetate using the Hnatowich technique [4] supplied by Amersham International. For imaging purposes 3 mCi (120 MBq) of ^{123}I labelled or ^{111}In labelled HMFG2 is used.

Imaging Using Radiolabelled HMFG2

The patient is selected as appropriate for the study by the gynaecological surgeon, usually as a step before a second-look operation, or by the medical oncologist usually to evaluate the effect of chemotherapy. The nature of the test is explained to the patient and informed signed consent is obtained as required by the Ethical Committee. Oral potassium iodide 60 mg is given the day before the test, during and for 3 days after the test. An intradermal skin test with 0.1 ml HMFG2 is given half an hour before the study and the result is compared with a saline control. No reactions to the skin test or to the injection have been observed in over ninety patients.

The patient lies supine on the scanning couch and a gamma camera is placed over the pelvis anteriorly. The injection of 3 mCi of ^{123}I labelled monoclonal antibody containing 0.5 mg antibody is given intravenously to the patient. Dynamic studies are recorded for the first 10 min directly into the computer. Static images are then taken, anteriorly and posteriorly of the whole of the abdomen together with marker scans. These are transferred directly into the computer.

Similar procedures occur at 4 h and 22 h. For [111]Indium imaging is also repeated at 48, 72 and 96 h.

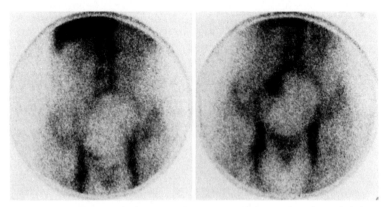

Fig. 1. Radioimmunoscintigraphy with ^{123}I HMFG2: anterior view of abdomen and pelvis at 10 min (*left*) and 4 h (*right*) after injection. Increased uptake in the right central abdomen and around a cystic mass is seen at 4 h as compared to 10 min. (Courtesy Nuclear Medicine Communications)

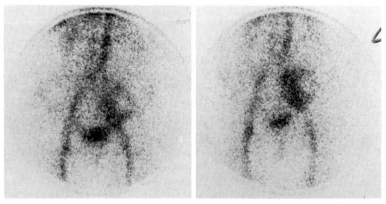

Fig. 2. Radioimmunoscintigraphy with ^{123}I HMFG2: anterior view of the abdomen and pelvis at 4 h (*left*) and 24 h (*right*). Uptake with a central defect is seen in a left ovarian mass shown to be adenocarcinoma with a necrotic centre at operation. (Courtesy Nuclear Medicine Communications)

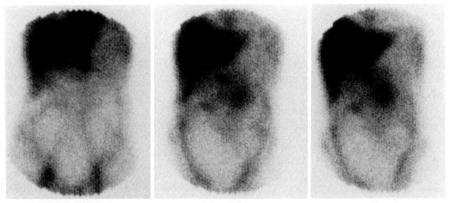

Fig. 3. Radioimmunoscintigraphy with ^{111}In HMFG2 in a patient with multiple abdominal recurrences of a previously resected ovarian adenocarcinoma. Anterior view of the abdomen at 10 min. Anterior view of the abdomen at 52 h and 96 h after injection. (Courtesy Blackwell Publications)

Typical examples of ^{123}I HMFG2 uptake in ovarian cancer are shown in Figs. 1 and 2, while an example of ^{111}In HMFG2 uptake in ovarian cancer is shown in Fig. 3.

In the European Nuclear Medicine Congress, Helsinki, a blind prospective study using ^{123}I HMFG2 in 30 patients presenting with a pelvic mass was reported [5]. Ten of the patients turned out not to have ovarian cancer when the study was finally analysed. Five of these ten patients without ovarian cancer showed the features which would be taken for ovarian cancer, with low initial and high late uptake.

There were two patients with large benign ovarian tumours and three patients with metastases from other cancers: stomach, colon and liver. In a further two patients there was poor uptake generally, true negatives, and in three patients there was high uptake initially followed by high uptake persisting at 24 h, indicating high vascularity. Two masses were due to fibroids and one to a tubo-ovarian abscess. Therefore, it is quite clear from this prospective study that this technique cannot be used to screen patients as to whether or not they have ovarian cancer when they present with a mass in the pelvis, because the antibody is not sufficiently specific for this purpose. However, in 18 of 20 patients with ovarian cancer, the distribution of activity demonstrated on the scans had a close correlation with the independently determined surgical findings.

In one patient the distribution was not as accurate although a positive diagnosis was made, giving an equivocal result, and in one patient, two 0.5-cm lesions were missed, a poor result. In order to improve these results which were obtained only using the conventional transparent film display, a number of methods of data analysis have been undertaken. First, an original technique whereby an early image is subtracted from a late image was introduced [6, 7]. However, the subtraction technique is somewhat subjective, since one has to decide how much of one image to subtract from the other. Nevertheless, using this technique we developed a repositioning protocol whereby both the patient and subsequently the computer images could be accurately aligned.

A new approach, using a more objective method of analysis is the development of a kinetic change detection algorithm by Nimmon et al. [9]. The basis of the differentiation of tumour from other tissue is that tumour uptake of the specific antibody increases with time, whereas the blood pool and other tissue activity decreases with time.

Thus, if a series of images are taken over a period of time and then analysed in such a way as to combine the temporal change, together with the count rate distribution, tumour sites will be clearly identified.

For example, in the comparison of a 10-min image and a 22-h image, the count rate content of each image is compared pixel by pixel as a frequency distribution. The pixels content of one image is plotted on the x-axis, and the other on the y-axis.

Comparison between the sets of pixel values defining the pair of aligned images is made using a weighted linear regression. Pairs of values with deviations greater than 1.2× the standard error of the estimate (SEE) are excluded and the regression analysis is continued iteratively. Each comparison is tested using a Chi-squared statistic and continues until no change occurs in the Chi-squared value. In order to allow for the occasional abnormal pixel, a cluster definition is also applied that requires that several pixels adjacent to each other must be shown to be significantly different. Assuming a normal distribution about this linear segment, a probability map is constructed with levels $P < 0.001$, $P < 0.01$ and $P < 0.05$. These levels are represented in three different colours or contours and correspond to SEE deviations of 3.29, 2.58 and 1.96, respectively. Simulation studies show that noise artefacts are minimised if a signal-to-noise ratio of over 20 is used for a cluster size of five pixels and that the technique can identify low contrast differences successfully. Accurate pre-alignment of images is essential in order to avoid the formation of edge artefacts. These new "probability" maps of the distribution of uptake of antibody in our hands have shown much higher sensitivity to the detection of abnormal uptake. In the same patient, the probability map usually shows more extensive disease than the simple subtraction image. Using this technique, the two 0.5-cm secondaries, proven by biopsy, were correctly identified in the patient misclassified in the prospective study described above.

In view of this success a small pilot study has been undertaken in six patients who had clinically no obvious disease at the end of their course of chemotherapy for ovarian cancer. They were all subjected to second-look operations. In each of the six patients, up to 14 biopsy sites were taken. Before the operation conventional ^{123}I HMFG2 antibody serial images were obtained and these underwent computer analysis using the kinetic change detection algorithm. These studies were then reported with no knowledge of the biopsy findings. The method was, that for each image the list of biopsy sites were given by the surgeon and from the image a statement was made as to whether each of the biopsy sites on the list was positive or negative. In addition, if the probability map showed other sites that were positive, even though they had not been biopsied, these sites were recorded. Finally, the histology at each biopsy site was revealed by the surgeon and the map was scored as being correct or incorrect. The results, which will be published elsewhere [10], may be summarised as follows:

There were good correlations between the 39 biopsy site findings and the probability maps. The specificity was 91% and the sensitivity 86% with an accuracy of 87%. In particular, the one disease-free patient and the five patients with recurrence were correctly identified and the probability map showed positive uptake at sites which were not normally accessible to biopsy such as under the left diaphragm.

In conclusion, imaging recurrences of ovarian cancer after chemotherapy is a clinically useful role for ^{123}I or ^{111}In HMFG2 in ovarian cancer. Kinetic analysis of the data with the construction of probability maps of significant uptake enable the detection of lesions not detectable at surgery, but proven to have viable cancer cells on biopsy. The technique is applicable in principle to all types of radioimmunoscintigraphy.

References

1. Arklie J, Taylor-Papadimitriou J, Bodmer WR, Egan M, Millis R (1981) Different antigens expressed by epithelial cells in the lactating breast are also detectable in breast cancers. Int J Cancer 28:23–29
2. Burchell J, Durbin H, Taylor-Papadimitriou J (1983) Complexity of expression of antigenic determination, recognized by monoclonal antibodies HMFG-1 and HMFG-2, in normal and malignant human mammary epithelial cells. J Immunol 131:503–513
3. Taylor-Papadimitriou J, Peterson JA, Arklie J, Burchell J, Ceriani RC, Bodmer WR (1981) Monoclonal antibodies to epithelium-specific components of the human milk fat globule membrane: production and reaction with cells in culture. Int J Cancer 28:17–21
4. Hnatowich DJ, Layne WW, Childs RL, Lanteigne D, Davis MA (1983) Radioactive labelling of antibody: a simple and efficient method. Science 220:613–615
5. Granowska M, Shepherd J, Mather S, Carroll MJ, Flatman WD, Nimmon CC, Taylor-Papadimitriou J, Ward B, Horne T, Britton KE (1984) A prospective study of radio-

immunoscintigraphy with 123-I monoclonal antibody in 26 patients with suspected ovarian cancer. Eur J Nucl Med 9:A61

6. Granowska M, Britton KE, Shepherd J (1983) The detection of ovarian cancer using ^{123}I monoclonal antibody. Radiobiol Radiother (Berl) 25:153−160

7. Granowska M, Shepherd J, Britton KE, Ward B, Mather S, Taylor-Papadimitriou J, Epenetos AA, Carroll MJ, Nimmon CC, Hawkins LA, Flatman WD, Horne T, Bodmer WR (1984) Ovarian cancer: diagnosis using 123-I monoclonal antibody in comparison with surgical findings. Nucl Med Commun 5:485−499

8. Carroll MJ, Flatman WD, Nimmon CC, Granowska M, Britton KE (1984) Congruent image registration as a prerequisite for detecting changes during radioimmunoscintigraphy. Nucl Med Commun 5:230−231 (Abs)

9. Nimmon CC, Carroll MJ, Flatman WD, Marsden P, Granowska M, Horne T, Britton KE (1984) Spatial probability mapping of temporal change: application to gamma camera quality control and immunoscintigraphy. Nucl Med Commun 5:231 (Abs)

10. Granowska M, Pring DW, Nimmon CC, Shepherd J, Ward B, Singh P, Mather S, Bomanji J, Slevin ML, Britton KE (1985) Kinetic analysis of radioimmunoscintigraphy, RIS, using probability mapping: comparison with multiple biopsy findings in ovarian cancer. Proc. Europ. Nucl. Med. Cong. London 1985. Eur J Nucl Med 11:A7 (Abs)

Immunoscintigraphy of Gynaecological Tumors

A. C. Perkins[1], M. C. Powell, M. V. Pimm, M. L. Wastie, E. M. Symonds, and R. W. Baldwin

Introduction

Neoplasms of the female genital tract present as a wide range of abnormalities and are the second most common source of fatal cancer in women after carcinoma of the breast [7]. Because of the diversity of gynaecological tumors, the diagnosis and followup of patients remains an important clinical problem. The application of techniques for early detection and successful treatment offers great prospects for the relief of suffering and extension of life. The targeting of monoclonal antibodies to tumors offers potential for both diagnosis and therapy and will hopefully improve the management of these patients.

Tumor antigenicity was first recognised by Witebsky [14], when a rabbit antiserum produced against a uterine carcinoma reacted poorly with normal tissues. More recently a range of both polyclonal and monoclonal antibodies have been used for the in vivo localisation of gynaecological cancers [3, 6, 8]. Antibodies against carcinoembryonic antigen (CEA), alpha fetoprotein (AFP), human chorionic gonadotropin and human milk fat globule (HMFG) have previously been used with reports of high diagnostic sensitivities — in some cases up to 90% [6]. More recently the tumor associated monoclonal antibody 791T/ 36, raised against a human osteogenic sarcoma has been used for the imaging of ovarian cancer [12]. This antibody has also been previously shown to localise in primary osteogenic sarcoma [5], colon carcinoma [1, 4] and breast cancer [13]. Further quantitative studies of the localisation of this antibody in tumors of the ovaries, cervix and uterine body have been undertaken. Of particular interest is the radiolabelling of antibodies with radionuclides having more favourable physical characteristics than ^{131}I for gamma camera imaging, which should improve the diagnostic accuracy and sensitivity of the technique. The 791T/36 antibody has been conjugated to the cyclic dianhydride of diethylenetriaminepentaacetic acid (DTPA) for radiolabelling with ^{111}In [10]. Preliminary in vivo studies in mice with human tumor xenografts gave a strong indication as to its suitability for clinical tumor localisation studies. Imaging studies of patients with gynaecological tumors have been carried out with the same antibody radiolabelled with either ^{131}I or ^{111}In and the results compared.

---

1 Medical Physics Department, Queen's Medical Centre, Clifton Boulevard, Nottingham NG7 2UH, UK

Nuclear Medicine in Clinical Oncology
Ed. by C. Winkler
© Springer-Verlag Berlin Heidelberg 1986

Materials and Methods

Monoclonal antibody 791T/36 (mouse IgG2b) was raised against an in vitro human osteogenic sarcoma cell line by the Cancer Research Campaign Laboratories of Nottingham University. Following isolation from hybridoma-culture supernatants using affinity chromatography on Sepharose-protein A, purified antibody was radiolabelled with either ^{131}I using an iodogen method [11] or ^{111}In after conjugation to DTPA dianhydride [10]. Labelled preparations were diluted in 10-ml saline and sterilised by terminal filtration. Between 200 μg and 1 mg of antibody radiolabelled with between 40 and 70 MBq of either ^{131}I or ^{111}In was injected into an antecubital vein of each patient following a subcutaneous test dose to test for anaphylaxis. Patients receiving ^{131}I-labelled antibody were also given oral potassium iodide throughout the study and for 10 days following injection, to block the thyroid uptake of free iodide.

The present study includes 63 patients with a strong suspicion of the presence of gynaecological malignancy at the time of the investigation. The nature of the study was clearly explained to each patient who gave their informed consent. Forty-three patients received ^{131}I-labelled antibody and twenty patients received ^{111}In-labelled antibody on a random basis. The diagnosis of the patients injected with ^{131}I-labelled antibody is indicated in Table 1. Table 2 shows the diagnosis of patients injected with ^{111}In-labelled antibody.

Images were acquired using an IGE 400T large field of view gamma camera and recorded by computer in a matrix of either 64×64 elements or 128×128 elements. Anterior and posterior views of the pelvis, abdomen and thorax were recorded between 18 and 72 h after administration of the antibody using a high energy parallel hole collimator (400 keV max.) for ^{131}I imaging and a medium energy collimator (300 keV max.) for ^{111}In imaging.

Blood pool subtraction was carried out for the studies of ^{131}I-labelled antibody using ^{99m}Tc-labelled erythrocytes and free pertechnetate to simulate the distribution of the nontumor labelled antibody. After acquisition of the two images and thresholding of the ^{131}I view, background subtraction was carried out as described by Perkins et al. [9]. Images of the ^{111}In-labelled antibody were compared with a blood pool view recorded 20 min after administration, which could also be used for subtraction if required.

Where appropriate, 360° emission tomography was carried out by acquiring counts over 64 increments each of 15 s duration. Data were reconstructed in a 64×64 matrix and the axial images were given a 9-point smooth in two dimensions.

Patients with primary tumors underwent surgery within 48 h of imaging and the resected tumor specimens were imaged by the gamma camera and then dissected. The tissues were then weighed and the radioactivity counted in a well scintillation counter. The count rates were then expressed as a percentage of the administered dose.

Table 1. Histology and results of patients imaged with ^{131}I-791T/36

Patient	Histology	Imaging result	
Ovary			
1. ST	Papillary adenocarcinoma	+	+H
2. IM	Inoperable mass (no histology)	+	+H
3. BA	Serous adenocarcinoma	+	+L
4. JN	Serous cystadenocarcinoma	+	
5. JL	Poorly differentiated adenocarcinoma	+	
6. GB	Poorly differentiated adenocarcinoma	+	
7. PU	Well-differentiated adenocarcinoma	+	
8. HL	Granulosa cell carcinoma	+	
9. MC	Granulosa cell carcinoma	+	
10. EK	Squamous cell carcinoma in a teratoma	+	
11. MS	Borderline carcinoma	+	
12. GP	Anaplastic carcinoma	+	
13. VQ	Cellular thecoma	+	
14. AT	Teratoma (containing thyroid tissue)	+	
15. DS	(Previous adenocarcinoma) normal laparoscopy	+	
16. PW	(Previous adenocarcinoma) normal laparoscopy	+	
17. JC	(Previous granulosa cell) normal laparoscopy	+	
18. MS	(Previous adenocarcinoma) normal laparoscopy	−	
19. LB-W	(Previous adenocarcinoma) normal laparoscopy	−	
20. BL	(Previous adenocarcinoma) normal laparoscopy	−	
21. PM	Serous cysts	−	
22. HS	Moderately differentiated adenocarcinoma	−	
Cervix			
23. LB	Poorly differentiated squamous cell carcinoma	+	
24. DF	Poorly differentiated squamous cell carcinoma	+	
25. YC	Poorly differentiated squamous cell carcinoma	+	
26. PD	Poorly differentiated squamous cell carcinoma	+	
27. TA	Poorly differentiated squamous cell carcinoma	+	
28. DH	Moderately differentiated squamous cell carcinoma	+	
29. MS	Recurrent carcinoma (histology not available)		
30. HN	Moderately differentiated squamous cell carcinoma	−	
31. EB	Moderately differentiated squamous cell carcinoma	−	
32. MW	Poorly differentiated squamous cell carcinoma	−	
33. MS	Previous squamous cell (in remission)	−	
34. SD	Previous adenocarcinoma (in remission)	−	
Uterine corpus			
35. JA	Moderately differentiated endometrial adenocarcinoma	+	
36. CW	Moderately differentiated endometrial adenocarcinoma	+	
37. CWL	Moderately differentiated endometrial adenocarcinoma	+	
38. PW	Poorly differentiated endometrial adenocarcinoma	+	
39. DS	Leiomyosarcoma	+	
40. DH	Leiomyomata	+	
41. PC	Benign cellular myoma	+	
42. MB	Benign cellular myoma	−	
43. EE	No abnormality	−	

+H, positive identification in liver metastases
+L, positive identification in lung metastases

Table 2. Histology and results of patients imaged with ^{111}In-791T/36

Patient	Histology	Imaging result	
Ovary			
1. LB	Poorly differentiated mucinous cystadenocarcinoma	+	
2. MW	Poorly differentiated adenocarcinoma	+	
3. JC	Endometrial carcinoma of the ovary	+	
4. HW	Poorly differentiated adenocarcinoma of the ovary	+	+ L
5. KJ	Dermoid cyst	+	
6. GD	Well-differentiated adenocarcinoma	−	
7. VW	Poorly differentiated adenocarcinoma	−	
8. ER	Cystadenocarcinoma	−	
9. CU	Cystic teratoma	−	
10. HH	Inclusion cyst	−	
11. FW	Cystadenofibroma	−	
12. MH	Mucinous cystadenoma	−	
13. GC	Mucinous cystadenoma	−	
14. DW	Ovarian fibroid	−	
15. DO	Previous carcinoma (in remission)	−	
16. MB	Dermoid cyst	−	
Cervix			
17. DG	Squamous cell (stage IV)	+	
Uterine corpus			
18. MF	Endometrial carcinoma	+	
19. SJ	Fibroids	+	
20. BW	Endometrial carcinoma	−	

+ L, positive identification of lung metastases

Results

All patients injected with labelled 791T/36 antibody tolerated the procedure well with no adverse reactions or side effects. Imaging studies with ^{131}I-labelled antibody showed a high detection rate for primary and recurrent malignancy. A small number of more extensive tumors could be visualised on the ^{131}I images alone, however in the majority of cases blood pool subtraction of the images was necessary for visualisation of tumor uptake. An example of a patient study with ^{131}I-labelled antibody is shown in Fig. 1. Imaging with ^{131}I-labelled 791T/36 antibody resulted in the detection of 94% of ovarian tumors, 60% of cervical tumors and 100% of tumors of the uterine body (overall detection rate of 80%). However, this high detection rate was also accompanied by the high incidence of false positive results. The imaging results together with tumor histology are given in Table 1. In two patients uptake of antibody was seen in liver metastases and in a further patient antibody uptake was demonstrated in lung metastases. The excretion of ^{131}I in the form of iodide was visualised in the urinary bladder of most patients despite micturition prior to imaging.

Studies with ^{111}In-labelled antibody showed a different in vivo biodistribution of tracer with high uptake into liver and spleen with additional bone

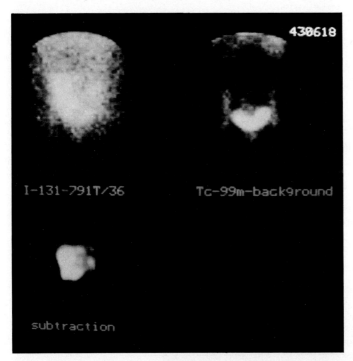

Fig. 1. Anterior planar images of the pelvis of a patient with ovarian carcinoma 48 h after injection of the ^{131}I-791 T/36 antibody, showing the ^{131}I-antibody image, the ^{99m}Tc-background image and the subtracted image showing the extent of tumor uptake

marrow and occasionally adrenal uptake. Accumulation of tracer was seen in the bowel of a number of patients. However tumor uptake could generally be seen above the activity in normal bowel. The blood clearance of ^{111}In-labelled antibody relative to the activity in the other tissues was increased compared with that of ^{131}I-labelled antibody, thus eliminating the need for image subtraction procedures. The presence of malignant tumor was correctly identified in 75% of the 20 patients studied, with two false positive results (Table 2). Uptake was seen in lung metastases of one patient using emission tomography of the thorax. A comparison of the detection rates for the localisation of pelvic malignancy using ^{131}I and ^{111}In-labelled antibody is given in Table 3.

The increased photon yield of ^{111}In over that of ^{131}I per unit of administered dose together with the use of a medium energy collimator provided count rates more suitable for single photon emission tomography. No additional sites of tumors were detected from the reconstructed axial views, however the tomographic studies did increase the confidence of tumour localisation particularly in determining tumor uptake from activity in normal bowel. An example of both planar and tomographic imaging with ^{111}In-antibody of a patient with an endometroid carcinoma of the ovary is shown in Fig. 2. This patient subsequently underwent surgery and the removed tumor showed intense uptake of the antibody. After dissection and weighing the tissues were counted in a well

Table 3. Detection of pelvic gynaecological malignancies by immunoscintigraphy using antibody 791T/36 (%)

	^{131}I-791T/36 Imaging	^{111}In-791T/36 Imaging
Overall detection rate	80	75
Accuracy	74	75
Sensitivity	86	67
Specificity	53	82

Accuracy   = true positive + true negative

$$\text{Sensitivity} = \frac{\text{true negative}}{\text{true negative} + \text{false positive}}$$

$$\text{Specificity} = \frac{\text{true positive}}{\text{true positive} + \text{false negative}}$$

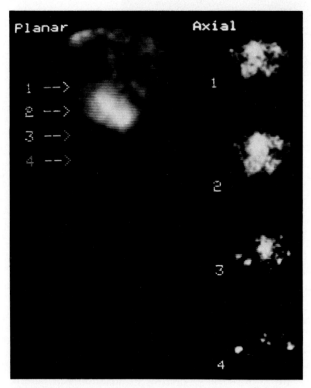

Fig. 2. Planar and tomographic images of the pelvis of a patient with an endometrial carcinoma of the left ovary 48 h following injection of ^{111}In-791T/36 antibody. The anterior image of the pelvis (*top left view*) indicating the position of the four axial slices, (*1*) through the upper region of the tumor, (*2*) through the centre of the tumor, (*3*) through the lower region of the tumor, also showing bone marrow uptake in femoral heads and activity in the femoral arteries and (*4*) through the femora

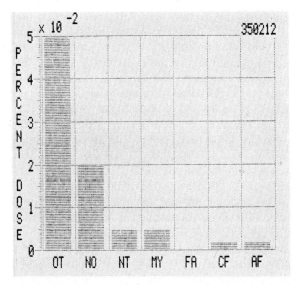

Fig. 3. Percent uptake of the administered dose of antibody per gram of tissue from the specimen in Fig. 3. *OT*, ovarian tumor; *NO*, normal ovary; *NT*, normal fallopian tube; *MY*, normal myometrium; *FA*, normal fat; *CF*, cystic fluid and *AF*, ascitic fluid

scintillation counter. The relative amount of activity per gram of tissue is shown in Fig. 3, thus confirming the preferential uptake of labelled antibody in the tumor tissues. The uptake of labelled antibody in ovarian tumor was found to be approximately 0.05% of the administered dose per gram of tissue. The tumor to normal ovary (taken from the contralateral side) uptake ratio was 2.8:1 and the tumor to fat uptake ratio was 185:1.

Repeat imaging studies with ^{131}I-labelled antibody have been carried out in 12 patients. The analysis of blood samples taken after the first injection of antibody has shown the presence of anti-mouse antibodies within 7 days of administration and remaining for over 10 months. Serial imaging studies in two patients demonstrated increased splenic uptake after the second and third administration. In each case the final imaging study was unsatisfactory.

Discussion

A preliminary study using the monoclonal antibody 791T/36 radiolabelled with ^{131}I has previously shown sufficient localisation of antibody in ovarian tumors to permit external imaging [12]. This study has demonstrated the uptake of this antibody radiolabelled with either ^{131}I or ^{111}In in malignant tumors of the ovary, cervix and uterine body. At the present time there are still relatively few monoclonal antibodies available for clinical in vivo imaging studies. However, as the range of suitable antibodies increases it is necessary to evaluate their relative potentials as both diagnostic agents and as carriers of cytotoxic drugs. The nature of expression of antigens defined by monoclonal antibodies is such that one antibody may localise in a variety of tumor types, providing widespread application as a radiopharmaceutical for tumor diagnosis. Its diagnostic ability must be compared with other available imaging modalities. The use of different antibody radiolabels also requires assessment, particularly with regard to the relative diagnostic sensitivities and specificities of tumor localisation.

Overall the detection rate of both primary and recurrent gynaecological cancer using ^{131}I-labelled 791T/36 antibody was 80%, whilst that of the same antibody when labelled with ^{111}In was 75%. Clearly the use of ^{111}In as the radiolabel with its superior physical characteristics to those of ^{131}I for gamma camera imaging, provided superior planar and tomographic images of antibody localisation, albeit with the disadvantage of uptake into normal liver, spleen and bowel. However, the relatively high detection rate of gynaecological malignancy with ^{131}I-labelled antibody and image subtraction was accompanied by a large number of false positive results, which if used as the only diagnostic criterion, may have resulted in unnecessary surgical procedures. These false positive results probably arise from the presence of ^{131}I in the urinary bladder which is not completely removed by image subtraction. A measure of the accuracy of the two techniques may be obtained by adding the numbers of true positive and true negative results yielding 74% and 75% accuracies for the ^{131}I and ^{111}In antibody studies, respectively. Further analysis of the sensitivity and specificity of the techniques for the detection of pelvic gynaecological malignancy resulted in ^{131}I-labelled 791T/36 antibody having a sensitivity of 86% and a specificity of 53%. The poor specificity resulted from the seven false positive studies out of a total of 43 investigations (16%). It would appear from the present study that ^{111}In seems to be a more suitable radiolabel for diagnostic imaging (despite the limitation of normal bowel uptake) with a sensitivity and specificity of 67% and 82%, respectively. Further studies are required to confirm these preliminary results.

Indium-111 has the additional advantage of providing good quality tomographic studies with acquisition times acceptable for the majority of patients. Although tomography did not demonstrate any improvement in either sensitivity or specificity of tumour detection, the axial slices did provide additional information regarding the extent of tumour spread within the pelvis.

No correlation between histology and antibody uptake has been demonstrated. The largest single group of patients where the technique failed to detect the presence of disease were those with carcinoma of the cervix. In these cases the tumor sizes were generally less than 2 cm in diameter which is a reflection of the relatively poor resolution of the gamma camera.

Counting of the activity contained in resected tissues provided a definitive measure of the preferential localisation of antibody in tumours. The varied nature of neoplasms of the female genital tract has necessitated the measurement of antibody uptake within the various tissue types. This should be considered particularly important in view of the use of a number of antibodies raised against oncofoetal antigens. Although the antibody 791T/36 is not known to be directed against an oncofoetal antigen, the uptake into normal ovary was slightly greater than that of the other normal tissues. This may be related in some way to the increased uptake of ^{111}In-labelled antibody seen in the testes of male patients with colorectal carcinoma [2].

The use of serial investigations for patient follow-up is currently under evaluation. The production of anti-mouse IgG antibodies in some patients [15] would appear to be a serious limitation for repeat imaging studies. Similar effects may also be observed should be antibody be used in serial therapeutic doses although the anti-mouse antibody response may vary with the amount of immunoglobulin administered on each occasion.

The development of new monoclonal antibodies and improved radiolabelling methods should improve both the sensitivity and specificity of the immunoscintigraphic technique for the detection of primary gynaecological cancer. Successful repeat imaging investigations will be of immense value in the follow-up of this type of patient. Monitoring the tumour localisation and in vivo distribution of antibody by imaging together with counting of the activity in resected tissues provides essential preliminary information prior to the use of monoclonal antibodies for reliable diagnostic imaging and effective immune-mediated therapy.

References

1. Armitage NC, Perkins AC, Pimm MV, Farrands PA, Baldwin RW, Hardcastle JD (1984) The localisation of an anti-tumour monoclonal antibody (791T/36) in gastrointestinal tumours. Br J Surg 71:407−412
2. Armitage NC, Perkins AC, Pimm MV, Wastie ML, Baldwin RW, Hardcastle JD (1985) Imaging of primary and metastatic colorectal cancer using an ^{111}In-labelled antitumour monoclonal antibody 791T/36. Nucl Med Commun (In press)
3. Epenetos AA, Mather S, Granowska M, Nimmon CC, Hawkins LR, Britton KE, Shepherd J, Taylor-Papadimitriou J, Durbin H, Malpas JS, Bodmer WF (1982) Targeting of iodine-123-labelled tumour associated monoclonal antibodies to ovarian, breast and gastrointestinal tumours. Lancet 2:999−1004
4. Farrands PA, Perkins AC, Pimm MV, Hardy JG, Embleton MJ, Baldwin RW, Hardcastle JD (1982) Radioimmunodetection of human colorectal cancers by an anti-tumour monoclonal antibody. Lancet 2:396−400
5. Farrands PA, Perkins AC, Sulley L, Hopkins JS, Pimm MV, Baldwin RW, Hardcastle JD (1983) Localization of human osteosarcoma by anti-tumour monoclonal antibody 791T/36. J Joint and Bone Surg 65-B:638−640
6. Goldenberg DM, DeLand FH (1982) History and status of tumour imaging with radiolabelled antibodies. J Biol Response Mod 1:121−136
7. Kraus FT (1977) Female genitalia. In: Anderson WAD, Kissane JM (eds) Pathology, vol 2. Mosby, St Louis
8. Mach J-P, Buchegger F, Forni M, Ritschard J, Berche C, Lumbroso J-D, Schreyer M, Giraoet C, Accolla RS, Carrel S (1981) Use of radiolabelled monoclonal anti-CEA antibodies for the detection of human carcinomas by external photoscanning and tomoscintigraphy. Immunol Today 2:239−249
9. Perkins AC, Whalley DR, Hardy JG (1984) Physical approach for the reduction of dual radionuclide image subtraction artefacts in immunoscintigraphy. Nucl Med Commun 5:501−512
10. Perkins AC, Pimm MV, Birch MK (1985) The preparation and characterisation of ^{111}In-labelled 791T/36 monoclonal antibody for tumour immunoscintigraphy. Eur J Nucl Med 10:296−301
11. Pimm MV, Embleton MJ, Perkins AC, Price HR, Robins RA, Robinson GR, Baldwin RW (1982) In vivo localisation of antiosteogenic sarcoma 791T monoclonal antibody in osteogenic sarcoma xenografts. Int J Cancer 30:75−85

12. Symonds EM, Perkins AC, Pimm MV, Baldwin RW, Hardy JG, Williams DA (1985) Clinical implications for immunoscintigraphy in patients with ovarian malignancy: a preliminary study using monoclonal antibody 791T/36. Br J Obstet Gynecol 92:270−276
13. Williams MR, Perkins AC, Campbell FC, Pimm MV, Hardy JG, Wastie ML, Blamey RW, Baldwin RW (1984) The use of monoclonal antibody 791T/36 in the immunoscintigraphy of primary and metastatic carcinoma of the breast. Clin Oncol 10:375−381
14. Witesbky E (1929) Disponibilität und Spezifität alkohollöslicher Strukturen von Organen und bösartigen Geschwülsten. Z Immunitaetsforsch 62:35−73
15. Pimm MV, Perkins AC, Armitage NC, Baldwin RW (1985) The production of antimouse-IgG antibodies in patients receiving labelled monoclonal antibody for diagnostic immunoscintigraphy. J Nucl Med 26:1011−1023

Radioimmunoscintigraphy by Means of Melanoma Antibody

S. M. Larson[1], J. A. Carrasquillo, J. C. Reynolds, I. Hellström, and K.-E. Hellström

Introduction

Disseminated malignant melanoma is incurable with presently available thera-peutic regimens. Average survival of patients with this disease ranges from a few months to 1 year. Frequently, the disease is disseminated before surgical therapy removes the primary lesion and this dissemination is frequently un-suspected [1]. Significant improvements are needed in both the therapeutic and diagnostic aspects of management of patients with disseminated melanoma.

The development of the hybridoma technique for producing monoclonal antibodies against specific antigens has opened up the possibility of using monoclonal antibodies to target human tumors in vivo [2]. In principle, anti-tumor antibodies can be used to carry radioactivity to tumors for both in vivo diagnosis and treatment of cancer. This strategy is shown in Fig. 1. First, for di-agnostic purposes, an antibody that targets a specific antigen (for example, the p97 antigen of human melanoma tumor) is labeled with a tracer amount of radioactivity. When this antibody radioisotope conjugate is injected into the bloodstream, the radioactive antibody travels throughout the body and in time percolates through all the tissues of the body. Because the tumor has specific antigens to which the antibody can bind, the radiolabeled antibody progressive-ly accumulates in the tumor. Using conventional nuclear medicine imaging equipment, the body of the patient is scanned for radioactivity content, and a map of the distribution of the radioactivity is displayed on photographic film. The tumor shows up as a dense area of radioactivity. In addition, if large amounts of radioactivity are employed, the same antibody radioisotope conju-gate can be used for therapy of tumors. In this case, there is sufficient locali-zation of radioactivity to the tumor to damage or destroy it.

Accordingly, in 1980, we began work employing monoclonal antibodies that recognize specific antigens on melanoma tumor for the purpose of targeting radioactivity to tumor deposits in vivo (Table 1). The antibodies employed tar-geted well-characterized antigens: p97, a 97,000 molecular weight glycoprotein, analogous to serum transferrin [3, 4] and the high molecular weight pro-teoglycan [5]. This work has resulted in a number of publications, involving both diagnostic and therapeutic applications, which will be summarized here [6 – 17].

---

1 Chief Department of Nuclear Medicine, CC, National Institutes of Health, NIH Building 10/RM. 1C 401 ACRF, 9000 Rockville Pike, Bethesda, MD 20205, USA

Nuclear Medicine in Clinical Oncology
Ed. by C. Winkler
© Springer-Verlag Berlin Heidelberg 1986

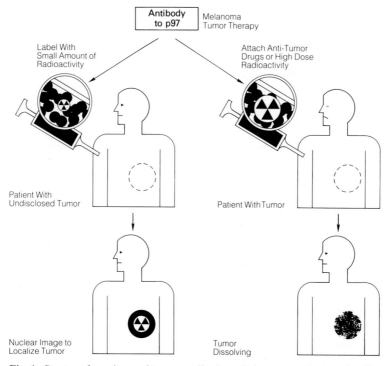

Fig. 1. Strategy for using antitumor antibody radioisotope conjugates for diagnosis and therapy of human tumor

Table 1. Selected radionuclides for radioimmunodetection

Nuclide	$t_{1/2}$	Decay characteristics
99mTc	6 h	IT (99%); = 141 keV (89%)
123I	13 h	EC (100%); = 159 keV (83%)
111In	68 h	EC (100%); = 171 keV (88%)
		245 keV (94%)
131I[a]	8.05 days	B⁻ (100%); = 364 keV
97Ru	69 h	EC (100%); = 216 keV (86%)
67Cu[a]	62 h	B⁻ (100%) = 91 keV (7%)
		93 keV (17%)
		184 keV (47%)

Technical Factors of Labeling

For success in targeting, as seen in Fig. 1, it is of very great importance to ensure that the radiolabel antibody continues to behave in a manner that reflects the biologic distribution of the radiolabeled protein. In particular, the antigen reactivity of monoclonal antibodies can be destroyed by the labeling process. It was necessary to develop techniques for labeling antibody to monoclonal anti-

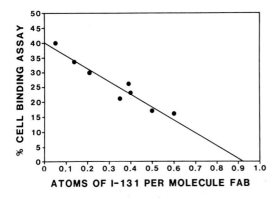

Fig. 2. Effect of I-131 labeling (chloramine-T) of anti-p97 Fab on immunoreactivity of the Fab molecule. $R = .97$; $P = < 0.001$

bodies which would not damage the protein [10]. Figure 2 shows the effect of increasing amounts of iodide on the immunoreactivity of a monoclonal antibody that is particularly sensitive to iodination. A test of immunoactivity was developed which assays the percent of the radiolabeled antibody which can still interact with antigen. In this particular example, degradation of immunoactivity begins to be seen at mass amounts of I-131 as low as 0.1 atoms of iodide per molecule of Fab. It is important, whether labeling for diagnosis or therapy, to ensure that the antibody is immunoactive, and thus, in general, labeling reactions must be carried out at relatively low specific activities.

Diagnostic Studies

Studies With Radiolabeled Whole Immunoglobulin

In early studies [6], we employed whole immunoglobulin radiolabeled with I-131 to target metastatic deposits in patients with disseminated malignant melanoma. For lesions greater than $1.5-2$ cm in diameter, about 85% were detected. This was in a study population which had been carefully screened to ensure the presence of reactive antigen on tumors. The 15% of metastases that were not seen had in general a position near a large vascular structure, which made it difficult to detect the presence of a nearby metastatic deposit (an example of one of our early studies is shown in Fig. 3). The patient had a metastatic melanoma to the right popliteal fossa. The lesion was bulky, about $2-3$ cm in diameter. The lesion is easily visualized as an accumulation of radioactivity in the region of the popliteal fossa. The image on the left in Fig. 3 shows the uncorrected scintiphoto, with the bulk of radioactivity in the tumor bed on the right knee. For comparison, an image was also taken of the popliteal fossa on the left. The major blood vessel in the left leg can be seen, but there is no focal accumulation evident in the popliteal on the left. A background subtracted image is shown on the right. This technique has the advantage of subtracting away radioactivity which is in the extracellular fluid surrounding the tumor and in the great vessels.

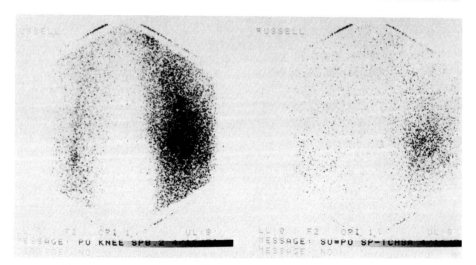

Fig. 3. Posterior scintigram of the popliteal fossa. In the right popliteal fossa, uptake is seen in metastatic melanoma. The scintigram was obtained 48 h after injection. The image on the *left* is unprocessed, and the image on the *right* has been subjected to a background subtraction technique to reduce the amount of blood pool activity

Although the sensitivity and specificity of the technique using I-131 whole immunoglobulin were acceptable, there were a number of disadvantages observed in this study. In the first place, a rather long time was required before sufficient radioactivity had been cleared from the blood pool to permit optimum imaging of tumor deposits. In addition, the whole immunoglobulin was quite immunogenic, and over 50% of patients developed human antimouse antibody response after a single injection. This immunogenic property of the mouse protein made repeat studies impossible.

Studies with Fab Fragments of Antimelanoma Antibody

Initial studies were performed with Fab fragments prepared from the anti-p97 antibody 96.5, and IgG2a, and 8.2, and IgG1. These two Fab preparations were approximately comparable in their ability to target tumor in vivo. Initial studies performed in nude mice [18] demonstrated the greater targeting of the immune Fab relative to a nonspecific Fab than was achieved with whole IgG. In selected patients, a similar proportion of metastases were seen − about 80% − 85% − [9]. I-123-labeled Fab fragments showed exceptionally good qualities for tomographic imaging [7]. In addition, it was observed that the amount of immune protein administered markedly altered the biodistribution of the immune protein. In general, larger mass amounts of antibody improved the targeting to tumor and shifted the activity away from liver. In a series of patients with skin nodules, the amount of specific localization to the tumor of an I-131 labelled, anti-p97 Fab, was shown to be proportional to the concentration of antigen in the tumor as measured by a radioimmunoassay [9].

Clinical studies were also performed with I-131 labeled Fab against the chondroitin sulfate proteoglycan or high molecular weight antigen of human melanoma. The sensitivity and specificity of this technique were approximately the same as for the previous immune preparations, except that the spectrum of cross-reactivity was different. In all of the studies, patients were preselected for the presence of either the high molecular weight or the p97 antigen, and the appropriate antibody was used in the clinical study [17].

In a group of five patients, a comparison was made between the biodistribution and plasma clearance of 8.2, a Fab fragment specific for the p97 antigen, and 1.4, a Fab fragment of the same subclass, but which was not reactive against any human antigen. This antibody reacts against a murine leukemia virus. The blood clearance of the two immune preparations was markedly different. The p97 specific antibody had an initial rapid phase of clearance, where approximately 40%−50% of the radioactivity was cleared from blood within the first 10 min after intravenous administration. On the other hand, 1.4 had a much smaller component that was rapidly cleared, and both Fabs had a longer component of clearance, with a half-time of about 83 min. It was also of interest to observe the percent of immunoactive 8.2 that was present in the blood as a function of time after intravenous administration. The average immunoreactivity of these five preparations was about 50%. Immediately after administering the antibody, there was a very rapid clearance of the immunoactive portion from the plasma. By 2 h after injection, less than 5% of the I-131 activity in plasma was immunoactive.

Figure 4 shows a comparison of the distribution of the Fab fragments in the region of the upper abdomen. I-131 Fab 96.5 is an anti-p97 Fab. This prep-

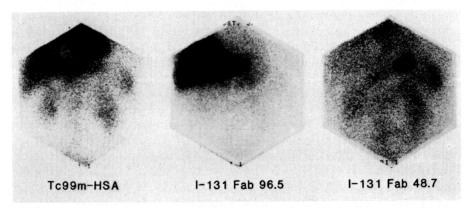

Tc99m-HSA   **I-131 Fab 96.5**   **I-131 Fab 48.7**

Fig. 4. Anterior projections of the upper abdomen in a patient with local recurrence of metastatic melanoma in supraclavicular lymph node, but with no known metastases elsewhere. The patient had comparison gamma camera images of the upper abdomen, obtained with I-131 Fab 96.5 (anti-p97) (*middle panel*), and 48.7 (anti-high molecular weight antigen) (*right panel*), with imaging performed 48 h after injection. In the *left panel*, an image of the same anatomic region is shown after ^{99m}Tc human serum albumin was given intravenously (5 mg) in order to image the location of blood pool of heart, liver, kidney, and spleen. There is a marked difference between the distribution of the anti-p97 Fab and the anti-high molecular weight Fab. The anti-p97 Fab is localized and retained in liver, whereas the high molecular weight Fab is not

aration is rapidly cleared in the liver and, in fact, the liver uptake accounts for the early rapid clearance which was seen on the plasma curves. There is prolonged retention of the radioactivity in the normal liver, so that by 48 h considerable persistent activity is seen. On the other hand, I-131 Fab 48.7 is the anti-high molecular weight preparation which was used in the clinical study reported [17]. In contrast to the anti-p97 preparations, the anti-high molecular weight Fab does not concentrate readily in liver, and instead is rapidly cleared from the body. It is an important general principle of use of these immune preparations that each immune protein has its own characteristic biodistribution in vivo.

Alternative Radiolabeling Methods

Each radionuclide, when used as a label for an immune protein, is more or less suitable as a label for tracing the biodistribution intact antibody in vivo. In the first incidence, as we have seen, radiolabeling methods themselves may disrupt the immunoactivity of the antibody. In addition to disrupting immunoactivity, the labeling procedure may alter the biologic behavior of the radiolabeled antibody radioisotope conjugate. This is particularly a problem for indium labeled antibodies, which increase the targeting of the antibody to the liver. Finally, the metabolism of the radiolabel itself will determine the final biodistribution of radioactivity within the body. For example, I-131 is subjected to deiodination and once cleaved from the immune protein, is distributed throughout the extracellular fluid, being concentrated by the glandular structures such as thyroid, salivary glands, and stomach, and ultimately excreted by the kidneys. The breakdown of such proteins is approx. 10% − 15% of the radioactivity per day. On the other hand, radioactive metals, such as indium-111 are also subjected to metabolism, and in this case, there is frequently a translocation of the radiolabeled metal from the immune protein to transferrin. Subsequently, the transferrin is metabolized with localization of the radiometal into marrow, and renal excretion is minimal. In some cases with indium-111, excretion into the gut may be observed.

Halpern and his associates [19] have championed use of indium-111 for protein labeling. In comparison to I-131, indium-111 is retained longer in the tissues which concentrate the antibody, both in the tumor and other sites such as liver. Figure 5 shows an image of indium-111 labeled 96.5 in the region of the chest. There is considerable localization in axillary and right superclavicular and infraclavicular lymph node chains. Notice also the large amount of concentration of indium-111 in liver. This is the major problem with the use of indium-111 as a label for antibodies, since detection of tumor localization in liver is virtually impossible because of the large background from "nonspecific" targeting of indium antibodies to this organ. Figure 6 shows an indium-111 scan in the same patient, clearly demonstrating a previously unsuspected cerebral metastasis. Note also the localization in cervical lymph nodes.

Indium-111-96.5 (an anti-p97 antibody), has shown considerable promise in clinical studies as an adjunct to Ga-67 citrate imaging for localization of malig-

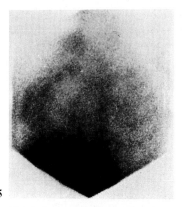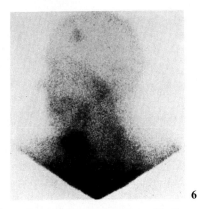

5   6

Fig. 5. Image of the anterior chest, of a patient after intravenous injection of indium-111 anti-p97 IgG. There is dense uptake in the liver (*6 o'clock*), and uptake along the right lateral chest in lymph nodes of the axilla, infraclavicular, and right supraclavicular nodes

Fig. 6. Indium-111 anti-p97 IgG from the same patient as in Fig. 5. There is uptake in a previously unsuspected brain metastasis of melanoma. The metastatic melanoma deposit was confirmed by Ct

nant melanoma and metastases. In a study reported by Neumann et al. [20], over 90% of malignant melanoma metastases were detected by a combination of Ga-67 citrate and indium-111 anti-p97 imaging. Each radiopharmaceutical, when used separately in this population, detected only 67% of the lesions.

This interesting finding suggests a possible biological link between the uptake of Ga-67 citrate uptake and the localization of indium-111 anti-p97. It is known that p97 is a transferrin-like substance on the membrane of melanoma. It is also known that the iron can be bound to the p97 molecule. It may be that the presence of the p97 protein in the membrane has something to do with the iron economy of trace metal metabolism by the tumor cells. Ga-67 citrate appears to be concentrated in tumor via the Ga-67 transferrin intermediate with the aid of a transferrin receptor. The reciprocal nature of uptake in these two populations suggests the possibility that in some tumor types there may be a sparing of the need for transferrin receptor utilization and p97 may be the means through which this is achieved. Of course this is pure speculation, but it is based on the interesting point that the tumor-specific protein p97 does have a biologic function; namely, iron binding, although its overall importance to the trace metal metabolism of the tumor cell is not known.

Studies using the IgG, indium-111 labeled 9.2.27, an anti-high molecular weight antibody, were performed to determine the effect of dose on localization of metastases [21]. There was a great improvement in the percent of metastases detected between the 1-mg dose, and the 50- or 100-mg dose.

Two of five patients receiving 1 mg of 9.2.27 had two of eight known sites which were scanned positive. All four patients receiving greater or equal to 50 mg had positive scans in 19 of 22 known sites (χ^2, $P < 0.005$). It was noted that patients receiving the greater or equal to 50-mg dose level had less "nonspecific" organ uptake, principally liver. A more prolonged plasma retention was seen at higher doses with 14% in plasma at 24 h at 50 mg or greater and only 14% at 24 h at the lower dose.

Preliminary Radiotherapy Studies

In some patients studied with I-131 Fab, there was sufficient concentration of radioactivity in the tumor so that larger amounts of radioactivity could be considered for therapy purposes. These studies are very preliminary, but it is clear that with the I-131 Fab preparations, repeated targeting of large doses of I-131 are possible to metastatic tumor deposits in patients with metastatic melanoma. Our most successful strategy has been to use patients who are heavily selected, first, by the presence of a large amount of reactive antigen in their tumors, and second, by demonstrating on a diagnostic level study, considerable concentration in their tumor.

In a preliminary study of 10 patients, up to five repeated doses of I-131 Fab preparations could be given with minimal toxicity. Patients received single doses for therapy, ranging up to 342 mCu, without life-threatening toxicity. Two of three patients treated with more than 400 mCu of antimelanoma Fab showed an effect from the treatment. One patient had a prolonged stabilization of disease (6 months), while the second patient had a partial regression of tumor. Estimates based on thyroid probe counts of superficial lesions suggested that uptake was sufficient to give Rad dose exposures in the range of $5-12\,000$ Rads. Toxicity was observed at the largest dose, with a nadir in hematopoetic function at 1 month following treatment.

We have concluded from our studies that although both technical and biologic problems remain, the use of radiolabeled antibodies that are directed against tumor-associated antigens holds future promise in a new therapeutic approach to solid tumors resistant to conventional treatment [16]. Preliminary studies with two separate antigen antibody systems for malignant melanoma indicate that this technique holds promise for both diagnosis and therapy. Some factors important to the in vivo localization of radiolabeled antibody are:

1. Mass amount of antibody administered (AB dose)
2. Type of antibody fragment (i.e., whole IgG, Fab, Fab', $(Fab')_2$)
3. Heterogeneity/concentration of antigen expression on tumor sites
4. Presence of nontumor reservoir of antigen
5. Metabolism/excretion of radiolabeled antibody
6. Route of antibody administration

It seems clear that the large number of anti-tumor antibodies which can be used in clinical studies, and the exquisite specificity of some of these agents for interacting with tumor specific antigens, will ultimately provide excellent reagents for the study of a large number of human tumors.

Summary

Several antitumor antibodies have been developed against two tumor-associated antigens of human melanoma. The first antigen, p97, is a 97,000 molecular weight glycoprotein on the surface of melanoma tumor cells. The second antigen, the chondroitin sulfate proteoglycan antigen or high molecular weight antigen, is a complex antigen, also on the surface of melanoma tumor cells. We have used both whole immunoglobulin and Fab fragments directed against these antigens to target tumors in vivo in patients. We have found that there is an improved detection rate for metastases, with increased mass amounts of the Fab or whole immunoglobulin preparation. We have also shown that Fab fragments, for the anti-p97 and the anti-high molecular weight antigen systems, show more effective ratios between tumor to normal tissue than the corresponding whole immunoglobulin preparation. The uptake in the tumor, and the clearance from nontumor-bearing tissues is also more rapid, so that for at least some applications the Fab preparations are preferred over the whole immunoglobulin preparations. ^{111}In 9.2.27, a whole IgG, directed against the high molecular weight antigen showed good sensitivity (85%) and specificity (95%) for nonhepatic sites of metastases, particularly with large mass mounts of antibody (50 mg per patient). Liver metastases were obscured by nonspecific uptake in hepatic parenchyma, however. In preliminary clinical trials with both anti-p97 and anti-high molecular weight Fab, labeled with I-131, the sensitivity of the technique for individual metastatic sites was 80% − 85%, with specificity that approached 100%. In some patients, localization was sufficiently intense to serve as a rationale for therapeutic trials using greater than 100 mCu doses of I-131 antimelanoma Fab. These therapeutic trials are currently underway.

References

1. Mastrangelo MJ, Rosenberg SA, Baker AR et al. (1982) Cutaneous melanoma in cancer. Principles and practice of oncology. In: De Vita VT Jr, Hellman S, Rosenberg SA (eds) Lippincott, Philadelphia, p 1137
2. Köhler G, Milstein C (1975) Continuous culture of fused cells secreting antibody of predefined specificity. Nature 256:495 − 497
3. Brown JP, Nishiyama K, Hellström I, Hellström KE (1981) Structural characterization of human melanoma associated antigen p97 using monoclonal antibodies. J Immunol 127:539 − 546
4. Woodberry RJ, Brown JP, Yeh M-Y, Hellström I, Hellström KE (1981) Identification of a cell surface protein, p97 in human melanomas and certain other neoplasms. Proc Natl Acad Sci USA 77:2183 − 2186
5. Hellstrom I, Garrigues HJ, Cabasco L et al. (1983) Studies of a high molecular weight human melanoma-associated antigen. J Immunol 130:1467 − 1472
6. Larson SM, Brown JP, Wright PW et al. (1983) Imaging of melanoma with I-131-labeled monoclonal antibodies. J Nucl Med 24:132 − 139
7. Larson SM, Carrasquillo JA, Krohn KA et al. (1983) Diagnostic imaging of malignant melanoma with radiolabeled anti-tumor antibodies. JAMA 249:811 − 812
8. Larson SM, Carrasquillo JA, Krohn KA (1982) Radiotherapy with "anti-p97" iodinated monoclonal antibodies in melanoma. In: Raynaud C (ed) Proceedings of the 3rd World Congress of Nuclear Medicine and Biology, August−September, 1982, Paris, vol IV. Pergamon, New York, pp 3666 − 3669

9. Larson SM, Carrasquillo JA, Krohn KA et al. (1983) Localization of ^{131}I-labeled p97-specific Fab fragments in human melanoma as a basis for radiotheapy. J Clin Immunol 72:1201−1221
10. Ferens JM, Krohn KA, Beaumier PL et al. (1984) High-level iodination of monoclonal antibody fragments for radiotherapy. J Nucl Med 25:367−370
11. Hellström I, Hellström KE, Brown JP et al. (1983) Monoclonal antibodies to human melanoma antigens − possible clinical applications. Clin Immunol Newsletter 8:71−74
12. Larson SM, Carrasquillo JA (1983) Nuclear oncology: Current perspectives. In: Freeman LM, Weissman HS (eds) Nuclear Medicine Annual. Raven, New York, pp 167−198
13. Larson SM, Carrasquillo JA (1984) Nuclear oncology 1984. Semin Nucl Med XIV:268−276
14. Carrasquillo JA, Larson SM, Hellström KE et al. (1983) Radioimmuno-detection of tumor melanoma with monoclonal antibodies and Fab fragments. In: Burchiel SW, Roades BA (eds) Radioimmunoimaging and Radioimmunotherapy. Elsevier, New York, pp 357−368
15. Larson SM, Carrasquillo JA (1984) Role of labelled antibodies in tumor detection and possible treatment. Curr Concepts Diagn Nucl Med 1:13−16
16. Carrasquillo JA, Krohn KA, Beaumier PL et al. (1984) Diagnosis and treatment of solid tumors with radiolabelled antibodies and immune fragments. Cancer Treat Rep 68:1984
17. Larson SM, Carrasquillo JA, McGuffin RW et al. (1985) Preliminary clinical experience using an I-131 labeled murine Fab against a high molecular weight antigen of human melanoma. Radiology 155:487−492
18. Beaumier PL, Carrasquillo JA, Krohn KA et al. (1985) Localization of I-125 anti-p97 monoclonal Fab fragments in nude mice implanted with human melanoma xenografts. J Nucl Med 26:1172−1179
19. Halpern SE, Hagen PL, Carver PR, Cosial JA, Chen AWN, Franke JM, Bartholomew RM, Davis GS, Adams TH (1983) Stability characterization and kinetics of indium-111 labeled monoclonal antitumor antibodies in normal animals and nude mice. Human tumor models. Cancer Res 43:5347−5355
20. Neumann RD, Kirkwood JM, Zoghbi SS et al. (1985) Ga-67 vs In-111-DTPA-anti-p97 monoclonal antibody (MoAb) for scintigraphic detection of metastatic melanoma. J Nucl Med 26:15
21. Carrasquillo JA, Abrams PG, Schroff RW, Keenan AM et al. (1985) Improved Imaging of metastatic melanoma with high dose 9.2.27 In-111 monoclonal antibody. J Nucl Med 26:67

Radioimmunoscintigraphy of CA 19-9/CEA Producing Tumors Using I-131 Labeled F(ab')₂ Fragments of Monoclonal Antibodies (19-9/Anti-CEA Radioimmunococktail)

R. P. BAUM[1], F. D. MAUL, R. SENEKOWITSCH, M. LORENZ, C. HOTTENROTT, J. HAPP, R. STANDKE, J. F. CHATAL, J. C. SACCAVINI, H. KRIEGEL, and G. HÖR

Recently, monoclonal antibody techniques have provided an opportunity to reevaluate the role of nuclear medicine for the diagnosis of malignant diseases by using the immunological approach. The pioneering studies of Köhler and Milstein [1] made it possible to prepare in vitro immortal cell lines by means of the chemically mediated fusion of lymphocytes from immunized mice and cells from a mouse myeloma tumor. Cloned hybrid cells produce individual monoclonal antibodies in a continuous and virtually endless supply with extremely precise specificity and uniform reaction. To obtain greater specificity in the interpretation of neoplastic masses by in vivo methods, the immunological approach appears to be most promising. About 90 years ago the first attempt to use antibodies produced against malignant tissues was reported by Hericourt and Richet [2]. They prepared antiserum against human osteogenic sarcoma and observed that these sera were effective in the treatment of a fibrosarcoma and a gastric cancer.

That antibodies are the carriers of immunity was discovered 95 years ago by von Behring [3]. Jerne developed the Jerne Plaque Test in 1963, which made it possible to analyze a single antibody-producing cell in vitro [4]. Edelman [5] and Porter [6] − also Nobel Price laureates − performed excellent studies resulting in the discovery of the antibody structure. Pressman and Keighley [7] using I-131 first reported on successful localization of labeled antibodies (without changing their affinity) in the rat kidneys in vivo. As early as 1954, Korngold [8] showed that antibodies labeled with radioactive iodine could be used in animals on a diagnostic basis and that the location of the tumor containing the sequestered antibodies could be defined by means of radionuclide imaging. Later Bale et al. [9] demonstrated that tumor-localizing antibodies could be used as a therapeutic agent for treating experimental neoplasms by means of the radioactivity.

Most of the studies performed with polyclonal antibodies showed preferential uptake of the labeled antibody in nontumor tissue, including the lungs, liver, spleen, and kidneys in addition to tumor localization. In some instances, even more activity was located within nontumor structure than in tumors. Tumor to blood ratios of labeled antibody derived from percent injected activity

---

1 Zentrum der Radiologie und Chirurgie, Klinikum der Johann-Wolfgang-Goethe-Universität, Theodor-Stern-Kai 7, D-6000 Frankfurt am Main 70

Nuclear Medicine in Clinical Oncology
Ed. by C. Winkler
© Springer-Verlag Berlin Heidelberg 1986

per gram tissue resulted in considerable variability. Certainly, success in detecting and treating tumors with radiolabeled antibodies depends on a sufficiently high tumor to nontumor target ratio. The reproducibility of the results obtained with polyclonal antibodies, however, was limited by the fact that the antibodies used were directed against poorly defined tumor antigens.

The identification of the carcinoembryonic antigen by Gold and Freedman [10], offered the possibility of using the antigen as target for tumor localization of radiolabeled antibodies against the carcinoembryonic antigen (CEA). Mach et al. [11] and independently Goldenberg et al. [12, 13] and Hoffer et al. [14] showed that anti-CEA antibodies were capable of specific localization in vivo within CEA-containing tumors and that the radiolabeled antibodies were detectable on external scanning in animals bearing xenografts of human carcinomas. Later [15], purified I-131 labeled goat antibodies against CEA were injected into patients with carcinoma, and tumor detection with external photoscanning was reported as well as specific antibody accumulation in the tumor, first by Goldenberg et al. [16] in 1978. In their initial series of 18 patients they reported that scanning performed 48 h after injection detected almost all the CEA-producing cancers and gave no false positive results in patients without demonstrable tumor or in patients with tumors apparently devoid of CEA. In contrast, Mach et al. [15] obtained positive scans in only 11 out of 27 patients (41%) with CEA-producing tumors after injecting highly purified goat anti-CEA antibodies, even when including computerized subtraction of bloodpool and secreted radioactivity as detected after injection of Tc-99m-HSA and Tc-99-pertechnetate. By the paired labeling method (simultaneous injection of I-131 labeled goat anti-CEA and I-125 labeled normal goat IgG) it was demonstrated that the specific uptake of antibodies in tumors was up to 5 times higher than that of control normal IgG. However, at the same time the measurement of radioactivity in tumors showed that only a very small amount $(0.5-2.0\,\mu\text{Ci})$ of the injected antibody radioactivity $(1000\,\mu\text{Ci})$ was recovered in the whole tumor $3-8$ days after injection. In a later study using affinity-purified goat CEA antibodies or their fragments, Mach et al. [17] had positive scans in only 42% (out of a series of 35 patients with CEA-producing tumors). The conclusion from this study was that this method of tumor detection was not yet clinically useful and that radioimmunoscintigraphy could not be recommended as a routine clinical test [15].

The identification of a new tumor-specific antibody by Koprowski and his group [18, 19] — designated 19-9 which recognized a monosialoganglioside [20] that is shed into the circulation where it can be detected in radioimmunometric assay [21] — opened a new field for radioimmunodetection of gastrointestinal carcinomas. Another antibody, designated 17-1 A, recognizing an as yet undefined antigen that is not shed into the circulation by tumor cells, is also capable of inhibiting tumor growth [22]. Chatal and his colleagues administered these antibodies or their $F\,(ab')_2$ fragments to 90 cancer patients [23] and succeeded in detecting colorectal cancer sites in 59% (17-1 A), 66% (19-9) and 77% (17-1 A + 19-9, or anti-CEA + 19-9).

We report on our first results by means of radioimmunodetection of CEA and CA 19-9 producing tumors using a cocktail of $F\,(ab')_2$ fragments of monoclonal antibodies to CA 19-9 and CEA labeled with I-131. Up to now we examined more than 90 patients. This report contains results of the first 40 patients. The aim of this study (performed retrospectively in most of the cases) was, to evaluate the role (in terms of sensitivity and specificity) of immunoscintigraphy in patients with colorectal and other cancers for diagnosis of local recurrences and metastatic disease.

Patients and Methods

Each patient was extensively informed and gave signed consent before the examination was started. Data on the number, age, and sex of the patients are given in Table 1, and the diagnoses are listed in Table 2.

Tumor markers in vitro were determined just before immunoscintigraphy started. The serum CA 19-9 concentration was measured with a radioimmunometric assay using monoclonal antibodies (ID-CIS Centocor kit, cutoff 37 U/ml). CEA was determined in serum with a commercial RIA kit (ID-CIS, Dreieich, FRG, cutoff 10 ng/ml).

All 40 patients received intra-arterial chemotherapy via an subcutaneously implanted drug infusion pump through the hepatic artery because of metastases to the liver from adenocarcinomas of the colon or on account of other primary tumors.

Potassium iodide (Kalium jodatum Compretten 0.1, Cascan, FRG) was administered (100−200 mg, 3 times daily) 2 days prior to the injection and continued for 14 days to prevent free I-131 uptake by the thyroid. Alternatively, perchlorate (Irenat) was administered (90−120 drops) 60 min before the injection and 30 drops 3 times daily for 10−14 days, in all patients in whom the thyroid had not been blocked adequately by potassium iodide.

Table 1. Patient data

Number of patients		Age	Sex
Total	40	13 − 81 years	$\delta = 22$
			$\varphi = 18$
Prospective study	20		
Retrospective study	20		

Table 2. Primary tumor

Colorectal carcinoma	30
Breast cancer	3
Pancreatic cancer	2
Pheochromocytoma	1
Carcinoid	1
Hepatocellular carcinoma	3

Antibodies. F (ab')$_2$ fragments (mol. wt. 100,000) of monoclonal antibodies to CA 19-9 (IgG1, affinity 3×10^7, 1 mg/ml) and CEA (IgG1, affinity 1.1×10^9, 1 mg/ml) labeled with I-131 (specific activity: 55.5 MBq/mg) by the iodogen method (yield of incorporation: 91% [CA 19-9] or 78% [CEA]) with proven proteinic purity (HPLC with a TSK 300 column) and an immunoreactivity of about 85% (CA 19-9) and 77% (CEA), after biological controls (sterility, pyrogens, abnormal toxicity, virus testing) were kindly provided by ID-CIS, Dreieich, FRG). The antibodies were received frozen (in dried ice) and first slowly defrosted (2 h).

An activity of 30−123 MBq (mean: 61 MBq) was injected intravenously during 30 min (as proposed by Chatal) in 50−100 ml saline solution (0.9 NaCl) via an infusion pump (0.5−1 mg of each antibody). Neither antihistaminic drugs nor corticosteroids were used (except for 1 patient).

Scintiscans in planar technique were recorded (Searle LFOV gamma camera interfaced to an Informatek Simis 3 [Sophia Medical data processing system]) 3, 5 and in some patients 7, 10, 14 and up to 20 days after the injection of the I-131 labeled antibodies. Anterior, lateral, and posterior view of the liver as well as posterior view of the pelvis were obtained in each patient as an I-131 antibody image. In some special patients we performed immunoscans of the lung (anterior and posterior views), and of the head (anterior and lateral view). Pinhole images (Picker 4/11 gamma camera, interfaced to Informatek Simis 3) were also done in several patients.

37 MB9 Tc-99m colloid (Nanocoll, Solco) were injected at D5 and later for *anatomical landmarking* of the liver, spleen, and bone marrow simultaneously, providing the opportunity of drawing regions of interest (isocontours) around the liver, spleen, and bone marrow (Fig. 1). Tc-99m-DTPA (100−150 MBq) for anatomical imaging of the kidneys and the urinary bladder (Fig. 2) were helpful in some patients for better localization of local recurrences, which is not necessary if Nanocoll is used. Gamma camera and the patient's position were unchanged so that Tc isocontours could be superimposed electronically to the I-131 antibody image. Thus we were able to localize exactly the malignant process with the double-nuclide double-compound Tc-99m I-131 scans. Acquisition time for immunoscans was 10−40 min (in most of the cases 10−15 min),

---→

Fig. 1. Anatomical landmarking: isocontour around liver and spleen (derived from the Tc-colloid scan) and multiple liver metastases (confirmed surgically) as seen by immunoscan (19-9/anti-CEA cocktail)

Fig. 2. Anatomical landmarks of the urinary bladder and the kidney (Tc-99m-DTPA radionuclide urogram)

Fig. 3. Immunoscintigraphy (D7 post inject., unprocessed image). Local recurrence of a rectal adenocarcinoma (confirmed 8 months later by surgery, not seen by CT scan)

Fig. 4. Immunoscan (D3 post inject., processed image, isocontour technique). Primary tumor (colon sigmoideum) and intraabdominal metastasis (both confirmed surgically)

Fig. 5. Immunoscan (D7 post inject., subtraction technique): Bone marrow metastasis (thoracic column) of an adenocarcinoma of the colon

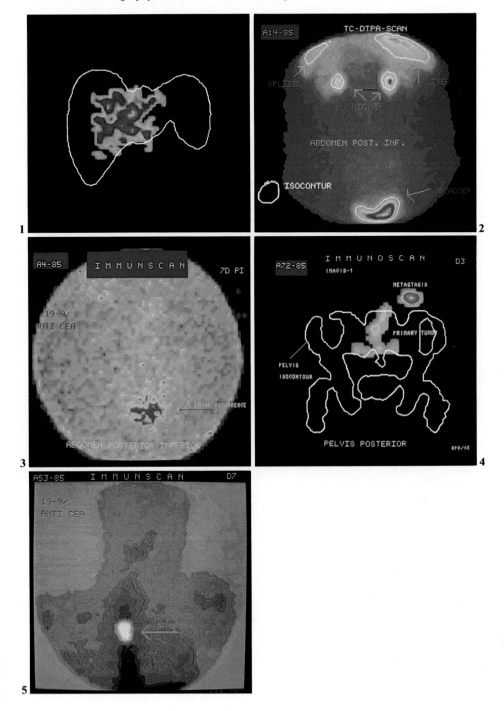

for Tc-scans 3 – 5 min. The nuclear medicine diagnosis was derived from the unprocessed I-131 images, and the findings were confirmed either by surgery/biopsy or by computed tomography (CT) and ultrasonography (US) and the clinical follow up for 6 months.

Results

In 40 patients suspected or proven to have a primary tumor, recurrence, or metastatic disease, immunoscintigraphy was positive in 36 out of the 40 patients (90%). A total of 54 tumor sites were visualized: 4 local pelvic recurrences (Fig. 3), 32 liver metastases (Fig. 1), 15 abdominal sites (Figs. 4 and 5) remote from the primary site, and 3 primary tumors (Fig. 4). The tumor size ranged from smaller than 1 cm (peritoneal carcinosis) to greater than 10 cm (liver metastasis) in diameter.

As the lung and the head were not studied systematically in all of the patients, they were excluded from the following analysis. CA 19-9 levels in serum were elevated in 19, CEA serum levels in 32 of the patients. Both tumor markers were increased in 19 patients. Normal CA 19-9/CEA concentration in serum was found in eight patients at the time of investigation.

The criteria for a positive or a false negative finding were:

Surgery performed in 31 of the patients
Confirmation by other diagnostic procedures (CT, US, X-ray, biopsy with histological examination) ($n = 9$).

The diagnosis were judged as true negative if:

Surgery could not find any tumor, *or*
CT, US (and other diagnostic approaches) were not able to detect any tumor and the clinical follow up for 6 months showed no evidence of recurrence or metastatic disease.

The criteria for a false positive finding in 1 patient was surgery. All doubtful cases were classified as negative. The results in terms of sensitivity and specificity are listed in Table 3.

Table 3. Immunoscintigraphy in patients receiving continuous hepatic artery infusion chemotherapy using 19-9/anti-CEA radioimmunococktail ($n = 40$[a])

Sensitivity	93%
Specificity	97%
Positive predictive value	96%
Negative predictive value	94%

[a] controlled by surgery ($n = 31$), CT/ultrasonography/biopsy. Follow-up 6 months

Discussion

High sensitivity and high specificity are prerequisites aimed at when using an "ideal" procedure for the diagnosis, staging, and follow up of primary tumors and their recurrences especially in colorectal cancer disease. Most of the diagnostic methods currently used for the detection of neoplastic masses provide indirect evidence (for example US and CT). To obtain greater specificity in the interpretation of neoplasias by in vivo methods, the immunological approach appears to be most promising. Two problems that interfered with progress in this field were the lack of tumor specific antigens and the lack of well-defined and reproducible antibodies. To improve the sensitivity and specificity of immunoscintigraphy as a technique for tumor localization 3 ways are reasonable:

The use of monoclonal antibodies
The use of fragments of antibodies
The use of single photon emission computerized tomography (SPECT)

The obvious advantages of *monoclonal* antibodies are their homogeneity, their specificity for the immunizing antigen, and the reaction with a single determinant − thus no large immunocomplexes with antigen are formed [24].

In radioimmunoimaging studies using a murine monoclonal antibody to CEA in a human colon carcinoma xenografted into hamsters, *F (ab')₂ fragments* were shown superior to F (ab) fragments and intact antibody. In double-label experiments with anti-CEA antibody and control monoclonal IgG, F (ab')₂ fragments were found to allow for better and more rapid specific tumor localization than intact antibody or F (ab) fragments. Thus F (ab')₂ fragments offer significant promise for tumor imaging and possible therapy [25].

As we have shown in previous studies in vitro [26−28], CEA and CA 19-9 are complementary in the diagnosis of recurrences of colorectal adenocarcinoma, and simultaneous determination of these tumor markers can increase the sensitivity. On the other hand, immunohistochemical studies showed positive staining of tumor cells for either CA 19-9 of CEA or both in some patients though the tumor markers in serum were normal [29]. We therefore used the *cocktail* of monoclonal antibodies for detecting recurrences. It remains to be proved, whether *SPECT* is capable of further improving the sensitivity without considerable loss of specificity. Previous studies by Berche [30] favour this assumption, since these authors concluded that "tumorscintigraphy showed tumors as small as a few cm³." On the other hand, the same group reported that − cutting out a piece of tumor tissue − they recovered only about 18 nCi/g 5 days after injection. Labeling of monoclonal antibodies with short-lived radionuclides (^{111}In, ^{123}I) should increase the detection level. Some of the problems involved in using these radionuclides are discussed by Larson in this book.

Conclusions

1. The use of *"monoclonals"* is superior to the use of polyclonal antibodies.
2. The use of *fragments* [F (ab')₂] increases the tumor/nontumor ratio [31, 32].

3. A *slow* infusion of the antibodies (as proposed by Chatal) is important to avoid formation of large complexes and accumulation in the spleen and bone marrow.

4. Using *planar* scintigraphic technique 1.5 (or less) to 2 mCi (55.5−75 MBq) of I-131 labeled monoclonal antibodies are sufficient for imaging most of the tumors. Using the SPECT technique, more activity might be necessary and useful.

5. *Late imaging* (later than 5 days after application of the antibodies) is a very important point and increases sensitivity as well as specificity (exclusion of nonspecific iodine accumulation) in the stomach and in the lung (blood-pool effect). A persisting contrast is typical for a malignant process [33, 34].

6. A second tracer technique is essential for tumor localization. These *anatomical landmarks* by the use of a double-nuclide scintigraphy and especially the isocontour technique (first proposed by us for routine use in immunoscintigraphy) are helpful and simplify the procedure *because*

7. Subtraction technique, a possible source of artifacts is no longer necessary when late imaging (beyond day 5) is performed [35].

References

1. Köhler G, Milstein C (1975) Continuous cultures of fused cells secreting antibody of predefined specificity. Nature 256:495
2. Hericourt J, Richet C (1895) Traitment d'un cas de sarcome par la sérotherapie. CR Hebd Seances Acad Sci 120:948
3. Behring v E, Kitasato S (1890) Dtsch Med Wschr 49:1113
4. Jerne NK, Nordin AA (1963) Plaque formation in agar by single antibody-producing cells. Science 140:405
5. Edelmann GM (1973) Antikörperstruktur und molekulare Immunologie. Angew Chem 85:1083
6. Porter RR (1973) Strukturuntersuchungen an Immunglobulinen. Angew Chem 85:1097
7. Pressman D, Keighley G (1948) The zone of activity of antibodies as determined by the use of radioactive tracers; the zone of a activity of nephrotoxic antikidney serum. J Immunol 59:141
8. Korngold L, Pressman D (1954) The localization of antilymphosarcoma antibodies in the Murphy lymphosarcoma of the rat. Cancer Res 14:96
9. Bale WF, Spar IL, Goodland RL (1960) Experimental radiation therapy of tumor with I-131-carrying antibodies to fibrin. Cancer Res 20:1488
10. Gold P, Freedman SO (1965) Demonstration of tumor specific antigens in human colonic carcinoma by immunological and adsorption technique. J Exp Med 21:439
11. Mach J-P, Carrel S, Merenda C, Sordat B, Cerottoni J-C (1974) In vivo localization of radiolabeled antibodies to carcinoembryonic antigen in human colon carcinoma grafted into nude mice. Nature 248:704
12. Goldenberg DM, Preston DF, Primus FJ, Hansen HJ (1974) Photoscan localization of GW-39 tumors in hamsters using radiolabeled anti-carcinoembryonic antigen immunoglobulin G. Cancer Res 34:1
13. Primus FJ, Wang RH, Goldenberg DM, Hansen HJ (1973) Localization of human GW-39 tumors in hamsters by radiolabeled heterospecific antibody to carcinoembryonic antigen. Cancer Res 33:2977
14. Hoffer PB, Lathrop K, Bekerman G, Fang VS, Refetoff S (1974) Use of ^{131}I-CEA antibody as a tumor scanning agent. J Nucl Med 15:323

15. Mach J-P, Carrell S, Forni M, Ritschard J, Donath A, Alberto P (1980) Tumor localization of radiolabeled antibodies against carcinoembryonic antigen in patients with carcinoma. A critical evaluation. N Engl J Med 303:5

16. Goldenberg DM, DeLand F, Kim EE, Bennett S, Primus FJ, van Nagell JR, Estes N, De Simone P, Rayburn P (1978) Use of radiolabeled antibodies to carcinoembryonic antigen for the detection and localization of diverse cancers by external photoscanning. N Engl J Med 298:1384

17. Mach J-P, Forni M, Ritschard J, Buchegger F, Carrel S, Wildgren S, Donath A, Alberto P (1980) Use and limitations of radiolabeled anti-CEA antibodies and their fragments for photoscanning detection of human colorectal carcinomas. Oncodev Biol Med 1:49

18. Koprowski H, Steplewski Z, Mitchell K, Herlyn M, Herlyn D, Führer P (1979) Colorectal carcinoma antigens detected by hybridoma antibodies. Somatic Cell Genet 5:957

19. Koprowski H, Herlyn M, Steplewski Z, Sears HF (1981) Specific antigen in serum of patients with colon carcinoma. Science 212:53

20. Magnani JL, Brockhaus M, Smith DF, Ginsburg V, Blasczyk M, Mitchell KF, Steplewski Z, Koprowski H (1981) A monosialoganglioside is a monoclonal antibody-defined antigen of colon carcinoma. Science 212:55

21. Del Villano BC, Brennan S, Brock P, Bucher C, Liu V, McClure M, Rake B, Space S, Westrick B, Schoemaker H, Zurawski VR jr (1983) Radioimmunometric assay for a monoclonal antibody-defined tumor marker, CA 19-9. Clin Chem 29:549

22. Herlyn DM, Steplewski Z, Herlyn MF, Koprowski H (1980) Inhibition of growth of colorectal carcinoma in nude mice by monoclonal antibody. Cancer Res 40:717

23. Chatal J-F, Saccavini JC, Fumoleau P, Douillard J-Y, Curtet C, Kremer M, Le Mevel B, Koprowski H (1984) Immunoscintigraphy of colon carcinoma. J Nucl Med 25:307

24. Mach J-P, Buchegger F, Forni M, Ritschard J, Berche C, Lumbroso J-D, Schreyer M, Girardet C, Accolla RS, Carrel S (1981) Use of radiolabelled monoclonal anti-CEA antibodies for the detection of human carcinomas by external photoscanning and tomoscintigraphy. Immunol Today 2:239

25. Wahl LR, Parker CW, Philpott GW (1983) Improved radioimaging and tumor localization with monoclonal F (ab')$_2$. J Nucl Med 24:316

26. Lorenz M, Maul FD, Hottenrott C, Encke A, Happ J (1985) CA 19-9 im Vergleich zu CEA in der Diagnostik gastrointestinaler Tumoren in der Chirurgie. In: Greten H, Klapdor R (eds) Neue tumorassoziierte Antigene − 2 Jahre klinische Erfahrung mit monoklonalen Antikörpern. Thieme, Stuttgart, p 332

27. Lorenz M, Happ J, Reimann-Kirkowa M, Hottenrott C, Maul FD, Encke A, Hör G (1985) CA 19-9 im Vergleich mit CEA in der chirurgischen Primär- und Rezidivdiagnostik. In: Greten H, Klapdor R (eds) Neue tumorassoziierte Antigene − 2 Jahre klinische Erfahrung mit monoklonalen Antikörpern. Thieme, Stuttgart, p 95

28. Lorenz M, Hottenrott C, Happ J, Reimann-Kirkowa M, Maul FD, Encke A, Hör G (1985) CEA und CA 19-9 als Verlaufsparameter bei der intraarteriellen Therapie von Lebermetastasen. In: Greten H, Klapdor R (eds) Neue tumorassoziierte Antigene − 2 Jahre klinische Erfahrung mit monoklonalen Antikörpern. Thieme, Stuttgart, p 112

29. Mach J-P (1985) Personal communication

30. Berche C, Mach JP, Lumbroso JD, Langlais C, Aubry F, Buchegger F, Carrel S, Rougier P, Parmentier C, Tubiana M (1982) Tomoscintigraphy for detecting gastrointestinal and medullary thyroid cancers: first clinical results using radiolabelled monoclonal antibodies against carcinoembryonic antigen. Brit Med J 285:1447

31. Senekowitsch R, Maul FD, Wenisch HJC, Kriegel H, Hör G (1985) Immunoscintigraphy of human pancreatic carcinoma in nude mice with I-131-F (ab')$_2$-fragments of monoclonal antibodies. J Nucl Med 26:P110

32. Senekowitsch R, Maul FD, Baum RP, Wenisch HJC, Schneidereit M, Moellenstaedt S, Kriegel H, Hör G (1985) Radioimmunoscintigraphy and immunohistochemical detection of different antigens in human pancreatic carcinoma xenografts with monoclonal antibodies. European Nuclear Medicine Congress, London (in press)

33. Baum RP, Maul FD, Lorenz M, Hottenrott C, Senekowitsch R, Happ J, Brandhorst I, Reimann-Kirkowa M, Encke A, Hör G (1985) Immunoscintigraphy with anti-CA 19-9/CEA

monoclonal antibodies: follow-up of liver metastases (colonic cancer) before/after regional intraarterial treatment. Nucl Med Commun 6:597

34. Baum RP, Maul FD, Klapdor R, Senekowitsch R, Lorenz M, Hottenrott C, Montz R, Happ J, Kriegel H, Chatal JF, Hör G (1985) Immunszintigraphie kolorektaler Tumoren mit ^{131}J-markierten monoklonalen Antikörpern (19-9/Anti-CEA): Erste Ergebnisse. Nuc Compact 16:121

35. Chatal J-F, Fumoleau P, Kremer M (1985) Complementary roles of immunoscintigraphy and ultrasonography. Eur J Nucl Med 10:464

Radioimmunodetection of Malignant Melanoma with Radiolabelled (^{131}I, ^{123}I, ^{111}In, ^{99m}Tc) Monoclonal Antibodies and F(ab')$_2$ Fragments

G. L. Buraggi[1] L. Callegaro, N. Cascinelli, S. Ferrone, A. Turrin,
A. Attili, E. Bombardieri, M. Gasparini, G. Deleide, G. A. Scassellati,
and E. Seregni

Introduction

Several research projects involving the production, the characterization and the utilization in clinical oncology of monoclonal antibodies (MoAb) to tumor-associated antigens expressed by different tumors, are currently in progress at the Istituto Nazionale Tumori of Milan (Italy). After the significant results obtained with immunoscintigraphy by Goldenberg et al. [1], Mach et al. [2], and Larson et al. [3], our group adopted this new approach to tumor imaging as a priority research field.

Our experience with the radioimmunoimaging of malignant melanomas is based on the use of monoclonal antibody 225.28S against a high-molecular-weight melanoma-associated antigen (HMW-MAA) with a restricted tissue distribution, which is expressed from more than 90% of melanomas [4]. This antibody, an IgG$_{2a}$, was isolated and characterized by Ferrone, Natali and others [5]. It was shown that the antibody localizes human melanomas transplanted in nude mice.

In early 1982, a pilot study was begun to investigate the potential applications of MoAb 225.28S in humans and to improve the technical methodology of tumor imaging [6–9]. A further step in our research involved applying the optimized technology to a large series of patients from several Italian and European nuclear medicine centers. The aim of the extensive study was to confirm our results and to compare different experiences. At present, a new ongoing project aims at evaluating the clinical usefulness of melanoma imaging in the management of patients bearing melanoma.

Materials and Methods

The anti-HMW-MAA MoAB 225.28S was purified from ascitic fluid and F(ab')$_2$ fragments were generated by digestion of purified IgG using pepsin. F(ab')$_2$ fragments were separated from undigested IgG and other digestion products by Sephadex G200 SF chromatography. The pool containing F(ab')$_2$ fragments was applied to a Protein A Sepharose CL6B column. The yield of F(ab')$_2$ fragments was 1 mg F(ab')$_2$/10 mg intact IgG.

---

1 Istituto Nazionale per lo Studio e la Cura dei Tumori, Via Venezian 1, I-20133 Milano

Nuclear Medicine in Clinical Oncology
Ed. by C. Winkler
© Springer-Verlag Berlin Heidelberg 1986

Five different immunoreagents were employed as radiolabelled IgG and F$(ab')_2$, namely ^{131}I-MoAb, ^{131}I-F$(ab')_2$, ^{111}In-F$(ab')_2$ and ^{99m}Tc-F$(ab')_2$. The purified MoAb 225.28S and F$(ab')_2$ fragments were radiolabelled with [131]I (ORIS-CEA, Saclay France) or with [123]I (IRE, Fleurus Belgium) at $40-50$ mCi/mg using the iodogen method [7].

[111]In (ORIS-CEA, Saclay France) was bound to F$(ab')_2$ fragments by means of the cyclic anhydride of diethylenetriamine pentaacetic acid (DTPA) [8]. The DTPA-bound antibodies were separated from unbound ones using gel filtration and then incubated with ^{111}In chloride (5 mCi). Unbound indium was separated from the conjugated compound by gel filtration on Biogel P6.

F$(ab')_2$ fragments were labelled with ^{99m}Tc after their lyophilization. Thirty minutes before injection lyophilized F$(ab')_2$ fragments (350 µg) were dissolved in $3-5$ ml of a sterile solution of sodium ^{99m}Tc-pertechnetate (ORIS-CEA, Saclay France). After 15 min incubation, free ^{99m}Tc was separated from the antibody-bound ^{99m}Tc by ion exchange chromatography through a sterile Sephadex DEAE-A 25 column [10].

The radiolabelled antibodies were filtered through a 0.22 µm filter. Sterility and pirogen tests were performed by standard techniques [8].

The antibody reactivity after labelling procedures was measured employing the binding test with cultured melanoma cells Colo 38 and cultured B lymphoid cells Victor.

Indirect immunofluorescence was performed as previously described [11]. The antiserum was adsorbed on AB Rh$^+$ erythrocytes and glutaraldehyde-insolubilized human plasma. Avidin-biotin peroxidase staining reagents were purchased from Vector Laboratories (Burlingame, California, USA). Technical steps were done following the manufacturer's instructions. Peroxidase activity was detected using 3-amino-9-ethylcarbazole (AEC) solution (20 µg/ml). Sections were counterstained with Mayer's hematoxylin.

Very strict criteria were established at the beginning of the study for patients' admission. Only patients with advanced malignant melanomas (stage III B and III AB aged more than 65 years, and stage IV) were admitted. Only after having verified the absence of adverse reactions was the study extended to all stages. Every patient had given his informed consent and declared any history of prior allergic disease.

Before intravenous injection of monoclonal antibodies patients were tested for hypersentitivity to mouse IgG with an intradermal injection of $2-3$ µg antibody. Routine clinical analyses to evaluate hematopoietic, hepatic, pancreatic, and renal functions were performed before injection and repeated 4 times during the subsequent 2 weeks.

Patients injected with [131]I- or ^{123}I-labelled antibodies had the thyroid previously blocked by potassium iodide administration (120 mg/die for 10 days, starting 3 days before injection). Patients injected with ^{99m}Tc-labelled antibodies were treated with 400 mg potassium perclorate on the day of F$(ab')_2$ injection.

All radiolabelled F$(ab')_2$ preparations were injected intravenously over a 2-min period. The amount of radioactivity injected in the patients and its correlated protein weight is summarized in Table 1. Serial blood samples were

Table 1. Characteristics of labelled antibodies utilized in immunoscintigraphy

Immunoreagent	Patients n	Antibody injected (µg)		Specific activitiy (mCi/mg)		Activity injected (mCi)	
		x̄	range	x̄	range	x̄	range
^{131}I-MoAb-AM	2	21	14– 28	52.1	50.7–53.6	0.92	0.70–1.42
	2	695	640–750	1.0	1.0		
^{131}I-F(ab′)2-AM	4	22	18– 30	41.7	31.0–57.2	1.01	0.93–1.04
^{123}I-F(ab′)2-AM	4	217	170–290	14.8	12.0–17.4	3.18	2.40–4.00
^{99m}Tc-F(ab′)2-AM	6	160	80–200	46.9	40.0–64.0	7.49	4.48–8.50
^{111}In-F(ab′)2-AM	6	37	32– 40	51.0	50.0–55.0	2.16	0.92–4.56
	9	288	106–420	11.6	3.9–18.6		
^{131}I-F(ab′)2-AHBs	6	20	15– 60	29.5	9.0–56.0	0.60	0.50–0.80

drawn from all patients at 5, 10, 20, 30, and 40 min, and then at 1, 3, 6, and 12 h after the injection. Furthermore, a blood sample was drawn after 25 h from patients injected with ^{111}In-F(ab′)$_2$ fragments. The plasma samples were assayed for radioactivity in a counter.

Scintigraphy and single photon emission computerized tomography (SPECT) were performed using a double-head whole-body camera (KR7/LB/GAMMA CAT 2 SELO, Milan, Italy) connected with a PDP 11/34 computer (Digital Equipment Corporation, Maynard Montana, USA). The camera was equipped with parallel hole medium-energy collimators of high sensitivity or of high resolution. Regional scans of the lesions were performed at the rate of 1 frame/min for the first 30 min. Then whole-body and regional scans were performed every 2 h during the first 8 h and 24 h after the injection. In patients injected with ^{111}In-F(ab′)$_2$ fragments, further scans were performed at 48 h after administration of antibodies. The biodistribution of radioactivity was studied by analyzing specific regions of interest at the appropriate times.

Image enhancement was achieved by the subtraction technique only if a tumor imaging was evident on the direct scan.

Results

Labelling the MoAb 225.28S F(ab′)$_2$ fragments with ^{131}I, ^{123}I, ^{111}In, ^{99m}Tc, even at the high specific activities that were generally used, did not affect their immunological activity. In fact, the in vitro tests on human melanoma cell lines Colo 38 confirmed their nearly unchanged affinity for cancer cells. On the other hand, the radiolabelled F(ab′)$_2$ fragments did not show any immunoreactivity with cultured B lymphoid cells free from HMW-MAA.

From May 1982 to October 1984, our group examined 42 patients bearing 74 melanoma localizations. From November 1983 to April 1985, an other 204 patients bearing 426 malanoma lesions were studied in 6 Italian nuclear medicine centers taking part in the multicenter trial supported by a research project of the Italian National Research Council. The results obtained by our group and some preliminary data of the multicenter trial will be summarized below.

The cases subjected to immunoscintigraphy, when surgical specimens were available, were evaluated by immunohistochemical staining to obtain a better interpretation of the results. Following this method we could know the expression of the melanoma antigen in neoplastic lesions and interpret the reason for negative results.

Table 2 shows the immunohistochemical findings obtained with different antimelanoma antibodies in a group of patients. It can be seen that negative scintigraphic results sometimes correlated with negative immunohistological patterns. All positive scintigraphic results corresponded to the lesions expressing the antigen. In contrast, not all lesions showing positive staining were imaged in vivo. In some cases, these controversial data were due to the small size of the lesion. Moreover, it must be noted that some large lesions that were histologically positive also had negative immunoscintigraphy.

The kinetic studies of the various radiocompounds in the whole body and in most important organs showed a differentiated behavior between the whole antibody and the $F(ab')_2$ fragments, and between the antibody labelled with iodine and the others. These differences affected the doses adsorbed by the patients. Table 3 indicates the dosimetry evaluated for each tracer. The most favorable dosimetric conditions were obtained with the radiotechnetium compounds: even the ^{99m}Tc uptake in the kidney was higher than with other compounds. We observed no difference in tumor uptake among the five different tracers used. In the positive cases, tumor uptake appeared immediately in the first minutes after the injection. This rapid accumulation probably correlates with a high degree of vascularization of lesions. This hypothesis was confirmed by the results obtained in patients bearing metastatic localization as previously described [8, 9].

Figure 1 shows an example of radioimmunoimaging.

The specificity of the antibody uptake was investigated by studying the tumor-background ratio of the radioactivity in 4 patients simultaneously injected with two different $F(ab')_2$: the specific HMW-MAA $F(ab')_2$ radiolabelled with ^{111}In or ^{99m}Tc, and an irrelevant $F(ab')_2$ labelled with iodine. A clear difference was obtained between the uptake of the two antibodies, measured as tumor:background ratio in each patient. The maximum value of tumor:background ratio was reached at different times after injection in each patient. This ratio often showed differences in different tumor localizations.

The kinetic studies showed that the best conditions for performing immunoscintigraphy, namely the highest tumor:background ratio values, were reached, as a rule, 6−24 h after injection. The evaluation of the antibody distribution and the consideration of the dosimetric measurements indicated that ^{99m}Tc was the most reliable tracer for immunoscintigraphy. Moreover, the ^{99m}Tc emission energy is easily detectable by camera. Therefore, a lyophilized preparation of $F(ab')_2$ fragments was studied to assemble a kit for labelling procedure for every nuclear medicine department.

The cumulative results obtained by this study are reported in Table 4. No false-positive results were observed: 73% of all examined lesions were imaged.

Table 2. Immunocytochemical staining with different antimelanoma monoclonal antibodies

Patient	Localization	Lesion size (cm)	Imaging	Monoclonal antibodies 225-28S	456	376-96	354-34
PM 1	Post. chest	3	+	+	∓	±	+
VB 2	Multiple superf. nodes	0.7	−	±	+	−	∓
CP 3	Frontal	1.2	−	∓	+	−	∓
CM 4[a]	L. axilla	1.2	−	−	−	ND	−
SP 5	L. groin	3	+	+	∓	−	+
GF 7	Abdomen	2	−	−	∓	−	+
SR 9	R. groin	4	+	±	∓	−	±
DV 10	L. axilla	5	−	+	ND	ND	ND
	R. groin	1.4	−	±	+	∓	∓
	Post. chest	4	−	+	+	±	∓
	Post. chest	0.7	−	±	+	+	+
DG 11	L. thigh	6	+	+	∓	+	+
PM 14	R. groin	1.5	+	+	ND	ND	ND
FG 26	Abdomen	10	+	+	ND	ND	ND
	Liver	9	−	+	ND	ND	ND
CA 27	R. chest	3	+	+	ND	ND	ND

[a] Benign lesion; ND, not done

Table 3. Dosimetric evaluation on different radiolabelled antibodies

Organ	^{131}I-MoAb	^{131}I-F(ab')$_2$	^{123}I-F(ab')$_2$	^{99m}Tc-F(ab')$_2$	^{111}In-F(ab')$_2$
Whole body	0.70	0.40	0.03	0.0003	0.37
Bone marrow	0.77	0.32	0.14	0.002	0.27
Kidneys	7.79	1.66	0.03	0.097	0.49
Spleen	25.00	10.01	0.60	0.030	2.45
Livr	2.02	1.44	0.86	0.010	1.15
Ovary	0.02	0.003	0.002	0.0009	0.002
Testicle	0.002	0.0003	0.00001	0.00004	0.003

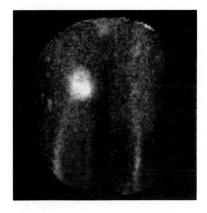

Fig. 1. Radioimmunoimaging performed 1 h after injection in a patient bearing a melanoma localization to the right thigh

Table 4. Incidence of positivity obtained by immunoscintigraphy with 225.28S antimelanoma MoAb and F(ab')$_2$ fragments labelled with different radioisotopes

Lesions	Iodine[a]		^{99m}Tc		^{111}In		Total	
	pos/tot	%	pos/tot	%	pos/tot	%	pos/tot	%
Liver	–	–	–	–	0/3	0	0/3	0
Lungs	2/6	33.3	1/2	50	3/7	42.9	6/15	40
Bone	–	–	–	–	1/1	100	1/1	100
Lymphatic nodes	4/5	80	13/13	100	7/7	100	23/25	92
Skin	7/12	58.3	4/5	80	12/12	100	23/29	79.3
Abdomen	–	–	0/1	0	–	–	0/1	0
Total lesions	13/23	56.5	18/21	85.7	23/30	76.7	54/74	73
Patient numbers	12		14		16		42	

[a] ^{131}I-MoAb, ^{131}I-F(ab')$_2$, ^{123}I-F(ab')$_2$

Table 5. Correlation between lesion size and scintigraphic positivity

Size (cm)	1	2	3	4	5	6	7	8	9	10	Total (n)	(%)
Lesions (pos/tot)	3/11	13/18	11/11	7/10	3/5	2/3	–	2/2	0/1	3/3	44/46	68.7

As to the different compounds used, the best results were obtained with ^{99m}Tc compounds (85.7%), followed by those obtained with ^{111}In tracers (76.7%).

Even if some lesions with a diameter of 1 cm or less could sometimes be visualized, an improvement of sensitivity of 80% for the whole series is reached if lesions of 2 cm or more are considered (Table 5). Nevertheless, this is not the only reason which explains negative scintigraphic results.

As far as the Italian multicenter trial is concerned, we are now completing the collection of the data. Results are under evaluation and will be published in the near future. A certain difference between the sensitivity obtained by the different centers can be observed, and this needs a more detailed analysis. Of the 500 tumor localisations examined, 64 were imaged by means of immunoscintigraphy before other diagnostic tools. ^{99m}Tc compounds seem to give better results.

It is too early to draw any conclusion about the prospective study which our group began in January 1985.

Discussion

Our study demonstrated that 225.28S MoAb is a suitable reagent for performing immunoscintigraphy in malignant melanomas. Of the 5 radiopharmaceuticals obtained with this antibody, the whole MoAb shows less favorable distribution than the F(ab')$_2$ fragments. In fact, a higher uptake was evident in different abdominal organs and in bone marrow. This behavior leads to an unfavorable dosimetry.

Of the $F(ab')_2$ fragments labelled with different radioisotopes, the ^{99m}Tc compound gave the best results. Its use is possible because of the rapid increase of radioactivity in tumor tissue after administration. The favorable dosimetry due to this compound allows the administration of higher activities.

It is known that ^{99m}Tc energy is very suitable for detection with a γ camera, and sophisticated techniques like single photon emission tomography can be used in the best technical conditions. These factors explain the rate of positivity which is higher with ^{99m}Tc than with other compounds. Several factors interfere with the positive rates of imaging. Some are due to physical and geometrical conditions of measurements, such as lesion size and site. In fact, lesions in deep organs are more difficult to visualize than superficial lesions because of the high background and the radiation attenuation. Other factors are due to the biological phenomena, such as lack of antigen expression by the tumor or the unusual blood pool modifications, and, as recently demonstrated, a basal membrane formation surrounding the metastatic lesions. The overall positive rate of imaging was 73% with a maximum for ^{99m}Tc compounds which corresponded to 85.7%. Nevertheless, in spite of the good results obtained in tumor imaging, other problems have to be solved for a clinical application of this appraoch. First of all, we must define if and when these methods can be used or preferred to other available examinations for diagnostic purposes. And this will be the first step in our research for the near future. The multicenter trial demonstrated that of the 500 localisations studied, 64 were unknown lesions, and it confirms that it is possibile to apply this method for a better definition of advanced studies.

Moreover, the most important diagnostic problems are to discover distant metastases in patients at stage II or to differentiate malignant from benign regional limphonodal alterations in patients with a primitive melanoma or during the follow-up. In January 1985, a prospective study was begun in our institute to give indications on these points. Another very important remark with regard to the clinical application of this method is that no immediate adverse reactions have yet been observed in any of the patients examined. This was also true when, as happened in some patients, the reagent was injected 2 or 3 times. A specific study performed with serial examinations of several functional parameters also confirmed the absence of late dangers.

References

1. Goldenberg DM, De Land F, Kim E, Bennet S, Primus FJ, Van Nagell JR, Estes N, De Simone P, Rayburn P (1978) Use of radiolabelled antibodies of CEA for the detection and localization of diverse cancers by external photoscanning. N Engl J Med 298:1384–1388
2. Mach JP, Chatal JF, Lumbroso JD, Buchegger F, Forni M, Ritschard J, Berche C, Douillard JY, Carrel S, Herlyn M, Steplewski Z, Koprowski H (1983) Tumor localization in patients by radiolabelled monoclonal antibodies against colon carcinoma. Cancer Res 43:5593–5600
3. Larson SM, Carrasquillo JA, Krohn KA, Brown JP, McGuffin RW, Ferens JM, Graham MM, Hill LD, Beaumier PL, Hellstrom KE, Hellstrom I (1983) Localization of ^{131}I-

labelled p97-specific Fab2 fragments in human melanoma as a basis for radiotherapy. J Clin Invest 72:2101–2114

4. Ferrone S, Giacomini P, Natali PG, Ruiter D, Buraggi GL, Callegaro L, Rosa U (1983) A human high molecular weight-melanoma associated antigen (HMW-MAA) defined by monoclonal antibodies. First Int. Meet. on Boron Neutron Capture MIT Boston, 12–14 October 1983, pp 174–183

5. Natali PG, Wilson BS, Imai K, Bigotti A, Ferrone S (1982) Tissue distributions, molecular profile and shedding of a cytoplasmic antigen identified by the monoclonal antibody 465.12S to human melanoma cells. Cancer Res 42:583–589

6. Buraggi GL, Callegaro L, Ferrone S, Turrin A, Cascinelli N, Attili A, Bombardieri E, Mariani G, Deleide G (1984) In vivo immunodiagnosis with radiolabelled anti-melanoma antibodies and F(ab')₂ fragments. Nuclear medizin: Proceedings of the 21 Int. Ann Meet SNME Ulm 13–16 Sept. 1983. Schattauer, Stuttgart, pp 713–716

7. Buraggi GL, Callegaro L, Mariani G, Turrin A, Cascinelli N, Attili A, Bombardieri E, Terno G, Plassio G, Dovis M, Mazzucca N, Natali PG, Scassellati D, Rosa U, Ferrone S (1985) Imaging with ¹³¹I-labelled monoclonal antibodies to a high molecular weight-melanoma: efficacy of whole Ig and its Fab2 fragments. Cancer Res 45:3378–3387

8. Buraggi GL, Callegaro L, Turrin A, Cascinelli N, Attili A, Emanuelli H, Gasparini M, Deleide G, Plassio G, Dovis M, Mariani G, Natali PG, Scassellati A, Rosa U, Ferrone S (1984) Immunoscintigraphy with ¹²³I, ⁹⁹ᵐTc and ¹¹¹In-labelled F(ab')₂ fragments of monoclonal antibodies to a human high molecular weight-melanoma associated antigen. J Nucl Med Allied Sci 28 [4]:283–295

9. Buraggi GL, Turrin A, Cascinelli N, Attili A, Terno G, Bombardieri E, Gasparini M, Seregni E (1986) Immunoscintigraphy with antimelanoma monoclonal antibodies. Immunoscintigraphy Proceedings of Saariselka Int. Meet. 1984. Gordon and Breach, London (in press)

10. Callegaro L, Ferrone S, Plassio G, Dovis M, Mariani G, Buraggi GL, Boniolo A, Rosa U (1983) Biochemical characterization of monoclonal antibodies and F(ab')₂ fragments against human melanoma associated antigen labelled with different radioactive isotopes. J Nucl Med Allied Sci 27:82–85

11. Natali PG, Cavaliere R, Matsui M, Buraggi GL, Callegaro L, Ferrone S (1984) Human melanoma associated antigens identified with monoclonal antibodies: characterization and potential clinical application. In: Cutaneous melanoma and precursor lesions. Nijhoff, Boston

Imaging of Bone and Soft Tissue Tumors
Using an Antitumor Monoclonal Antibody

N. C. Armitage[1], A. C. Perkins, M. V. Pimm, R. W. Baldwin,
and J. D. Hardcastle

Introduction

Imaging of malignancy in patients using radiolabelled antibodies has now been successfully demonstrated in various tumor types. These include colorectal cancer [2, 11, 14], breast cancer [7], malignant melanoma [13], and ovarian cancer [22]. However, although rodent sarcomas were among the first tumors to be localised using specific antitumor antibodies in animals [12, 18], there is little clinical data concerning immunoscintigraphy in bone and soft tissue tumors. In 1981 a monoclonal antibody raised against an osteosarcoma cell line, 791T, was described by Embleton et al. [4]. This monoclonal antibody showed no reaction with fibroblasts, human red blood cells or peripheral mononuclear cells. However, it reacted strongly against the immunizing osteosarcoma cell line and other osteosarcoma cell lines. It was demonstrated that with the addition of iodine as a radiolabel the antibody maintained its activity against osteosarcoma cell lines. In vivo studies using 791T tumors xenografted into immunodeprived mice showed that radiolabelled 791T/36 localised within the tumors, demonstrated both by external gamma scintigraphy and by direct measurement of uptake when a localisation index of between 4 and 5.6 was found compared with radiolabelled normal mouse immunoglobulin (NMI) [17]. This localisation prompted clinical studies using this radiolabelled antibody in patients with bone and soft tissue and a single case was reported showing clear localisation in a patient with osteosarcoma [8].

Although bone and soft tissue sarcomas are uncommon, staging is important since management decisions as to surgery, chemotherapy or radiotherapy will depend on accurate staging. With standard bone scanning using ^{99m}Tc-labelled polyphosphate skip metastases are often missed [6]. Using computerised axial tomography (CAT) up to 30% of patients with osteosarcoma have pulmonary metastases at the time of presentation which are often missed using plain chest X-rays and even whole lung tomography [1, 21]. One potential advantage of immunoscintigraphy is that in a single investigation bone and soft tissue deposits can be imaged simultaneously. Many soft tissue sarcomas, particularly osteosarcoma, have a high recurrence rate, and overall approximately 50% of patients die of their tumors within 5 years of presentation [3]; the use of monoclonal antibodies specifically to target antitumor agents may represent a significant step forward in improving patient survival.

1 The University of Nottingham, Department of Surgery, Floor E, West Block, University Hospital, Nottingham NG7 2UH, UK

Nuclear Medicine in Clinical Oncology
Ed. by C. Winkler
© Springer-Verlag Berlin Heidelberg 1986

Patients Studied

Twenty patients with proven or suspected bone or soft tissue tumors were studied; five had osteosarcomas, three had malignant fibrous histiocytomas, one had Ewing's sarcoma and one had a small cell tumor of the chest wall. Two patients were studied with chondromata, one of which had been traumatised. One patient had an osteoblastoma and one an osteoclastoma. Six other patients were studied with lesions thought radiologically suspicious of malignancy, which were later found to be non-neoplastic. Three of these patients had stress fractures, one of which was through a bone cyst; two had chronic inflammation, one due to polyarteritis nodosa and one to infection, and one patient had Paget's disease. All these diagnoses except that of Paget's disease were confirmed on biopsy.

Antibody and Labelling

The monoclonal antibody used was 791T/36. This is an IgG_2b antibody and was obtained from ascitic fluid from BALB/C mice maintained ascites. It was purified as previously described [17], tested for toxicity and pyrogenicity. It was labelled initially with ^{131}I using the iodogen method [9]. Briefly 300μl aliquots of iodogen (1,3,4,6-tetrachloro-3,6-diphenyl-glycouryl, Pierce Chemical, Chester, UK) in methylene chloride were evaporated in conical tubes. 791T/36 at 1 mg/ml was added with $Na^{131}I$ (Amersham International, UK) and incubated at room temperature for 15 min. The mixture was removed and free iodine was separated from the mixture by passage through a Sephadex G25 column [17]. The antibody was filtered using a 0.22 μm millipore filter and diluted in sterile normal saline.

In two patients the antibody was labelled with ^{111}In. Since indium is a metal ion, it requires conjugation via a chelating agent. This labelling has been fully described previously [16]. Briefly the antibody was allowed to react with DTPA anhydride for 5 min at room temperature, after which excess DTPA anhydride was removed by passage through a Sephadex G25 column. ^{111}In-indium chloride was diluted 1 in 1 with sodium acetate and added to the antibody conjugate. Any unbound ^{111}In was removed by passage down a Sephadex G50 column and 10 mg EDTA was added to the dose to promote excretion of any unbound ^{111}In following administration to the patient. The labelled antibody was filtered in a similar way to the iodine-labelled antibody.

Imaging

All patients had the procedure fully explained to them and in the case of minors this was explained to the parents. For ^{131}I imaging the patients were started on potassium iodide 60 μg daily 24 h prior to the imaging. This was continued for at least 10 days subsequently. This was unnecessary in patients receiving the indium-labelled antibody. After a subcutaneous dose to test for anaphylaxis, the antibody was infused intravenously. The dose given was 70 MBq of indium or iodine (200 − 1000 µg protein). In the case of one small child only 30 MBq was administered. Depending on the radiolabel, two different protocols were used for imaging. For iodine the patients were imaged at 48 − 72 h using an IGE 400T gamma camera with a high energy collimator (400 keV). Views taken were of the affected and contralateral limb, the abdomen and the thorax. Following acquisition of the iodine image, a blood pool image was obtained. This was achieved either by labelling the patient's red blood cells in vivo by the injection of stanous pyrophosphate, the dose calculated by nomogram, followed by 200 MBq ^{99m}Tc pertechnetate or by labelling circulating transferrin by injection of 200 MBq ^{113m}In-indium chloride. Blood pool images were acquired for the same views as the iodine image to simulate the distribution of radiolabelled antibody in the circulation. After normalisation of count rates within the images, the blood pool images were subtracted from the iodine image using computer, to leave a resultant antibody image [15]. For indium, images were obtained at 20 min after administration of the radiopharmaceutical to show distribution of the antibody in the circulation, using an IGE 400T gamma camera with a medium energy collimator (300 keV). Similar views were obtained 72 h to show the resultant antibody distribution. The images were displayed onto nuclear medicine film and interpreted without computer subtraction. In one patient using ^{111}In-labelled antibody, 360° emission tomography of the thorax was performed. All patients except one had bone imaging using ^{99m}Tc methylene diphosphonate. In one patient only, tumor and normal tissue was obtained within 4 days of injection of antibody; this was weighed and counted for radioactivity in an LKB well counter.

Establishment of Xenograft

In one patient with an osteosarcoma, tumor was obtained at surgery and implanted subcutaneously into CBA immunodeprived mice [17]. Six of these implanted tissue samples developed tumors and this was demonstrated histologically to be very similar to the primary tumor despite several passages. From the fourth passage a culture line was established. In order to determine expression of the 791T/36 defined antigen on the tumor cells, a direct immunofluorescence test was performed; 2×10^5 sorted cells were reacted with 1 µg of FITC 791T/36 and the cellular fluorescence measured using a FACS IV flow cytometer (Becton Dickinson, Sunnyvale, Ca). From this, a mean fluorescence intensity was calculated. Specificity of 791T/36 binding was measured by competition assay; between lug of FITC 791T/36 mixed with increasing amounts (0.1 − 2 µg) of unlabelled 791T/36. As a positive control 791T cells were used in parallel. Antibody localisation in vivo was shown in the mice xenografted with this tumor both by direct measurement whereby mice received a mixture of ^{131}I-791T/36 and ^{125}I NMI by intraperitoneal injection. They were sacrificed after 4 days and samples of tumor, blood and normal organs were weighed and counted using a well counter. Localisation was also assessed by gamma camera imaging. The mice were injected with 4 MBq of ^{131}I-labelled antibody and imaged at 2 days using a gamma camera fitted with a pinhole collimator. Blood pool subtraction was performed after administration of 10 MBq of ^{99m}Tc.

Results

All five patients with osteosarcomas gave positive images at the site of the primary tumor (Fig. 1). Patient 5 was known to have pulmonary metastases at the time of presentation which were not demonstrated by planar imaging. Three patients have undergone follow-up imaging. In patient 2, six months following excision of the right inominate bone, further uptake was noted in the pelvis, correctly predicting local recurrence which became obvious clinically some weeks later. This patient subsequently developed pulmonary metastases which were not detected by planar imaging. Patient 3 was imaged after a course of chemotherapy; the follow-up image showed no antibody activity at the site of her tumor. She subsequently underwent resection, and histological examination of the tumor showed the vast majority of the tumor cells to be dead. Patient 4 underwent amputation and follow-up imaging was negative. These results are summarised in Table 1.

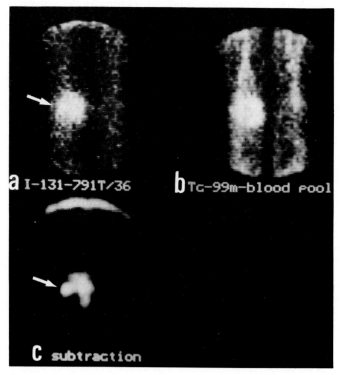

Fig. 1. a ^{131}I-791T/36 images (anterior lower limbs) or patient 1 with an osteosarcoma of right lower femur (*arrow*). **b** Blood pool image. **c** Subtracted image showing "hot" area (*arrow*) corresponding with tumor site

Table 1. Results of imaging patients with osteosarcoma

Patient no.	Age (years)	Sex	Site of primary tumour	Image result	Site of secondary tumour	Image result
1	16	F	Lower femur	+		−
2	26	M	Innominate bone	+		−
	Postsurgery			−	Pelvis	+
					Lung	−
3	24	F	Upper tibia	+		−
	Postchemotherapy			−		−
4	16	F	Lower tibia	+		−
5	57	M	Upper humerus	+	Lung	−

Table 2. Results of imaging patients with bone and soft tissue tumours

Patient no.	Age (years)	Sex	Histology	Site of primary tumor	Image result	Site of secondary tumor	Image result
6	60	M	Malignant fibrous histiocytoma	Thigh	+		−
7	72	F	Malignant fibrous histiocytoma	Thigh	+	Lung	+
8	49	M	Malignant fibrous histiocytoma	Thigh	−	Local recurrence (microscopic)	−
9	35	M	Ewing's sarcoma	Femur	+		−
	Postchemotherapy				−		−
10	12	M	Small-cell tumour	Chest wall	+		−
	Postchemotherapy			Chest wall	+		−
11	24	F	Osteoblastoma	Tibia	+		−
12	53	F	Osteoblastoma	Tibia	−		−
13	20	M	Chondroma	Femur	+		−
14	46	M	Chondroma	Inominate	−		−

Two of the three patients with malignant fibrous histiocytomas gave positive images. Two patients had large lesions in the thigh which were clearly seen. In one of these, patient 6, normal and tumor tissue was obtained at excision 4 days after injection of ^{131}I and a tumor:nontumor uptake ratio was calculated at 2.8:1. Patient 7, in addition to the large primary tumor in the thigh, also had pulmonary metastases. When ^{111}In was used as the radiolabel, these were not detected on planar imaging. However, on emission tomography these deposits were detected, one of which was 1.5 cm in diameter. The primary tumor of patient 8 was not imaged, but views were taken when the patient was about to undergo further excision for recurrence. A negative image was obtained. However, on histological examination only one microscopic focus of tumor could be found.

Both the patient with Ewing's sarcoma and the patient with the small-cell tumor of the chest wall gave positive images. Of the other tumors, one patient with an osteoblastoma gave a positive image although the patient with an os-

Table 3. Results of imaging non-neoplastic disease

Patient no.	Age (years)	Sex	Histology	Site	Image result
15	5	F	Stress fracture	Tibia	−
16	17	F	Stress fracture	Fibula	−
17	24	F	Stress fracture (through bone cyst)	Femur	−
18	55	M	Paget's disease	Spine	−
19	50	M	Osteitis (polyarteritis nodosa)	Tibia	+
20	65	F	Osteitis (suppurative)	Femur	+

teoclastoma was negative. One of the two chondromas gave a positive image, although this was the condroma which had been traumatised. These results are summarised in Table 2. Three cases of stress fracture were negative as was the case of Paget's disease. Both cases of chronic osteitis, however, gave clear positive images. These are shown in Table 3.

Xenograft Studies

With binding assay using FITC 791T/36 with xenograft cultured cells and 791T cultured cells, it was found that there was strong binding of 791T/36 to the cultured tumor cells which was suppressed by the addition of increasing concentrations of unlabelled antibody. On injection of ^{131}I 791T/36 and ^{125}I-NMI into immunodeprived mice bearing xenografts, it was found that the antibody level in the tumor was 2.5 times that of control IgG_2b. This localisation was confirmed by gamma camera scintigraphy, which gave clear images of the tumor site.

Discussion

We have shown that radiolabelled 791T/36 localises in osteosarcomas and in other malignant sarcomas as demonstrated by gamma camera imaging. In one patient, we were able to confirm preferential uptake by direct counting of tumor and normal tissue. In addition, from one of the osteosarcomas established both as a xenograft and as a cultured cell line, we were able to show in vitro binding which was shown to be suppressed on competition assay with unlabelled 791T/36 indicating a specific antibody antigen reaction, and in vivo localisation in xenografts of the tumor with a specific localisation index of 2.5:1 compared with normal mouse immunoglobulin. Roth found binding of this particular antibody in osteosarcomas to be significant in 15 of 22 extracts of both primary and secondary osteosarcomas, but no binding to normal adult or foetal tissues [19].

It was disappointing that pulmonary metastases in two patients were not demonstrated by immunoscintigraphy; however, in these studies we used planar imaging. It was heartening, therefore, that in the one patient on whom emission tomography with ^{111}In-labelled antibody was performed, the presence of pulmonary metastases were demonstrated. It may be that the failure to detect the pulmonary metastases in the other two patients was related to the limitations of planar imaging and to the use of ^{131}I as a radiolabel rather than failure of localisation of the antibody. Where there was sufficient tumor bulk, the other malignant sarcomas gave positive images, and in one of these tumors direct measurement of the uptake of antibody into tumor was possible and demonstrated a T:NT ratio of 2.8:1. The patient with an osteoblastoma gave a positive image, while the image of another patient with an osteoblastoma was negative. The reason for this is not clear, but may be related to the fact that the osteoblastoma is a bone-forming rather than bone-removing tumor.

Of the nonmalignant lesions studied, it was interesting that all three cases of stress fracture gave negative images, although they showed clear hot areas on standard bone scanning. Thus, the production of a positive image would seem not to be related simply to increased hyperaemia. Of the two chondromas studied, one patient gave a positive image and one a negative image. The reason for this is unclear, although the patient with a positive image had received some trauma to this tumor. Both patients with chronic osteitis and suppuration gave positive images, and it is possible that the immunoglobulin becomes pooled in pus, thus giving local areas of increased uptake and, consequently, positive images.

Iodine-131 has a number of disadvantages as a radiolabel which include urinary excretion, a long half-life, inefficient detection by conventional gamma camera and thyroid uptake. As a result we have had to employ computer subtraction techniques with the possibility of artefact formation and have been unable to effectively use emission tomography. Having now successfully labelled the antibody using ^{111}In, it appears that this radiopharmaceutical is particularly suitable for immunoscintigraphy in the limbs and in the thorax, although intense hepatic and spleen uptake limit its ability to detect liver metastases. The major advantages however have been that computer subtraction is no longer necessary and emission tomography is possible within acquisition times acceptable to most patients. Thus immunoscintigraphy may have a place in the detection and staging of bone and soft tissue sarcomas, though the resolution of the technique still needs to be increased.

However, it is in the prospect of targeting antitumor agents that the tumor monoclonal antibodies may have their greatest part to play. Conjugates between 791T/36 and various cytotoxic drugs including vindesine [5] and methotrexate [10] have been produced which have been shown to be cytotoxic to osteosarcoma target cells (791T/36). In addition, the vindesine and methotrexate conjugates [17, 20] have been shown to suppress to growth of 791T xenografts without producing the same degree of toxicity as the free drug. We have been able to show uptake of antibody into tumors in patients by immunoscintigraphy. This uptake may be employed in the delivery of specific antitumor agents to this type of tumor with the prospect of improving survival.

References

1. Bacci G, Picci D, Caldreni P, Figus E, Borgh A (1982) Full lung tomograms and bone scanning in the initial work up of patients with osteosarcoma: a review of 126 patients. Eur J Cancer Clin Oncol 18:967–971

2. Chatal JF, Saccavini J-C, Fumoleau P, Douillard J-Y, Curtet C, Kremer M et al. (1984) Immunoscintigraphy of colon carcinoma. J Nucl Med 25(3):307 – 314

3. Eilber FR, Eckhardt J, Morton DL (1984) Advances in the treatment of sarcomas in the extremity. Cancer 54:2695 – 2701

4. Embleton MJ, Gunn B, Byers VS, Baldwin RW (1981) Antitumour reactions of monoclonal antibody against a human osteogenic sarcoma cell line. Br J Cancer 43:582 – 587

5. Embleton MJ, Rowland GF, Simmonds RG, Jacobs E, Marsden CH, Baldwin RW (1983) Selective cytotoxicity against human tumour cells by a vindesine-monoclonal antibody conjugate. Br J Cancer 47:43 – 49

6. Enneking WF, Kagan A (1975) 'Skip' metastases in osteosarcoma. Cancer 36(6): 2192 – 2205

7. Epenetos AA, Mather S, Granowska M, Nimmon CC, Hawkins LR, Britton K et al. (1982) Targetting of iodine-123-labelled tumor-associated monoclonal antibodies to ovarian, breast and gastrointestinal tumors. Lancet ii:999 – 1004

8. Farrands PA, Perkins AC, Sully L, Hopkins JS, Pimm MV, Baldwin RW, Hardcastle JD (1983) Localisation of human osteosarcoma by antitumour monoclonal antibody. J Bone Joint Surg 65-B:638 – 640

9. Fraker PJ, Speck JC (1978) Protein and cell membrane iodination with a sparingly soluble chloroamide 1,3,4,6-tetrachloro-3,6-diphenyl-glycouril. Biochem Biophys Res Commun 80:849 – 857

10. Garnett MC, Embleton MJ, Jacobs E, Baldwin RW (1983) Preparation and properties of a drug-carrier-antibody conjugate showing selective antibody-directed cytotoxicity in vitro. Int J Cancer 31:661 – 670

11. Goldenberg DM, DeLand F, Kim E, Bennett S, Primus FJ, Van Nagell JR, Estes N et al. (1978) Use of radiolabelled antibodies to carcinoembryonic antigen for the detection and localisation of diverse cancers by external photoscanning. N Engl J Med 298(25):1384 – 1388

12. Korngold L, Pressman D (1954) The localisation of anti-lymphosarcoma in the Murphy lymphosarcoma of the rat. Cancer Res 14:96 – 99

13. Larson SM, Brown JP, Wright PW, Carrasquillo JA, Hellstrom I, Hellstrom KE (1983) Imaging of melanoma with I-131 labelled monoclonal antibodies. J Nucl Med 24(2):123 – 129

14. Mach JP, Buchegger F, Forni M, Ritschard J, Berche C, Lumbroso JD et al. (1981) Use of radiolabelled monoclonal anti-CEA antibodies for the detection of human carcinomas by external photoscanning and tomoscintigraphy. Immunol Today 2(12):239 – 249

15. Perkins AC, Whalley DR, Hardy JG (1984) Physical approach for the reduction of dual radionuclide image subtraction artefacts in immunoscintigraphy. Nucl Med Commun 5:501 – 512

16. Perkins AC, Pimm MV, Birch MK (1985) The preparation and characterisation of ^{111}In-labelled monoclonal antibody for tumour immunoscintigraphy. Eur J Nucl Med 10:296 – 301

17. Pimm MV, Embleton MV, Perkins AC, Price MR, Robins RA, Robinson GR, Baldwin RW (1982) In vivo localisation of antiosteogenic sarcoma 791T monoclonal antibody in osteogenic sarcoma xenografts. Int J Cancer 30:75 – 85

18. Pressman D, Korngold L (1953) The in vivo localisation of anti-Wagner osteogenic sarcoma. Cancer 6:619 – 623

19. Roth JA, Restropo C, Scuderi P, Baldwin RW, Reichert CM, Hosoi S (1984) Analysis of antigenic expression by primary and autologous metastatic sarcoma using monoclonal antibodies. Cancer Res 44:5320 – 5325

20. Rowland GF, Axton CA, Baldwin RW, Brown JP, Corvalan JRF, Embleton MJ et al. (1985) Antitumor properties of vindesine monoclonal antibody conjugates. Cancer Immunol Immunother 19:1 – 17

21. Simm FR, Pritchard DJ (1980) Computer tomography for the detection of pulmonary metastases in patients with osteosarcoma. Proc Am Assoc Cancer Res 21:148

22. Symonds EM, Perkins AC, Pimm MV et al. (1985) Clinical implications for immunoscintigraphy in patients with ovarian malignancy. A preliminary study using monoclonal antibody 791T/36. Br J Obstet Gynaecol 92:270 – 276

V. Nuclear Magnetic Resonance Imaging and In Vivo Spectroscopy

Current Status of Magnetic Resonance Imaging of the Central Nervous System

B. S. WORTHINGTON[1]

At the present level of development, clinical trials of magnetic resonance imaging have established that for the brain and spinal cord its depiction of gross structure now rivals those of computed tomography (CT) and is superior in its ability to detect pathological change in normal tissue. Magnetic resonance, however, is not a generic technique, but by manipulation of the applied spin sequences a whole range of different image classes can be generated which have varying weightings by proton density, the relaxation times T_1 and T_2 and bulk flow. It has to be realised that in practical terms the use of an inappropriate sequence may fail to disclose pathology and the application of even a representative selection of sequences may be precluded by considerations of time. Much work is now being directed towards both defining the optimal sequence for a given pathological condition and exploring the specificity of the information which can be derived from the images. The hope has long been expressed that magnetic resonance imaging would allow a more precise prediction of tissue type than is possible with computed tomography. Pathological tissues, particularly in tumours, are seldom homogeneous and it is not surprising, therefore, that a wide range of spin relaxation values can be found in a single tumour. The biophysical basis underlying such changes in the relaxation times observed in pathological tissues is imperfectly understood. The major factor is undoubtedly the ordering of water molecules, but the presence of lipids and paramagnetic substances can also be important. It now seems apparent that precise tissue characterisation will prove impossible; nonetheless, several approaches are being made to determine the degree to which this will be possible. The most obvious method is an empirical correlation of the scan appearances and the clinical findings with the subsequently identified pathology.

This corresponds with they way in which CT was originally evaluated and, in a similar fashion with MRI, the description of several appearances has preceded an understanding of the underlying mechanism resulting in the scan findings. The short T_1 relaxation values associated with recent haematoma (Fig. 1) are now known to be due to the formation of methaemoglobin in the clot and the short T_1 relaxation values of metastatic melanoma deposits reflect the presence of paramagnetic compounds. An alternative approach is to prepare a calculated proton density and relaxation time map, and these are calculated from the results of applying different spin sequences. To obtain accu-

---

1 Diagnostic Radiology, The University of Nottingham, University Hospital and Medical School, Clifton Boulevard, Nottingham NG7 2UH, UK

Nuclear Medicine in Clinical Oncology
Ed. by C. Winkler
© Springer-Verlag Berlin Heidelberg 1986

rate measurements is difficult and time consuming. The wide range of values associated with different pathological tissues probably accounts for the relatively poor results achieved so far by this means. It has proved fruitful, however, in assessing the water content of the nucleus pulposus in intervertebral discs as a means of determining the changes which occur with age and degeneration. It may prove a useful means for monitoring the effects of treatment on individual tumours and in detecting recurrences. The most fruitful approach to tissue characterisation will probably lie in the study of the relative change in the contrast between a lesion and the adjacent normal tissue when several different spin sequences are applied. By this means, for example, bulk flow of blood within angiomas and giant aneurysms can be highlighted by the application of a saturation recovery sequence. If the relaxation characteristics of a tissue are known in advance, for example, in the case of CSF with its very long T_1 value, then a sequence can be chosen to highlight it on scans and this is the basis of long T_R, long T_E spin-echo sequences to produce the equivalent of an MR myelogram in the study of pathology such as disc protrusions which encroach on the spinal theca. Such a sequence is also of value in the identification of arachnoid cysts and loculations of CSF.

Comparison of magnetic resonance imaging with CT shows that space-expanding intrinsic tumours produce recognisable displacements and deformity of the ventricular system and subarachnoid cisterns on transverse axial scans. The multiplanar facility of MRI allows precise volumetric assessment, the demonstration of secondary brain herniations and facilitates accurate location of pathology. In high-convexity mass lesions, for example, a parasagittal scan can make localization certain. The precise size and position of supra- and infratentorial components in tentorial meningiomas can be elegantly shown. This additional information is difficult to quantify, but it has proved of great value to our neurosurgical colleagues in planning the operative approach to tumours. The sagittal perspective has had a considerable impact on the assessment of tumours of the corpus callosum, those within or impinging on the midline ventricular system, those involving the brain stem or lying adjacent to the craniovertebral junction. There is no doubt that the requirement for invasive procedures in assessing such tumours will be diminished in units which have access to MRI. Unlike CT, the maximal proximity of irregular bone and air does not give rise to partial volume artefacts, and this is of particular significance in studying tumours close to the skull base (Fig. 2). Furthermore, the lack of signal from cortical bone has allowed even small intracanalicular acoustic neuromas to be imaged directly. The better display of topographical anatomy provided by multiple planes and the substantially reduced bone artefact make

---

Fig. 1. Transverse axial NMR scan (T_R 2000 ms; T_E 500 ms)showing a haematoma in the right frontal pole with an associated mass effect on the adjacent lateral ventricle

Fig. 2. Transverse axial NMR scan (T_R 1500 ms; T_E 80 ms) showing a cholesteatoma within the right petrous bone in a patient with facial palsy

Fig. 3. Transverse axial NMR scan (T_R 1200 ms; T_E 80 ms) showing an acoustic neuroma which has grown forwards and medially deforming the brain stem

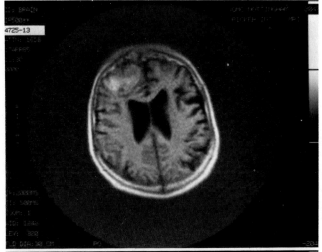

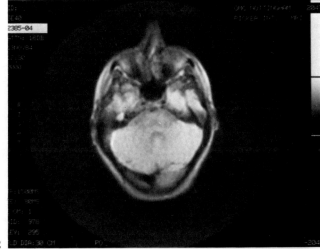

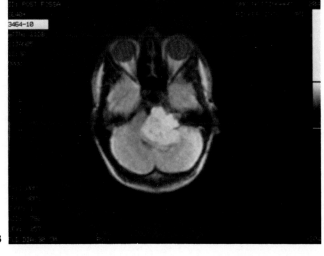

the distinction between intrinsic and extrinsic tumours, particularly in the posterior fossa, easier with MRI than with CT (Fig. 3).

In NMR imaging, inversion recovery images give an exquisite differentiation of the gray and white matter, and this has been exploited in the evaluation of demyelinating disorders, as well as the study of delays and deficits in myelination in the child. It is now well established that MRI is more sensitive than CT in the detection of plaques of multiple sclerosis which appear as focal areas of long T_1 and T_2, and follow-up studies have shown reduction in size of lesions during remissions. The use of surface coil data acquisition to provide improved image quality over a small imaging volume has been exploited to advantage in the orbit. The quality of images which can now be obtained competes favourably with that obtained by CT, and the multiplanar facility and avoidance of ionizing radiation make this a particularly attractive application.

Using inversion recovery T_1 weighted sequences, the whole length of the spinal cord can be visualised without the use of contrast media and the additional perspective of direct sagittal and coronal views is particularly useful in the assessment of pathology, such as hydromyelia and intrinsic tumours which extend over several segments. By using spin-echo sequences with a long T_R and T_E, the CSF pool can be highlighted, which allows the assessment of extradural mass lesions that encroach on the spinal canal and deform the theca. The vertebral bodies are well visualised on account of the high signal from the central marrow cavity; the outline of the posterior vertebral elements is defined by the signal from tissues adjacent to their margins. Although the cortical bone around the exit foramina is not seen on MRI, the emerging nerve roots can be visualised on account of a surrounding sleeve of fat. In the normal disc, the nucleus pulposus has a higher water content than the surrounding annulus fibrosus, and the two components can be separated, especially in the lumbar region, by the use of T_2 weighted spin-echo sequences. Following disc degeneration, the signal intensity from the nucleus pulposus diminishes and eventually becomes the same as that from the annulus. Disc protrusions are readily identifiable by their encroachment on the theca in long T_R, long T_E sequences. At the present time, the greater slice thickness and lack of oblique sections mean that assessment of osteoarticular and disc disease is more readily assessed in the transverse axial plane by CT than MRI.

One of the few drawbacks to MRI is its inherently low sensitivity, and this coupled with the wide range of potential spin sequences which can be employed means that in practical terms it is a very time-consuming examination. Methods have been developed which allow multiple slices to be acquired during a single exposure, and this effectively reduces the data acquisition time for each section. Even with multislice and multiecho data acquisition, MRI remains a relatively slow examination requiring an experienced operator to choose the appropriate plane or planes and sequences for each examination. It is doubtful whether a throughput of more than two patients per hour will be achieved when optimum studies are carried out. It may well be that diagnostic efficacy may be sacrificed in order to achieve higher throughput by using sequences which give faster data acquisition, but are not necessarily the most sensitive in the detection of pathology.

NMR Imaging of Tumors in the Body Stem

R. Schwarzrock[1], J. Kotzerke, and H. Hundeshagen

In the diagnosis of CNS disorders, NMR has already gained widespread acceptance as a routine tool due to its unique image quality and the fact that the disadvantages of transmission computerized tomography (TCT) are not present. This is not yet true for the tumor diagnosis of the body stem, because there are some special shortcomings and a lack of extensive experience [15].

In the following we will discuss the disadvantages and advantages of NMR in diagnosing tumors (TU) of the body stem. Its clinical value now, and its probable use in the future, for the various organs or organ systems will be outlined.

Disadvantages of NMR Imaging in the Body Stem

1. Lower Spatial Resolution and Thicker Slices Compared with Modern TCT. Where the whole-body spool has to be used, slice thickness up to now has not been under 10 mm and pixel size not under 2 mm within reasonable imaging time. Often enough the high contrast resolution overcomes this disadvantage. In many situations, however, tumors and their spread to neighboring tissues are only detectable if spatial resolution is high.

With the use of surface coils, spatial resolution is comparable to, or even better than, TCT. This is true for the neck, mamma, spine, and the extremities. With higher field strength and the development of faster pulse sequences, spatial resolution comparable to TCT will be achieved even for the whole-body spool. Imaging time will not be prolonged.

2. Loss of Image Quality Due to Cardiac and Respiratory Motion. Cardiac motion can be overcome by ECG trigger without prolongation of the imaging time. The only problems are arrhythmias and the fact that repetition time cannot be freely determined since it is given by the heart rate. ECG trigger is necessary in the imaging of the heart itself, but also in the mediastinum and the thoracic spine. The loss of image quality due to respiratory motion is tolerable in most cases. It can be prevented by respiratory gating. But with the techniques developed so far [23] it triples imaging time and requires that the patient breathe deeply and regularly. Its use is therefore very limited. New techniques

---

1 Institut für Nuklearmedizin und Spez. Biophysik der Med. Hochschule Hannover, Konstanty-Gutschow-Straße 8, D-3000 Hannover 61

Nuclear Medicine in Clinical Oncology
Ed. by C. Winkler
© Springer-Verlag Berlin Heidelberg 1986

might bring the same results in much shorter imaging time. It would then be of use in the imaging of the liver, kidneys, adrenals, pancreas, and, of course, the lung itself. The combination of ECG trigger with respiratory gating, which offers the best results, would then also be possible within reasonable imaging time.

3. Long Imaging Time. In more simple diagnostic problems with a standardized sequence of only a few pulse sequences, imaging time is in the range of 30 min and is thus comparable to TCT when the multislicing method is used. In the more complicated case with many different sequences and slice orientations, imaging time can easily reach 90 min. However, the vast majority of patients are able to tolerate the time.

4. Limited Experience. To define the value of NMR properly, careful comparison with TCT and US in a large number of patients is needed. Up to now there has been a certain lack of experience concerning tumors of the body stem, because CNS diagnosis has so far received the most attention. This might be the main reason why NMR has not gained acceptance as a routine tool in the body stem.

5. No Positive Display of Calcium. This is a disadvantage when the impact of tumors on bony structures is of diagnostic importance. Furthermore, calcium may help in the differential diagnosis of tumor type. In cortical bone, however, tumor is easily seen due to the loss of the bright signal of fatty bone marrow.

Advantages of NMR Imaging in the Body Stem

1. High Contrast Between Different Tissue Types. The high tumor-nontumor contrast inside parenchymatous organs results in a high sensitivity in tumor detection. This is especially true for the liver and thyroid. Outside parenchymatous organs the high contrast between fat, air, fluid, flowing blood, and tumor tissue provides for the better diagnostic quality of NMR compared to TCT.

2. Absence of the Typical TCT Artifacts. There are neither streak artifacts arising from air in the bowel or metallic clips nor are there beam-hardening artifacts in the subcostal region. This makes NMR the method of choice in cases of significant TCT image degradation.

3. Direct Display of Sagittal, Frontal, and Axial Slices as well as Any Angle Thereto. This allows a much better definition of tumor origin, extension, and spread into the neighboring organs than axial slices alone. Especially the surgeon profits from this illustrative manner of presentation (Fig. 1).

4. Display of Major Blood Vessels Without Contrast Agents. This is a major advantage for the detectability of a tumor with low contrast and for tumor staging.

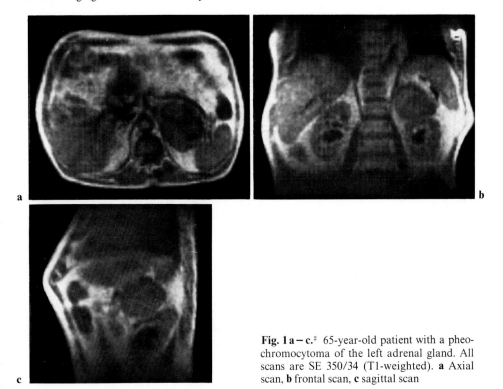

a

b

c

Fig. 1 a − c.[2] 65-year-old patient with a pheochromocytoma of the left adrenal gland. All scans are SE 350/34 (T1-weighted). **a** Axial scan, **b** frontal scan, **c** sagittal scan

Involvement of vessels can be clearly demonstrated. Therefore, as has already been shown, NMR is more successful than TCT in the staging and/or detection of renal, cardiac, mediastinal, and cervical masses.

5. Possibility of Tissue Typing Through the Analysis of the NMR Parameters T1, T2 and the Proton Density Together with the Shape of the Lesion. Differentiation between TU, parenchymal, or connective tissue as well as air and fluid is easy with NMR. Definition of tumor histology and differentiation between benign and malignant tumors or inflammation is much more difficult than was believed in the early days of NMR. Especially analysis of T1, T2, and rho alone is not reliable enough. This is not only due to technical problems involved in the reliable and exact calculation of these parameters, but also to the significant overlap of the values between the different entities.

The classification through T1/T2 value in combination with the shape of the lesion, however, can give good results. This will be shown later in the text with the example of liver tumors.

---

2 The figures are made by a prototype resistive magnet of 0.2-T field strength. Despite their lower spatial resolution compared to modern superconducting magnets, they show the unique advantages of NMR.
In the explanation to the figures, SE is spin echo and IR is inversion recovery. The first number is the repetition time in ms, the second the echo delay in ms, and the third the inversion time if the IR mode is used.

Diagnostic Value of NMR in Relation to other Noninvasive Imaging Modalities

The diagnostic value in clinical practice in relation to the other noninvasive imaging modalities ultrasound (US), TCT, and X-ray will now be discussed on the basis of our own experience and the recent literature.

NMR is of clearly superior value:

In the nasopharynx region. The presentation of the region is clear, as it is free of bony artifacts, and since direct multiplanar views are possible [4].

In cardiac tumors. By the means of ECG trigger a clear presentation of the heart without movement blur is possible. Thrombus, lipom, aneurysm, and TU can be differentiated [8] (Fig. 2).

In prostate and bladder tumors. Here detection and staging are superior due to sagittal presentation and the high contrast between different tissues and urine [16] (Fig. 3).

In bone tumors. Here the spread inside the marrow but also outside the cortical bone is clearly defined. TU tissue can be differentiated from edema, inflammation, and hematoma. Even the differentiation of scar tissue from recurrent TU seems to be possible [2, 3] (Fig. 4).

NMR is of comparable value in the majority of the tumors not mentioned above. In these cases NMR is not the method of first choice because of high cost, long imaging time, and lack of general availability. However, when results with the other methods are equivocal or not thoroughly descriptive, NMR can provide ultimate clarity and is then indicated.

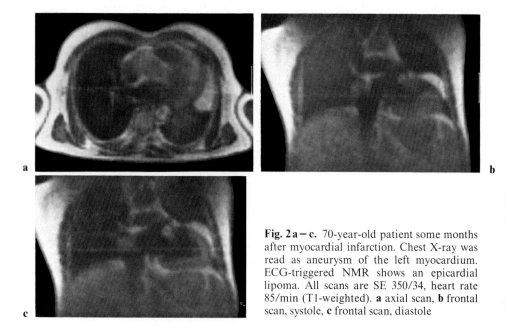

Fig. 2a–c. 70-year-old patient some months after myocardial infarction. Chest X-ray was read as aneurysm of the left myocardium. ECG-triggered NMR shows an epicardial lipoma. All scans are SE 350/34, heart rate 85/min (T1-weighted). **a** axial scan, **b** frontal scan, systole, **c** frontal scan, diastole

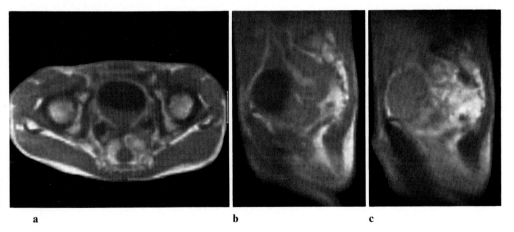

a   b   c

Fig. 3a–c. 49-year-old patient with a bladder carcinoma. In the T1-weighted image (a) it appears as a thickening on the dorsal bladder wall. In the sagittal plane (b) the spread of the tumor is clearest. In the T2-weighted sagittal plane (c) the tumor is bright. **a** Axial scan, SE 350/34, **b** sagittal scan, SE 350/34, **c** sagittal scan, SE 1600/68

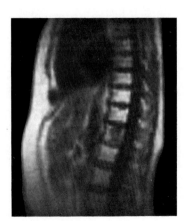

Fig. 4. Patient with a metastasis of a mammacarcinoma in a vertebral body of the thoracic spine. The negative contrast of the lesion in the T1-weighted image results from the loss of fatty bone marrow. Sagittal scan in SE 350/34

Some Special diagnostic areas are:

The cervical region. US and scintigraphy are very efficient. TCT is of use in showing subternal spread and involvement of the esophagus and trachea, but differentiation between TU, blood vessels, and muscle is difficult. With a special neck spool, NMR has the same spatial resolution but a superior contrast resolution. It thus overcomes these disadvantages of TCT [21].

Whether NMR is able to differentiate between benign and malignant thyroid nodules is not yet clear. The probability is low, as even the pathologist has problems with the highly differentiated follicular carcinoma. The papillary type, on the other hand, is composed of heterogeneous tissue material and thus should give no typical picture in a number of cases.

The mediastinum. If TCT is done by a very experienced radiologist, its results are similar to NMR in most cases. NMR images, however, show the tumor more clearly due to the excellent contrast between TU, blood vessels, and fat and the presentation in the frontal view [8].

Lymph nodes (LN). Outside the mediastinum the better spatial resolution of TCT is advantageous in the detection of lymph node enlargement. On the other hand, NMR provides for the better distinction between LN and blood vessels. So in general, each method gives similar results but they are complementary [5, 21]. Differentiation between inflammation and malignant infiltration is not yet possible with NMR because of a lack of spatial resolution.

Kidney and adrenals. TCT is better in the detection, NMR in the staging [10, 17].

Pelvis. Other than the prostate and the bladder, there is in most cases no clearly proven advantage [1].

Mamma. With the special mamma spool, NMR has high spatial resolution and is able to differentiate reliably between fatty degeneration and cysts. Solid tumors cannot be differentiated through T1/T2 alone. Differentiation is possible when shape and contour are also considered. Yet the results are not clearly better than with the mammography. More experience is needed [7].

NMR is of less value in the pancreas and lung. Alone it has brought inferior results so far, although it has been complementary in some cases [12, 20].

Our Own Results in Liver Tumors

Up to now, it has been difficult to define the ultimate value of NMR, because the number of patients with one single diagnostic problem or TU examined by NMR is low. Therefore, most papers can report only initial experiences. Our own experience with 145 patients with 169 liver tumors can serve as an example for the possibilities and shortcomings of NMR in TU diagnosis.

A total of 95% of the TU could be clearly detected. Extent, configuration, origin, and spread to neighboring structures were shown clearly, although our NMR device used for this study was a prototype resistive magnet of only 0.2-T field strength and had a pixel size of 3.5×3.5 mm. In contrast to TCT, there were no streak artifacts obscuring the left lobe of the liver and the dome. The impact on larger vessels could be shown more clearly. Contrast in most cases was superior. Only 5 cases of focal nodular hyperplasia (FNH) could not be detected, due to the fact that there was no contrast between the benign liver-like tissue of FNH and the normal liver tissue. With the better spatial resolution, as is provided for by the new superconducting machines which allow for the detection of small capsules or distortion of even smaller blood vessels, we would have probably detected them.

To analyse the reliability of tissue typing, we calculated T1 and T2 in all tumors with a diameter of more than 2 cm, classified them into the five clinically important groups and analysed them statistically [11, 18]. The results are graphically shown in the Figs. 5 and 6. A significant overlap between the enti-

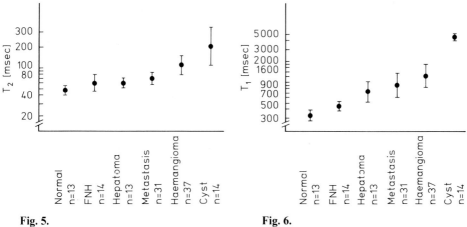

Fig. 5.   **Fig. 6.**

Table 1. Classification of 109 tumors with a diameter of more than 2 cm in the liver by T1 and T2

	Number of tumors		
	Correct	False	Total
Cyst	13	1	14
Hemangioma	24	13	37
Malign TU	41	3	44
FNH	5	9	14
Total (%)	83 (76)	26 (24)	109 (100)

FNH, focal nodular hyperplasia

Table 2. Classification of 93 patients with tumors in the liver through qualitative parameters (see text)

	Number of patients			
	Correct	Equivocal	False	Total
Cyst	12	–	–	12
Hemangioma	25	3	–	28
Malign TU	37	3	1	41
FNH	7	5	–	12
Total (%)	81 (87)	11 (12)	1 (1)	93 (100)

FNH, focal nodular hyperplasia

ties can be seen. All of them except the FNH have a clearly prolonged T1 compared to normal liver tissue. This explains the good detectability with T1-weighted pulse sequences. To differentiate TU type T2, weighted pulse sequences were also necessary.

If TU type is classified only by T1/T2, the results shown in Table 1 are received. In only 76% of tumors could the type be correctly determined. If we classify the tumors qualitatively, we obtain the results shown in Table 2. We estimated T1 and T2 on the basis of 4 different pulse sequences, and considered such factors as shape, homogeneity, contour, and multiplicity. In this way we were able to reliably differentiate among tumor types in an astonishingly high number of cases. In only one case was the classification clearly wrong: in 11 cases the classification was equivocal; in 87% of the cases, however, the classification was correct.

Our results obtained through the analysis of 145 patients with 169 liver tumors show that the presentation is characteristic enough to classify tumor type reliably. It can thus be used in clinical practice. This is in contrast to some of the experience of others with a smaller number of patients [6, 12−14, 22]. With a more exact calculation of T1/T2 than was possible with our device, even better results should be obtainable. Some of the latest literature supports our results and conclusions [9, 14]. It can be assumed that with more experience similar results will be obtained in other parts of the body stem. Intravenous contrast enhancement in NMR might bring further improvement in tumor-type differentiation. It has already been used successfully in brain tumors.

Summary

NMR is a unique noninvasive imaging modality with a very high contrast resolution; direct imaging in multiple planes and tissue typing are possible. TCT artifacts are absent. However, the technology used so far has the following disadvantages when the body stem is imaged: less spatial resolution, image degradation through respiratory and cardiac motion, and long imaging time. Stronger magnetic fields, the use of surface coils, and respiratory and cardiac gating will improve image quality without necessitating a prolongation of imaging time. Another disadvantage is the lack of widespread experience and general availability. Thus, NMR of the body stem has not yet become a routine method of choice in most diagnostic situations.

However, it can provide additional information when TCT or US are not sufficient. In the diagnosis of the nasopharynx region and in cardiac, prostata, bladder, and bone tumors it is superior to TCT and could already be used prior to, or instead of, TCT at this stage. In addition to the developments already mentioned, there are other advantages that will be gained through the use of intravenous contrast enhancement and through the separate display of the water-bound and the fatty-acid-bound protons.

It is highly likely that in the future due to its unique diagnostic possibilities NMR will replace or complement TCT examination for a large number of problems despite the high cost and complicated technology.

References

1. Bies JR, Ellis JH, Kopecky KK, Sutton GP, Klatte EC, Stehman FB, Ehrlich CE (1984) Assessment of primary gynecologic malignancies: Comparison of 0.15-T resistive magnetic resonance imaging with CT. AJR 143:1249–1257
2. Brady JT, Rosen BR, Pykett IL, McGuire MH, Mankin HJ, Rosenthal DI (1983) Nuclear magnetic resonance imaging of leg tumors. Radiology 149:181–187
3. Cohen MD, Klatte EC, Baehner R, Smith JA, Martin-Simmerman P, Carr BE, Provisor AJ, Weetman RM, Coates T, Siddiqui A, Weisman SJ, Berkow R, McKenna S, McGuire WA (1984) Magnetic resonance imaging of marrow disease in children. Radiology 151:715–718
4. Dillon WP, Mills CM, Kjos B, DeGroot J, Brant-Zawadzki M (1984) Magnetic resonance imaging of the nasopharynx. Radiology 152:731–738
5. Dooms GC, Hricak H, Crooks LE, Higgins CB (1984) Magnetic resonance imaging of the lymph nodes: Comparison with CT. Radiology 153:719–728
6. Doyle FH, Pennock JM, Banks LM, McDonnell MJ, Bydder GM, Steiner RE, Young IR, Clarke GJ, Pasmore T, Gilderdale DJ (1982) Nuclear magnetic resonance imaging of the liver: Initial experience. AJR 138:193–200
7. El Yousef SJ, Duchesneau RH, Alfidi RJ, Haaga RJ, Bryan PJ, LiPuma JP (1984) Magnetic resonance of the breast. Work in Progress. Radiology 150:761–766
8. Gamsu G, Stark DD, Webb WR, Moore EH, Sheldon PE (1984) Magnetic resonance imaging of benign mediastinal masses. Radiology 151:709–713
9. Glazer GM, Aisen AM, Francis IR, Gyves JW, Lande I, Adler DD (1985) Hepatic cavernous hemangioma: Magnetic resonance imaging. Radiology 155:417–420
10. Hricak H, Demas BE, Williams RD, McNamara MT, Hedgcock MW, Amparo EG, Tanagho EA (1985) Magnetic resonance imaging in the diagnosis and staging of renal and perirenal neoplasms. Radiology 154:709–715
11. Kotzerke J (1984) Die Bedeutung der Kernspinotomographie für die Differentialdiagnose bei raumfordernden Prozessen der Leber. Dissertation, Hanover
12. Kressel HY, Axel L, Thickman D, Alavi A, Pollack H, Arger P, Edelstein W, Bottomley P, Redington R, Baum S (1983) NMR imaging of the abdomen at 0.12 T: Initial clinical experience with a resistive magnet. AJR 141:1179–1186
13. Moss AA, Goldberg HI, Stark DB, Davis PL, Margulis AR, Kaufman L, Crooks LE (1984) Hepatic tumors: Magnetic resonance and CT appearance. Radiology 150:141–147
14. Ohtomo K, Itai Y, Furui S, Yashiro N, Yoshikawa K, Iio M (1985) Hepatic tumors: Differentiation by transverse relaxation time (T2) of magnetic resonance imaging. Radiology 155:421–423
15. Paushter DM, Modic MT, Borkowski GP, Weinstein MA, Zeman RK (1984) Magnetic resonance. Principles and applications. Med Clin North Am 68:1393–1421
16. Poon PY, McCallum RW, Henkelman NM, Bronskill MJ, Sutcliffe SB, Jewett MAS, Rider WD, Bruce AW (1985) Magnetic resonance imaging of the prostate. Radiology 154:143–149
17. Schultz CL, Haaga JR, Fletcher BD, Alfidi RJ, Schultz MA (1984) Magnetic resonance imaging of the adrenal glands: A comparison with CT. AJR 143:1235–1240
18. Schwarzrock R, Kotzerke J, Hundeshagen H, Tiffe HW (1984) Die Wertigkeit der NMR-Tomographie bei der Differentialdiagnostik von Lebertumoren. In: Höfer R, Bergmann H (eds) Radioisotope in Klinik und Forschung, vol 16/2. Gasteiner Internationales Symposium 1984, pp 727–734. Eggermann, Vienna
19. Smith FW, Mallard JR (1984) NMR imaging in liver disease. Br Med Bull 40:194–196
20. Stark DD, Moss AA, Goldberg HI, Davis PL, Federle MP (1984) Magnetic resonance and CT of the normal and diseased pancreas: A comparative study. Radiology 150:153–162
21. Stark DD, Moss AA, Gamsu G, Clark OH, Gooding GAW, Webb WR (1984) Magnetic resonance imaging of the neck. Part II: Pathologic findings. Radiology 150:454–461
22. Steiner RE, Bydder GM (1984) Nuclear magnetic resonance in gastroenterology. Clin Gastroenterol 13:265–279
23. Tiffe HW, Hagemann H, Schwarzrock R, Jordan K, Hundeshagen H (1984) Vermeidung von Bewegungsartefakten in KST-Bildern durch atem- und herzsynchrone Datenerfassung. In: Schmidt T (ed) Medizinische Physik 1984. Nuernberg, pp 487–490

NMR In Vivo Spectroscopy in Tumor Diagnosis

V. R. McCready[1], P. A. Hammersley, M. O. Leach, and J. Griffiths

Introduction

Although most interest in nuclear magnetic resonance (NMR) centres around its imaging capability, the technique was originally used in the laboratory to determine the relative concentrations of metabolites and intracellular pH. Subsequently, in vivo studies in animals demonstrated that it could be used to study metabolism of muscle, various organs and tumours. Its noninvasiveness and lack of radiation hazard has led to its introduction into clinical practice, especially for the study of muscle disorders. It is now hoped that the technique will also be of value in the monitoring of tumour response to drug therapy. This has been made possible by the introduction of higher strength magnets in which the whole body or limbs can be placed.

Principle

Although in theory any nucleus with an odd number of protons or neutrons can be studied by nuclear magnetic resonance, e.g. ^1H, ^{13}C and ^{17}O, in practice only ^1H and ^{31}P have been the subject of any detailed research in vivo. The sensitivity for detection is related both to the natural abundance and the NMR characteristics. Protons (^1H) have the highest sensitivity and therefore are used for NMR imaging. However, there are a vast number of hydrogen-containing molecules, and so it is difficult to distinguish one from another, especially in the presence of high concentrations of water and fat. Of more interest is ^{31}P, which occurs in fewer sites in biological molecules and so produces fewer, but more resolvable, spectral lines.

Technique

The technique of NMR spectroscopy is rather complicated, as indeed is NMR imaging. However, it can be simplified sufficiently to explain the results obtained in clinical practice.

---

1 The Royal Marsden Hospital, London & Surrey, Dept. of Nuclear Medicine, Downs Road Sutton, Surrey SM2 5PT, UK

Nuclear Medicine in Clinical Oncology
Ed. by C. Winkler
© Springer-Verlag Berlin Heidelberg 1986

Nuclei with angular momentum ("spin") can be considered as small bar magnets. These magnets line up when placed in a uniform magnetic field. Each nucleus spins in the magnetic field rather like a top with a resonant frequency dependent both on the magnetic field strength of the magnet and on the particular molecule to which the nucleus is bound. The nucleus can absorb and emit electromagnetic radiation at this resonant frequency, which is in the radio frequency (RF) user band. The nuclei can be excited by a pulse of RF radiation and this will stimulate a measurable RF signal at the same frequency.

By analysing the returning signal into its separate frequencies, it is possible to display the presence of molecules that contain the particular element under study. In the case of phosphorus, this includes compounds such as adenosine triphosphate (ATP), phosphocreatine (PCr), inorganic phosphate (Pi) etc. The radio frequency is transmitted and recieved through a surface coil; in the case of the following experiments this lies on the surface of the skin close to the tumor under examination.

Tumor Metabolism

It is fortunate that the spectra obtainable from phosphorus-containing molecules can yield information concerning the metabolic state of tumor. This is because ATP is the energy source for a range of biochemical reactions. Under conditions where ATP concentration is diminished, it may be replenished from the high-energy phosphate source, phosphocreatine.

Thus,

$$\begin{array}{rl} ATP & \rightarrow ADP + Pi \\ PCr + ADP & \rightarrow ATP + Cr \\ \hline PCr & \rightarrow Cr \quad + Pi \end{array}$$

So the overall result is the conversion of PCr to Pi. This ratio can be measured from the NMR spectrum. Growing tumors are often hypoxic, the cells deriving their energy by anaerobic glycolysis. To compensate for the lesser efficiency of this pathway, the tumor cells convert ADP to ATP using PCr. This results in a decrease in PCr intensity and an increase in the Pi peak of the NMR spectrum. Confirmation of this has been seen in enlarging tumors, where the PCr peak decreases and the Pi peak increases.

Similar results found in a human rhabdomyosarcoma have been published elsewhere [1]. The authors showed that when chemotherapy was unsuccessful in controlling tumor growth the PCr peak diminished in height. Our present studies concern the effect of chemotherapy on animal tumors and the possible application of the results to the human situation.

NMR Studies on Animal Tumors

We have obtained NMR spectra from mouse tumors using surface coils. The spectra were measured at 32 MHz in an Oxford Instruments TMR 32 spec-

trometer using 8-µs pulses with a 2-s repetition time. Usually 500−1000 scans
are obtained and the mice are anaesthetised with Nembutal during the
measurements.

Results

A typical spectrum from a mouse transplantable tumor (PM sarcoma) is shown
in Fig. 1. This tumor has a doubling time of approximately 2.5 days, and all the
tumors examined histologically show necrotic centres and other foci of cell
death.

However, in general the tumor is well vascularised. The spectrum in Fig. 1
shows strong ATP, Pi and monophosphate (MP) peaks.

More typical of this type of tumor and showing a greater degree of necrosis
is the spectrum seen in Fig. 2. This shows a strong Pi peak with reduced MP
and ATP peaks. Note, however, that there is still a strong PCr peak. With
further necrosis (Fig. 3) the spectrum demonstrates an intense Pi peak, whereas
the other ATP and monophosphate peaks are minimal.

Similar studies were carried out on a plasmacytoma (ADJ/PC6) transplanted mouse tumor. This is well vascularised with a doubling time of 2.6 days. The
tumor only rarely shows gross necrosis, although histologically some individual
dead cells may sometimes be seen. A typical NMR spectrum from this tumor is
shown in Fig. 4. It is characterised by strong MP and ATP peaks and less intense peaks for Pi and PCr.

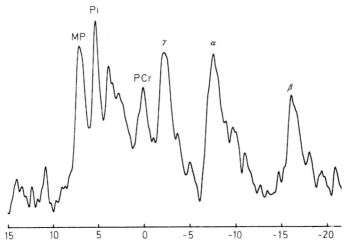

Fig. 1. PM sarcoma − typical spectrum. This spectrum of well-vascularised tumor with little
sign of necrosis shows strong ATP (α, β, γ) peaks, a low PCr, and clear Pi and monophosphate
(*MP*) peaks

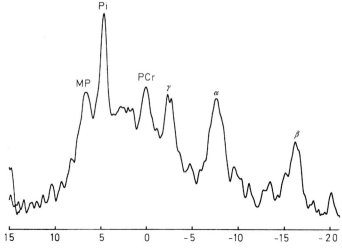

Fig. 2. PM sarcoma necrotic. As the tumor grows, more necrosis appears. The ATP peaks are smaller, the PCr and MP peaks are smaller while the Pi peak rises

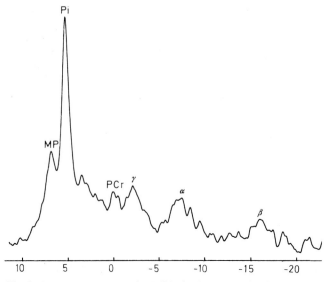

Fig. 3. PM sarcoma necrotic. With further necrosis the ATP peaks and PCr become even smaller while the Pi peak grows

Effect of Chemotherapy

A single dose of 200 mg/kg cytosine arabinoside (Ara-C) is known to shut off DNA synthesis completely. The NMR spectrum (Fig. 5) from a PC-6 tumor shows that 1½ h after administration of the drug all ATP and PCr peaks are greatly reduced. The MP and Pi peaks remain strong.

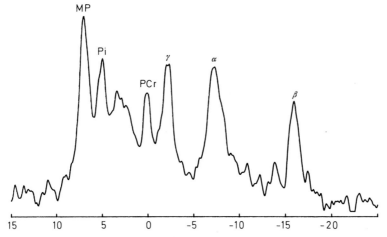

Fig. 4 PC-6 plasmacytoma – typical spectrum. This tumor rarely shows necrosis. The ATP peaks are prominent while the PCr and Pi peaks are small

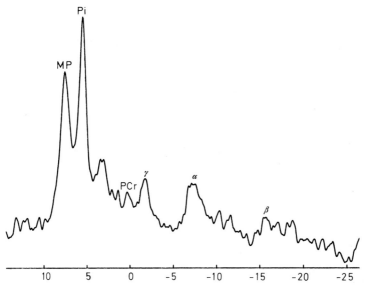

Fig. 5. PC-6 plasma 1.5 h after cytosine arabinoside. After a lethal dose of Ara-C the ATP and PCr peaks are greatly reduced while the Pi peak increases

Three days after Ara-C (Fig. 6), the Pi peak is reduced to normal and the ATP peaks are stronger, which suggests renewed cell growth. Similar results were also found in the PM sarcoma.

The dramatic increase in Pi shortly after Ara-C may be transient since it was not always observed. However, it may be noted that PCr was almost zero both immediately after administration of the drug and 3 days later.

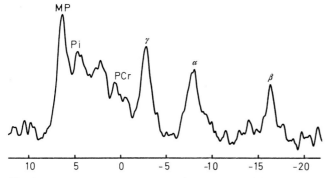

Fig. 6. PC-6 plasmacytoma 3 days after cytosine arabinoside. After 3 days the ATP peaks reappear, while the PCr and Pi diminish in height indicates return of metabolism

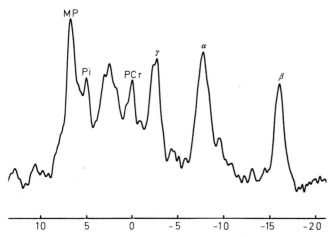

Fig. 7. PC-6 histologically dead. Although histologically dead, this tumor spectrum shows strong ATP peaks. The Pi and PCr peaks are smaller. This result could be explained by the presence of macrophages or of normal tissue in the sensitive volume

The results of chemotherapy are not always clear. A single dose of 20 mg/kg cyclophosphamide produces regression of the PC-6 tumor. NMR spectra from the PC-6 tumor taken 3 days after this therapy (Fig. 7) showed strong ATP peaks, although histologically the tumor consisted of dead cells. It could be that macrophages move in rapidly and that the spectrum reflects their presence, or more likely that the sensitive volume of the surface coil includes normal tissue.

The results are summarised in Fig. 8 for the PM sarcoma and Fig. 9 for the PC6. These show that ^{31}P NMR spectroscopy can be a useful technique for assessing the metabolic state of tumors. In particular, the Pi/PCr and MP/PCr ratios are good indicators of the presence of tumor necrosis and thus of the effectiveness of chemotherapy.

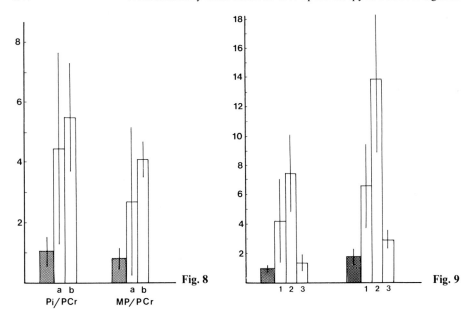

Fig. 8. PM sarcoma – Pi/PCr and MP/PCr ratios. This histogram shows the Pi/PCr ratios in control animals (*hatched*), necrotic tumors (*a*) and 2 h following cytosine arabinoside (*b*). The Pi/Cr ratio increases with necrosis and effective chemotherapy

Fig. 9. PC-6 plasmacytoma. Pi/PCr ratios (*left*) and MP/PCr ratios (*right*). Pi/PCr ratios in control animals (*hatched*), 2 h (*1*) and 3 days (*2*) following cytosine arabinoside show an increasing ratio as the tumor dies. 3 days following an injection of 20 mg/kg cyclophosphamide (*3*) both Pi/Cr and MP/PCr ratios are close to normal, which may reflect the inclusion of normal tissue or perhaps an increase in the macrophage content

Conclusion

In conclusion, the fact that this noninvasive technique can be used to monitor animal tumors encourages optimism for its use in the human situation. Until now our experiments have been limited to tumors involving limbs which could be placed in the available small-bore magnets. However, the whole-body magnets should greatly facilitate the study of tumors in other parts of the body, and this technique can be used to monitor the effects of chemotherapy at a much earlier stage than has been possible previously.

Reference

1. Griffiths JR, Cady E, Edwards RHT, McCready VR, Wilkie FR, Wiltshaw E (1983) ^{31}P NMR studies of a human tumor in situ (letter). Lancet, 18th June 1983

VI. Positron Emission Tomography

Production and Use of Positron-Emitting Test Substances for Tumor Diagnosis

W. H. KNAPP[1]

Introduction

New therapeutic regimes like combinations of radio- or chemotherapy with hyperthermia have given rise to growing interest in methods for the in vivo assessment of tumor physiology and metabolism [1]. These methods usually require the use of radioactive compounds which undergo well-defined processes in the organism. Therefore, the attempt to monitor biologic properties of tumors necessitates considering organic radiopharmaceuticals and, in particular, positron emitters. This paper deals with the application of organic radioagents for the assessment of microcirculation and cellular integrity in tumors, and for therapeutic research.

Radioagents

The precursors for synthesis of positron-emitting organic compounds were produced with the 21.0 MeV German Cancer Research Compact Cyclotron. $^{11}C-CO_2$ was produced via the ^{14}N (p, α) ^{11}C reaction by irradiation of pure nitrogen gas with 14.0 MeV (the incident proton energy is reduced by the target material which consists of 1.1 mm aluminium foil). With a beam current of $15-20\ \mu A$ and an irradiation time of $30-40$ min $700-900$ mCi $^{11}CO_2$ were produced. NH_3 was another precursor used; it was produced via the ^{16}O (p, α) ^{13}N reaction. For a 15-min irradiation with a beam current of $10\ \mu A$, typical yields were approximately 100 mCi $^{13}NH_3$.

Two labeled organic compounds were used for injection in humans or animals. ^{11}C-butanol was employed for regional blood flow imaging [2] and ^{13}N-glutamate for the assessment of metabolic substrate uptake. The synthesis of $(1-^{11}C)$-butanol was based on the carboxylation of N-propylmagnesium chloride with $^{11}CO_2$ and subsequent reduction of the resulting free $(1-^{11}C)$ butyric acid with $LiAlH_4$ dissolved in anhydrous ether [3]. ^{13}N-L-glutamate was enzymatically produced by converting α-ketoglurate in a buffered solution of $^{13}N_3$ (pH $7.5-8.0$) with glutamic acid dehydrogenase [4].

1 Deutsches Krebsforschungszentrum, Institut für Nuklearmedizin,
  Im Neuenheimer Feld 280, D-6900 Heidelberg 1
Present address: Institut für Nuklearmedizin, Herzzentrum NRW, D-4970 Bad Oeynhausen

Nuclear Medicine in Clinical Oncology
Ed. by C. Winkler
© Springer-Verlag Berlin Heidelberg 1986

With these radioagents the following questions were pursued:

1. Does the amino acid uptake correlate with the degree of malignancy in different processes?
2. Is the uptake governed by perfusion or by tissue transport and/or metabolism?
3. Is separate monitoring of effects of chemo- and radiotherapy on tumor blood flow and metabolism achievable?
4. Do the methods promote the realization of new therapeutic concepts?

Results

1. Five different homologous tumor lines were implanted in one hind leg of 25 rats. ^{13}N-glutamate uptake of tumors was related to that of muscle. This relationship was 6.2 ± 1.7 (SD) in the most rapidly growing and metastasizing tumor line (adenocarcinoma), whereas a neurogenic sarcoma (nonmetastasizing and slowly growing) showed an average ratio of 2.5. ± 0.5. Five rats with fractured tibiae showed lesion-to-muscle uptake ratios of 1.7. ± 0.3. Clinical data were obtained in 40 patients having untreated and treated malignant and benign processes. The tumor-to-muscle uptake ratio ranged from 2.8 ± 12.0 in untreated malignant tumors ($n = 18$), from 1.3 − 3.2 in tumors treated < 2 weeks ($n = 10$), from 2.0 − 8.0 in metastases ($n = 3$) and from 1.0 − 3.5 in benign bone lesions. Clinical and experimental data suggest that ^{13}N-glutamate uptake reflects the degree of proliferative activity.

2. ^{13}N-glutamate uptake was correlated with that of ^{121}I-microspheres ($n = 10$) and with that of ^{11}C-butanol ($n = 24$) resulting in $r = 0.88$ and $r = 0.98$ respectively. In nine patients with untreated processes ^{13}N-glutamate uptake was correlated with that of ^{201}Tl resulting in $r = 0.97$ ($y = 0.33 ± 0.98 x$). Thus, ^{13}N-glutamate uptake in untreated tumors reflects perfusion (flow-limited uptake).

3. Investigations in 92 cases were based on subsequent i.v. injections of 1 − 5 mCi ^{13}N-glutamate and ^{11}C-butanol in 38 rats bearing Walker carcinomas in the hind leg. Before irradiation, the ^{13}N-glutamate tumor-to muscle uptake averaged 4.30 ± 0.66 (SEM, $n = 14$), 30 min after a single dose of 800 rd 3.06 ± 0.36 and 2 days later 4.04 ± 0.67 ($n = 10$). The corresponding ^{11}C-butanol uptake values were 4.69 ± 0.75, 5.52 ± 0.89 and 5.40 ± 1.28. Before methotrexate (mtx) ^{13}N-glutamate uptake (tumor-to muscle was 6.43 ± 0.68 ($n = 20$), 1 h after 10 − 50 mg/kg mtx 3.43 ± 0.33 ($n = 9$), 4 h after mtx 3.53 ± 0.77 ($n = 11$) and 2 days later 1.20 ± 0.13 ($n = 5$). The corresponding ^{11}C-butanol values were 6.91 ± 0.76, 6.52 ± 0.87, 4.23 ± 0.89 and 1.16 ± 0.11. 4 mg/kg 5-hydroxytryptamine (5-HT) i.p. [5] produced immediate reduction (10 min p.i.) of ^{13}N-glutamate and ^{11}C-butanol by 64 ± 19% (67 ± 19% respectively). The data show that radio- and chemotherapy change ^{13}N-glutamate uptake independently of flow. Flow limitation is turned into transport (or metabolic) limitation. The procedure allows the differentiation between indirect tumor response mediated by a reduction of blood flow (as exemplified with 5-HT) and direct action on the tumor cells.

4. The precondition for a therapeutic gain using hyperthermia is that the increment of tumor tissue temperature exceeds that of the surrounding normal tissue. In those tumors which cannot be heated selectively, it is assumed that tumor blood flow is as effective as that of the host tissue. Using ^{11}C-butanol as flow tracer, the effect of a calcium antagonist and a physiologic amine on tumor and muscle perfusion were investigated with the aim of improving the preconditions for external hyperthermia treatment of cancer. Nisoldipine (0.04−4.0 mg/kg) and 5-hydroxytryptamine (5-HT) (0.2−8.0 mg/kg) were administered i.p. in Sprague-Dawley rats bearing Walker 256 carcinoma, Yoshida sarcoma or a homologous tumor transplant derived from a spontaneous leiomyosarcoma of the uterus. Tumor-to-muscle uptake ratios of ^{11}C-butanol fell from 5.63 ± 1.98 to 3.32 ± 1.21 and from 5.3 ± 0.56 to 2.98 ± 0.30, after injection of 2.0 mg/kg nisoldipine and 4 mg/kg 5-HT, respectively. Similar reaction patterns and percentage changes were observed in different tumor lines at constant doses of 0.2 mg/kg nisoldipine and 4 mg/kg 5-HT. In eight rats bearing Walker carcinomas 2 mg/kg 5-HT caused an increase of tumor temperature from 41.2 ± 0.8 °C to 44.2 ± 1.3 °C by ultrasound at a constant temperature level of 41 °C within the surrounding normal tissue. By analogy, 0.2 mg/kg nisoldipine produced changes from 41.3 + 0.8 °C to 43.4 + 1.4 °C. Both drugs representing two different rationales of vasomotor action were able to reduce blood flow specifically in transplanted tumors; nisoldipine increased muscle blood flow and decreased arterial blood pressure, wheres 5-HT acted without substantial systemic effects. The methods designed to monitor these effects can be readily applied to transfer and validate this new therapeutic concept under clinical circumstances.

References

1. Reimann RE, Rosen G, Gelbard AS, Benua RS, Yeh SDJ, Laughlin JS (1985) Diagnostic demands in clinical and experimental oncology: application of substrates labeled with positron-emitting radionuclides. In: Knapp WH, Vyska K (eds) Tumor cell physiology and positron emission tomography. Springer, Berlin Heidelberg New York Tokyo, pp 73−85
2. Knapp WH, Helus F, Oberdorfer F, Layer K, Sinn HJ, Ostertag H, Matzku S (1985) ^{11}C-butanol for imaging of the blood-flow distribution in tumor-bearing animals. Eur J Nucl Med 10:540−548
3. Oberdorfer F, Helus F, Maier-Borst W et al (1982) The synthesis of (1-^{11}C)-butanol. Radiochem Radioanal Lett 53:237−252
4. Knapp WH, Helus F, Sinn H, Ostertag H, Georgi P, Brandeis W-E, Braun A (1984) ^{13}N-L-glutamate uptake in malignancy: its relationship to blood flow. J Nucl Med 25:989−997
5. Knapp WH, Debatin J, Layer K, Helus F, Altmann A, Sinn HJ, Ostertag H (1985) Selective drug-induced reduction of blood flow in tumor transplants. Int J Radiat Oncol Biol Phys 11:1357−1366

Uptake of ^{11}C-Aminocyclopentane Carboxylic Acid (ACPC) and ^{13}N-Ammonia in Malignant Tumors A Comparative Clinical Study

K. Schelstraete[1], K. De Vis, F. L. Vermeulen, J. Deman, J. Sambre, P. Goethals, D. Van Haver, G. Slegers, C. Vandecasteele, and A. De Schryver

Introduction

Positron emission tomography (PET) can be used advantageously in oncological patients to study the in vivo biochemical properties in tumors and to monitor their metabolic response to therapy [1]. Among the potential agents which are available for this purpose are ^{11}C-aminocyclopentane carboxylic acid or ACPC (a non-metabolized amino acid) and ^{13}N-ammonia, both of which show tumor affinity in humans [2 – 5].

After intravenous injection, ^{13}N-ammonia is cleared from the vascular compartment very rapidly, with only 1.4% remaining in the circulation after 200 s [6]. In the cells, ^{13}N-ammonia is converted into glutamine, a key intermediate product of nitrogen metabolism. Since most of the tissue uptake of [13]NH$_3$ results from first-pass extraction, regional blood flow undoubtedly plays a major role in its tissue uptake.

ACPC is a non-natural alicyclic amino acid which, after its entrance into the cell, is neither metabolized nor incorporated into proteins [7, 8]. Although maximal tissue uptake of ACPC is reached early (within 5 min), activity in the circulating blood remains quite stable at about 20% of the dose during the first 20 min after i.v. injection [2]. Therefore, regional blood flow is not likely to be a decisive factor in its tissue accumulation.

The present work was initiated to investigate which one of these agents was superior as a tumor tracer, and whether the existence or absence of differences in the uptake of [13]NH$_3$ and ^{11}C-ACPC in normal and neoplastic tissues might provide some indications as to the mechanisms involved in their accumulation.

Materials and Method

Twenty-eight patients suffering from known neoplastic lesions of various types were examined with ^{13}N-ammonia and ^{11}C-ACPC successively, using PET (Ecat II). Both tracers were produced at the University of Ghent Cyclotron Unit [9, 10]. The first scan was started 2 min after i.v. injection of 5 – 26 mCi (185 – 962 MBq) [13]NH$_3$. After a 45-min interval, 6 – 27 mCi (222 – 999 MBq) ^{11}C-ACPC were injected intravenously, and imaging was started 5 min later.

---

1 Department of Radiotherapy and Nuclear Medicine, University Hospital, De Pintelaan 185, B-9000 Gent

Nuclear Medicine in Clinical Oncology
Ed. by C. Winkler
© Springer-Verlag Berlin Heidelberg 1986

Since the patient's position remained unchanged during the entire procedure, a regional comparison of the two scans was possible.

To take full advantage of the potentials of PET, the tracer uptake in tumors and in assumedly normal tissues was calculated in absolute values, concentrations being expressed as a fraction of the injected dose per cm³ tissue (FID/cm³).

Results and Discussion

Overall, a parallelism was found between the 2 tracers as to their uptake in a given tumor, although the ACPC concentration was often higher. Highest ACPC uptakes were found in sarcomas and in cancer of the breast, with typical values for breast cancer ranging from 2.49 to 5.56 × 10⁻⁵ FID/cm³ and from 2.98 to 4.70 × 10⁻⁵ FID/cm³ for sarcomas. In normal tissues, the ACPC concentration was either lower than, or at most nearly equal to, ammonia uptake. However, this advantage was somewhat offset by the high ACPC activity in the circulating blood, whereas ammonia levels were extremely low (Fig. 1). Regional particularities of tracer concentration in normal tissue surrounding a cancer may have important consequences. For instance, the high uptake of ^{13}NH$_3$ in the normal brain may mask intracerebral lesions, whereas with ACPC a high tumor to non-tumor ratio is observed due to the low concentration of ACPC in the normal brain (Fig. 2).

At the thoracic level, the high ACPC blood activity interferes with the interpretation of lesions close to large blood pools, e.g. the mediastinum. Conversely, because of its very rapid clearance from the blood, ammonia is superior to visualize (juxta)mediastinal tumors.

Breast cancer was more evident with ACPC than with NH$_3$ for 2 reasons: higher ACPC levels in the tumor and lower ACPC concentration in adjacent organs, such as the lungs, myocardium and liver (Fig. 3).

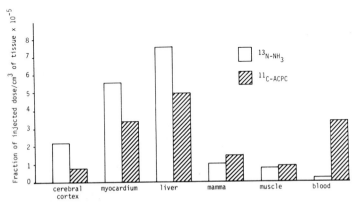

Fig. 1. Comparative concentration of ^{13}NH$_3$ and ^{11}C-ACPC in some normal organs and in the circulating blood

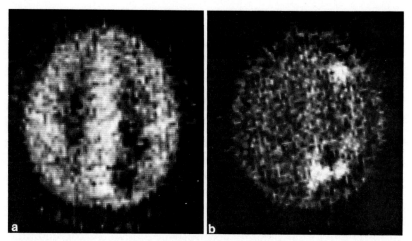

Fig. 2a, b. Cerebral metastases of breast cancer. **a** On the $^{13}NH_3$ scan the lesions are masked by high tracer uptake in the normal cerebral cortex. **b** With ^{11}C-ACPC, metastases are clearly visible in the frontal and occipital region, whereas ^{11}C-ACPC concentration in normal brain is low. In the occipital lesion a central necrotic area can be seen

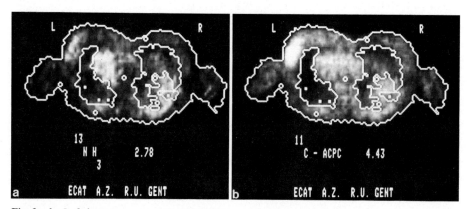

Fig. 3a, b. Left breast cancer. **a** On the $^{13}NH_3$ scan the tumor can be recognized but contrast is poor due to the relatively high tracer activity in the myocardium and liver dome. Absolute ammonia uptake in the tumor reached 2.78×10^{-5} of the injected dose (FID) per cm^3. **b** Same scan with ^{11}C-ACPC. Tumor contrast is better due both to higher absolute tracer concentration in the tumor (4.4×10^{-5} FID/cm^3) and lower activity in liver and lungs. The myocardium is not outlined, but the activity in the cardiac blood pool is rather high

In analogy to what has already been published for ^{13}N-glutamate [11], changes in the accumulation of ^{11}C-ACPC most probably may be used to follow a tumor's metabolic response to treatment.

As to the mechanisms involved in ACPC and NH_3 accumulation, speculations revolve around some differences which can be observed in their uptake. For instance, in normal lung tissue, ammonia uptake was much higher in patients who had received chemotherapy or radiation treatment involving the thoracic area. Under the same circumstances, only a slight tendency towards increase of ACPC was noticed. This observation suggests that non-specific changes, such as of blood flow or capillary permeability, play only a minor role in ACPC uptake. Furthermore, since ACPC levels do not reach the blood concentration in some well-perfused organs, such as the brain and the myocardium, and since the uptake of ACPC in tumors ranges from levels below to levels above the blood concentration, tumor cells seem to be able to selectively control the entrance of ACPC.

As to NH_3, the conclusion was reached in a previous paper that the accumulation of ammonia by tumors is to be regarded as the result of a complex interaction of regional blood flow and metabolic influences at the cellular level [4, 5].

Conclusion

As a rule, ^{11}C-ACPC is superior to $^{13}NH_3$ as a tumor tracer because of both is higher accumulation in many neoplastic lesions and its lower uptake in non-tumorous tissues, its only disadvantage being a slower clearance from the blood.

There is some evidence that tumor cells can selectively control their uptake of ^{11}C-ACPC. We feel that it is a promising tool for the monitoring with PET of therapy-induced changes in the metabolic behaviour of tumors.

References

1. Beaney RP (1984) Positron emission tomography in the study of human tumors. Semin Nucl Med 14:324−341
2. Hübner KF, Andrews GA, Washburn L, et al. (1977) Tumor location with 1-amino-cyclopentane (^{11}C) carboxylic acid: preliminary clinical trials with single-photon detection. J Nucl Med 18:1215−1221
3. Hübner KF, Strauss S, Washburn LC, et al. (1981) Tumor detection with 1-amino-cyclopentane and 1-aminocyclopentane C-11-carboxylic acid using positron emission computerized tomography. Clin Nucl Med 6:249−252
4. Schelstraete K, Simons M, Deman J, et al. (1982) Uptake of ^{13}N-ammonia by human tumours as studied by positron emission tomography. Br J Radiol 55:797−804
5. Schelstraete K, Deman J, Vermeulen FL, et al. (1985) Kinetics of ^{13}N-ammonia incorporation in human tumours. Nucl Med Comm 6:461−470
6. Phelps ME, Hoffman EJ, Huang S-C, et al. (1976) Tomographic images of blood pool and perfusion in brain and heart. J Nucl Med 17:603−612
7. Berlinguet L, Bégin N, Babineau LM (1962) Autoradiographic studies of distribution of 1-aminocyclopentane carboxylic acid in normal and cancerous mice. Can J Biochem 40:1111−1114
8. Sterling WR, Henderson JF, Mandel HG, et al. (1962) The metabolism of 1-amino-cyclopentane-carboxylic acid in normal and neoplastic tissues. Biochem Pharmacol 11:135−145
9. Slegers G, Vandecasteele C, Sambre J (1980) Cyclotron production of ^{13}N-labelled ammonia for medical use. J Radioanal Chem 59:585−587
10. Sambre J, Vandecasteele C, Goethals P, et al. (1985) Routine production of H^{11}CN and (^{11}C)-1-aminocyclopentane carboxylic acid. Int J Appl Radiot Isot 36:275−278
11. Reiman RE, Huvos AG, Benua RS, et al. (1981) Quotient imaging with N-13 1-Glutamate in osteogenic sarcoma: correlation with tumor viability. Cancer 48:1976−1981

Analysis of Brain Tumor Physiology by Positron Emission Tomography

O. Schober[1] and G.-J. Meyer

Malignant tumors are generally characterized by uncontrolled cell proliferation. The increased metabolic activity of neoplasms has been proven by in vitro studies and by in vivo administration of radiotracers to animals bearing various kinds of tumors followed by quantitative autoradiography. However, the results from in vitro studies and from animal experiments with chemically, virally or by transplantation induced tumors may not be applicable to tumor physiology in man. Consequently the increased metabolic activity of rapidly growing tissue has become a target for measurements with positron emission tomography (PET), which has been proven to be a sensitive tool for the assessment of local brain function in both, normal and pathological states.

A positive correlation was found between 2-^{18}F-2-deoxy-D-glucose (^{18}FDG) uptake and the histological grade of gliomas. This finding is interpreted as an enhanced rate of glycolysis in fast growing neoplasms. According to Di Chiro [4], in a number of cases the FDG-PET method has eventually proven to be more accurate than biopsy.

The anaerobic metabolic pathway was further substantiated by the finding that tumor regional cerebral blood flow, as measured by the $C^{15}O_2$ inhalation technique, is comparable to that of the contralateral cortex, whereas regional $^{15}O_2$ consumption on the tumor region is markedly depressed [8, 9]. Thus PET has provided a quantitative measurement of the energy demand of carcinogenic processes and the mechanism of its satisfaction.

Recently attempts have been made by Phelps et al. [12] and Bustany et al. [3] to set up quantitative kinetic models for the determination of protein synthesis in brain tissue. However, because of the complexicity of the physiologic models, metabolic turnover rates for brain protein synthesis have not been determined quantitatively up to now. Furthermore the models rely on an intact blood brain barrier and are therefore not directly applicable to protein synthesis rates in tumors.

For the quantification of metabolic processes in brain tumors and other brain disorders by PET measurements, a major difficulty stems from the uncertaincy of uptake contribution due to blood brain barrier (BBB) damage. Measurements with ^{68}Ga-EDTA and ^{82}Rb have clearly shown the possible use of these tracers for the localization of tumors with BBB disruption. While these early findings are very similar to the results obtainable by contrast enhanced CT imaging, a quantitative analysis of the BBB leak rate which varies signifi-

---

1 Medizinische Hochschule Hannover, D-3000 Hannover

Nuclear Medicine in Clinical Oncology
Ed. by C. Winkler
© Springer-Verlag Berlin Heidelberg 1986

cantly in different types of tumors and with their grade of malignancy is highly desirable. The use of different tracers, which are not metabolized but enter the brain by defined transport mechanisms as, e.g., 3-^{18}F-2'-deoxyglucose, ^{11}C-methylglucose, or non-natural synthetic amino acids, may allow a quantification of the diffusive contribution to the uptake and a more detailed analysis of various degrees of BBB damage.

The additional limitations which are imposed on the measurement of protein synthesis rates in tumors may then be overcome. However, if it can be shown that the diffusive uptake via BBB leakage is relatively slow compared with the active metabolic processes under study, an approximate measurement of protein synthesis rates may be obtainable even without such correction terms.

As long as accurate models and procedures for the quantification of protein synthesis rates in tumors are not available, simple uptake ratios of amino acids in tumor to non-tumor tissue may prove usefull for both, the semiquantitative understanding of the biochemical process in vivo and the clinical need for differential diagnosis.

Hübner et al. [5] have used ^{11}C-labelled D,L-valine, D,L-tryptophane, and D,L-1-aminocyclohexane-carboxylic acid (D,L-ACHC) to image brain tumors. The uptake contribution by BBB damage in these studies was not evaluated, however, Bergström et al. [2] demonstrated discrepancies in a brain tumor extent as determined by CT and PET using ^{68}Ga-EDTA, ^{11}C-glucose, and ^{11}C-L-methionine, thereby showing a limited influence of BBB damage on the amino acid accumulation. New results of this group, transmitted to us by private communication, corroborate this finding. Our very recent results show a clear uptake defect of ^{11}C-L-methionine in stroke patients with a proven BBB damage at least for the first half hour p.i. This also corroborates the hypothesis of a minor influence of a BBB damage, especially in view of the results of Barrio and Phelps (1985), who reported a very fast uptake of ^{11}C-L-leucine in brain tumors which gave high contrast images already after 5−10 min p.i.

In our own PET investigation on brain tumors [13, 10] ^{11}C-L-and D-methionine were chosen as the amino acid because it is known from in vitro studies and from nutritional support that methionine exhibits the highest tumor to nontumor ratios in gliomas and metastatic brain tumors. In normal brain the uptake of methionine in single pass extraction measurements is quite high and is surpassed only by phenylalanine, leucine, and tyrosine [11]. When compared with other amino acids, the amount of free methionine in brain tissue is small. This indicates a high utilisation rate of methionine which should make it a suitable tracer for protein synthesis. A recent comparison of ten amino acids for tumor uptake in an animal model (rat hepatoma AH109A) confirmed the high uptake of methionine [7]. Finally the routine production of optically pure ^{11}C-labelled stereoisomeres imposed no problems.

Tomographic imaging was performed on 7 patients with brain tumors prior to surgery. None of the individuals had undergone radiation or chemotherapy before. Final verfication of the diagnosis and the grading of the tumors was obtained from histological data subsequent to surgery. The results are summarized in Table 1.

Table 1. Accumulation of ^{11}C-methionine in brain tumors

No.	Diagnosis	Tumor/contralateral non-tumor ratio		L/D ratio tumor	L/D ratio pancreas	BBB breakdown
		L	D			
1	Calcified microangioma	1.01	0.98	1.02	–	pos
2	Metastatic brain tumor (partly necrotic)	1.28	1.28	1.00	>3	pos
3	Astrocytoma grade II	1.40	1.30	1.08	>3	neg
4	Metastatic brain tumor	1.86	–	–	>1.5	–
5	Meningioma	1.88	1.50	1.25	–	–
6	Glioblastoma	–	1.82	–	–	–
7	Astrocytoma grade IV	2.40	2.60	0.92	–	–

In reconstructed slices which contained no tumor tissue according to the final diagnosis, the left over right hemisphere ratio was 1.0 ± 0.09 ($n = 50$). Although some brain structure could be seen in these cases, a rather homogenous activity distribution predominated except for the mucosa of the nasal cavity, which accumulated both forms of the amino acid. The L/D ratio in these slices was close to unity.

The uptake of both forms of methionine increased with the malignancy of the tumor with the highest uptake ratio of 2.6 in an astrocytoma IV. In most cases the L/D ratio in tumor was slightly increased; in the astrocytoma IV, however, the ratio was reversed.

In two of the cases where the abdomen was investigated, the pancreas showed a high selectivity for the L-form methionine with L/D ratios of >3. In one case (patient no. 4) with a bronchial carcinoma, the L uptake was decreased leading to a L/D ratio of only 1.5.

In three patients conventional ^{99m}Tc-DTPA studies were performed in order to investigate the BBB. Two patients with a positive ^{99m}Tc-DTPA scan accumulated no or only very small amounts of ^{11}C-methionine, while one patient with an astrocytoma II, who showed no ^{99m}Tc-DTPA uptake, had a positive ^{11}C-methionine accumulation.

In one patient with a meningioma, which showed a marked contrast enhancement in the CT image, the ^{99m}Tc-DTPA scan was omitted, since the damage to the BBB seemed to be verified sufficiently. Two corresponding NMR, CT, and PET images at two adjacent levels (1 cm apart) of this patient are presented in Fig. 1.

Because usually the diffusive uptake is a relative slow process and typically BBB brakdown can be visualized in ^{99m}Tc-DTPA scans in late images only, the present findings which were obtained within 30 min after injection seem to refer to an active metabolic process. The strongest support for this interpretation stems from the observation that in two cases the positive ^{99m}Tc-DTPA scan was accompanied by no or only slight ^{11}C-methionine uptake while no astrocytoma II with no BBB breakdown showed a distinct methionine uptake. Furthermore our latest results on methionine uptake in patients with

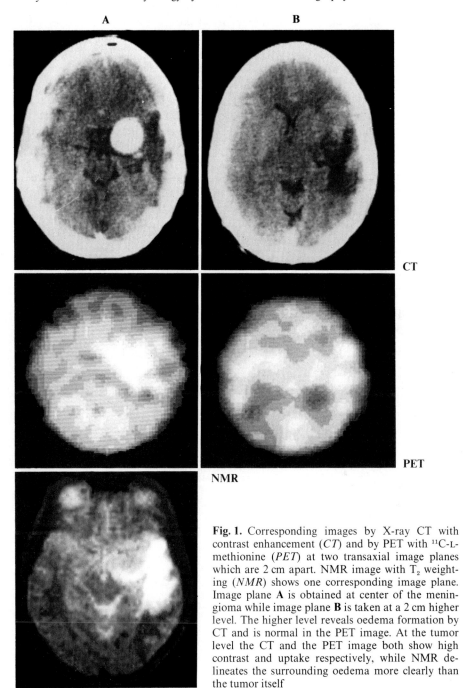

Fig. 1. Corresponding images by X-ray CT with contrast enhancement (*CT*) and by PET with ¹¹C-L-methionine (*PET*) at two transaxial image planes which are 2 cm apart. NMR image with T_2 weighting (*NMR*) shows one corresponding image plane. Image plane **A** is obtained at center of the meningioma while image plane **B** is taken at a 2 cm higher level. The higher level reveals oedema formation by CT and is normal in the PET image. At the tumor level the CT and the PET image both show high contrast and uptake respectively, while NMR delineates the surrounding oedema more clearly than the tumor itself

cerebrovascular disease indicate that in stroke patients with proven BBB damage early PET scans with ^{11}C-methionine reveal accumulation defects in the affected region rather than a positive uptake.

A similar finding was reported in ^{18}FDG uptake studies for CNS tumors. In this investigation a correlation was found for uptake and tumor grade also with mismatch of CT contrast enhencement (due to BBB disrupture) and ^{18}FDG uptake. Further evidence that active metabolic processes govern the amino uptake rather than diffusive processes, stems from the observation by Knapp et al. [6], that soft tissue tumors exhibit both, enhanced perfusion and a concomitant glutamate uptake [6].

Although a contribution to the uptake of ^{11}C-L-methionine and ^{11}C-D-methionine by BBB damage can not be ruled out from the current data, the missing uptake in proven BBB damage cases indicates that the amount of contribution by diffusive processes is relatively small, at least in the early phase after tracer administration.

References

1. Barrio JR, Keen RE, Huang SC et al. (1985) J Nucl Med 26:6 – 7
2. Bergström M, Collins PV, Ehrin E, et al. (1983) J Comput Assist Tomogr 7:1062 – 1066
3. Bustany P, Henry JF, Sargent T, et al. (1983) In: Heiss WD, Phelps ME (eds) Positron emission tomography of the brain. Springer, Berlin Heidelberg New York
4. Di Chiro G, Oldfield E, Bairamian D et al. (1985) In: Greitz T et al. (eds) The metabolism of human brain studied with positron emission tomography. Raven, New York, 351 – 361
5. Hübner KF, Purvis JT, Mahaley SM et al. (1982) J Comput Assist Tomogr 6:544 – 550
6. Knapp WH, Helus F, Sinn H et al. (1984) J Nucl Med 25:989 – 997
7. Kubota K, Yamada K, Fukada H et al. (1984) Eur J Nucl Med 9:136 – 140
8. Lammertsma AA, Wise RSJ, Jones T et al. (1983) Acta Neurochir 69:5 – 13
9. Lammertsma AA, Wise RSJ, Heather JD et al. (1983) J Cerebr Blood Flow Metab 3:425 – 431
10. Meyer GJ, Schober O, Hundeshagen H (1985) Eur J Nucl Med 10:373 – 376
11. Oldendorf W (1981) In: Marks N, Rodnight R (eds) Research methods in neurochemistry. Plenum, New York, pp 91 – 112
12. Phelps ME, Barrio JR, Huang SC et al. (1984) Ann Neurol [Suppl] 15:192 – 202
13. Schober O, Meyer GJ, Stolke D et al. (1985) J Nucl Med 26:98 – 99

VII. Use of Tumor Markers In Vitro

Overview of the Development of Tumor Markers

K. B. BJÖRKLUND

The first attempt to apply bacteriological serology to the problem of malignant tumors was probably made in 1895 by Richet and Hericourt [1] at the Pasteur Institute in Paris. They immunized a donkey and two dogs with human osteosarcoma tissue and injected the resulting immune sera into patients, with no favorable results. Other attempts followed, and one investigator after another became interested in the search for antigens in cancer cells. Between 1895 and 1911 about 55 papers were published on the subject [2−7]. During the next 10 years, there was little interest in the pursuit of this type of research.

After the First World War researchers started to look for possible tumor antigens all over again. A new wave of optimism could be seen, and among the numerous papers which followed, particularly those by Lumsden [8−12] should be mentioned. This British researcher worked for more than 12 years on the hypothesis that it should be possible to find substances in immune sera that have a specific effect against tumor cells. He also thought that it should be possible to stimulate the organism to produce similar substances. Contemporary cancer authorities, however, did not like Lumsden's ideas. He was heavily criticized, and finally he was deprived of the necessary resources for continued work.

In 1929, Woglom [13] summarized some 600 papers on cancer immunology in the following pessimistic way, "... of these communications a small number are of permanent value and far too large a proportion are merely ridiculous ... immunity to transplantable tumors ... appears to be entirely unrelated to other forms of immunity ... nothing ... may be hoped for at the present in respect to a successful therapy from this direction."

Very few people doubted the correctness of Woglom's statement, and interest in immunology and cancer gradually disappeared. The subject became positively unpopular and remained so until the fifties and sixties. It became established knowledge that immunology had nothing to do with cancer. Everybody knew that.

This state of affairs was saddening, because Lumsden and others had reached conclusions of importance, even though they were hampered by the lack of adequate techniques.

Both immunology and biochemistry were in a stage prior to great development as was the art of cell culture in vitro. Antibodies could not be analyzed

Cancer Immunology Section, The National Bacteriological Laboratory, Lundagatan 2, Solna, S-105 21 Stockholm

Nuclear Medicine in Clinical Oncology
Ed. by C. Winkler
© Springer-Verlag Berlin Heidelberg 1986

and measured, except by very crude and nondiscriminatory techniques. Therefore, we should admire Lumsden for being able to fractionate serum globulin by means of CO_2 precipitation and isolating antibodies which destroyed tumor cells in vitro in the absence of complement [12]. Lumsden also found a correlation between certain serum antibodies and the resistance to tumors in rats, but he admitted that he was totally unaware of the nature of the other factors which he considered must also play an important role [12]. Histoincompatibility antigens, for instance, were relatively unknown at that time.

Before and after the Second World War, the science of immunology was gradually developed. The quantitative theory of antigen and antibody reactions had been developed by Heidelberger and Kendall [15], the nature of complement was elucidated [16 – 19], and immunologic specificity became understood [20 – 22]. Subdisciplines of immunology were developed. Clinically, immunological techniques and concepts became increasingly popular.

Immunochemistry and biochemistry advanced rapidly, and radiolabelling of antibodies was developed by Pressman and his group at the Sloan-Kettering Institute in New York [23, 24]. The work by Heidelberger and Pressman created, among other things, the basis for radioimmunoassay.

Cell culture in vitro was transformed from an exclusive work by a few to become a useful aid for many. Murray and Kopech at Columbia University compiled a bibliography of 29,000 publications on cell culture in vitro which appeared between 1884 and 1950 [25]. During the period 1950 – 1955, however, more papers were published than during all previous years taken together.

When I started to become interested in cancer in 1951, the necessary tools were just about to be developed. The field was rather empty, and had it not been for our studies of antibodies to rabbit bone-marrow [26], I would probably never have found reason to work on human cancer. We had observed that horse antiserum to rabbit bone marrow, when injected i.v. into rabbits, caused severe, selective necrosis of the bone marrow. The immune serum was rendered nontoxic by absorption with the insoluble residue of rabbit bone marrow [27, 28], but no soluble components had such an effect. It struck me that these findings could be applied to cancer, because practically every paper on tumor antigen I had read had in its methods section a note saying, "The insoluble residue was discarded." Only the soluble fraction had been used for studies of tumor antigenicity.

If the insoluble residue of tumors had not yet been studied, there was still a possibility, just as in the bone marrow case, that antibodies to components of the insoluble residue might selectively react with, and perhaps damage, cancer cells. In any case, Woglom's gloomy words no longer seemed to be the last said on the matter.

Pathologists had long held the view that various types of cancer resembled each other more than they resembled normal tissues, and more than normal tissues resembled each other. This was true also from the biochemical standpoint [29]. It was difficult to reject the idea that the organism sometimes could rid itself of cancer. There were scattered cases of presumed spontaneous regression. Boyd [30, 31] wrote that, ". . . they suggest the development of an immunity which is at least partially successful. If only we could do something to make the success complete!" In 1956 and 1961 Everson and Cole [32, 33] reported 125 cases of spontaneous regression, which appeared to withstand the strictest scrutiny, i.e., no significant therapy, positive biopsy, etc. All this pointed to the existence of some sort of biologic control of cancer.

At the beginning of the fifties, I tried to combine the views of Boyd, Greenstein, and others with my own observations, by formulating the hypothesis that all human carcinoma tumors contain some principle in common, detectable by immunologic techniques, and which should differ qualitatively or quantitatively from normal tissues.

If the idea of a common human tumor antigenic principle were true, it should be possible to pool a large number of human carcinoma tumors without diluting out the common principle. Immunization with such a pool of tumors should lead to antibodies which should recognize the hypothetical common principle, but much less so the multiplicity of individual antigens, which also must be assumed to exist [34].

In 1952, the insoluble residue of 56 carcinoma tumors from the most common sites was injected into a horse, who was immunized for an extended period of time [35]. The resulting antiserum was heavily absorbed with the insoluble residues from large pools of various normal tissues. There was still reactivity left, as seen by immunological techniques, such as cytotoxicity inhibition [35, 36], tanned red cell agglutination inhibition [37], quantitative precipitation, and diffusion in gel. Absorption with pooled tumor residue or single tumors, on the other hand, readily absorbed out all detectable activity. The quantitative difference between carcinoma and normal tissue was about 23-fold [35].

The general approach to differentiating tumors from normal tissues is schematically illustrated in Fig. 1. In this approach, pooled tumor tissues and pooled normal tissues were subjected to an identical array of biochemical separation procedures. The fractions obtained were used to label aliquots of tannic acid treated sheep red cells, whereupon the agglutinability of the red cells was tested with the aid of specific immune sera which had been absorbed by normal antigens, tumor antigens, or by both normal and tumor antigens. If a difference in reactivity was observed, then the separation procedure was varied until the difference between the tumor and normal fractions reached a maximal level. At that point the separation procedure was adopted and another procedure was subsequently applied to the active fractions from tumors and the corresponding inactive fractions from normal tissues. In this way a number of purification methods were tried out, eventually resulting in a complete separation program.

By this approach the principle of common human carcinoma antigenicity was established. The antigenic principle seemed to consist of three major antigens, one of which was studied by us and later called tissue polypeptide antigen or TPA [38]. We now know that TPA is present in all types of carcinomas [39] and also in normal epithelial, nonepidermal cells [40] with special reference to duct cells [41].

It is significant that at the beginning of the fifties, two other groups set out to look systematically for antigens in human cancer tissue. They were Southam,

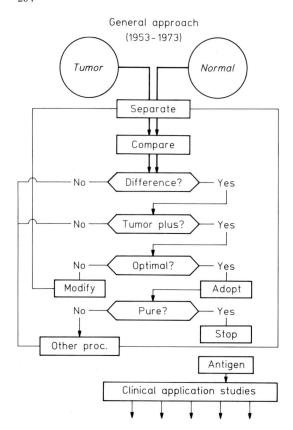

Fig. 1. Programmed search for qualitative or quantitative systematic differences between tumors and normal tissues. (Modified from Björklund [38])

Moore, and Rhoads at the Sloan-Kettering Institute in New York and Zilber at the Gamelaya Institute in Moscow.

The New York group studied homotransplantation of tumor cells and various cell lines and suggested that there are common antigens in cancer cell lines, and that resistance to proliferation of transplanted cells is weakened in cancer patients [42–44]. Controversy broke out, and the work was discontinued.

In Moscow, Zilber startled his colleagues by claiming that human gastric cancer contained antigens not detectable in normal tissue [45, 46]. He used weakly alkaline solutions to immunize rabbits, and performed tests by the method of sensitization-desensitization anaphylaxis in guinea pigs.

Zilber's results were distrusted but later confirmed by investigators assigned to his laboratory. On his sixtieth birthday Zilber was honored with a symposium and in 1959 the symposium book on the pathogenesis and immunology of tumors was published [47]. Zilber, however, lost his interest in tumor immunology.

The initial situation for my group in Stockholm resembled that of Southam and Zilber. To believe in tumor antigens was considered a sign of poor judgement. Action was taken to stop funding, but after international intervention, the theme became a matter for the Swedish Government. After consultation with domestic and foreign experts, the Government reached the conclusion that the work should continue.

An increasing number of laboratories became interested in tumor antigens. Similar and related findings were made, and it became increasingly evident that human tumor cells possess important and useful antigenic components. The works of Lang [48], Day et al. [49], Buinauskas et al. [50], Abramoff et al. [51], Aizawa and Southam [52], Bashkaev and Rosenbaum [53], Gorodilova and Shershul'skaia [54], Itoh and Southam [55], McKenna et al. [56], Perez-Cuadrado et al. [57], Hirai et al. [58], and Blaney et al. [59] are significant in this connection. They all used immunological techniques to demonstrate the antigenicity of tumor cells. Two of the most significant findings will be mentioned.

In 1963, Abelev and coworkers [60] found that an antigenic protein, called alpha-fetoprotein or AFP, was produced by hepatocellular hepatomas, and this fetal protein has since been demonstrated in the serum of patients with primary liver cancer [61]. It serves as a marker for germ cell tumors and is elevated in teratocarcinoma of the ovary and testis [62].

AFP was first studied by techniques which had been used in our laboratory in Stockholm. Descriptions were sent to Abelev and, according to him, they helped him to find AFP. At the beginning of the sixties, Gold had observed our findings and became interested. In 1965, Gold and Freedman, with reference given to our work, reported that they had pooled colonic carcinoma tumors and absorbed the resulting immune sera with normal tissues and found an antigenic activity they named carcinoembryonic antigen (CEA) [63, 64]. By using only colon cancers, they thought that their antigenic fraction should be specific for that type of cancer. It is, however, now known that CEA is present in a wide variety of cancers [65]. Gold also introduced extraction with perchloric acid, which destroys TPA but leaves CEA intact. Therefore, he did not find TPA.

CEA was important and became rapidly marketed worldwide. It stimulated great interest in the field. From our point of view, it represented the second member of the common human tumor antigenic principle.

After this brief and sketchy review of the story of tumor antigens, let us look at how the antigens were promoted to markers.

The term marker describes an important function of the antigen, just as other antigens are vaccines or allergens. Tumor markers have not been with us for long; the expression has gradually become accepted in conjunction with increased clinical use of tumor-derived antigens as markers of clinical events.

The name tumor marker is in common use today and it seems to be properly understood by most people. One should keep in mind, however, that whatever the terminology, no antigen has been described which is tumor specific in the strict sense of the word, i.e., present in tumors only. I should like to underline this statement.

In the past, considerable time was lost in arguments dealing with terminology as to whether an antigenic fraction, derived from tumor tissue or cells, should be called tumor associated, distinctive, related, typical, or tumor specific, nearly specific, really, really specific, or absolutely specific [66]. In fact, adequate terminology was just not invented and this led to misunderstanding and confusion. This still happens.

Table 1. Tumor growth products, applications, and references. (From Björklund [39])

Tumor growth product	Application	References
Tumor-associated antigens		
Carcinoembryonic antigen (CEA)	General (colorectal, breast, lung)	Gold and Freedman (1965), Hansen et al. (1974), Zamcheck (1981), Martin et al. (1977), Lokish et al. (1978), Vincent and Chu (1973)
Tissue polypeptide antigen (TPA)	General (colorectal, breast urinary bladder)	Björklund und Björklund (1957), Björklund (1981), Schlegel et al. (1981), Lüthgens and Schlegel (1981)
Alpha-fetoprotein (AFP)	Endodermal sinus tumor of the testis and ovary, liver cancer	Abelev (1968), Nørgaard-Pedersen et al. (1975), Talerman (1981)
Pancreatic oncofetal antigen (POA)	Pancreas cancer	Gelder et al. (1978)
Tennessee antigen (TAG)	General	Potter et al. (1980)
Human casein	Breast cancer	Zangerle et al. (1978)
Gastric fetal sulfoglyco-protein antigen (FSA)	Gastric cancer	Häkkinen (1966, 1978)
Ferritin	Hodgkin's disease, AML, myeloproliferative diseases, hepatoma, germ cell tumors, breast and lung cancer	Lamerz (1981)
Lung tumor-associated antigen (LTAA)	Lung cancer	Braatz et al. (1979) McIntire et al. (1979)
Serum β_2-microglobulin (β_2-m)	Leukemia, lymphoma, myelomatosis	Cooper and Plesner (1980)
Pregnancy-specific β_1-glyco-protein (SP$_1$) (also TBG, PAPP-C, PSβG)	Choriocarcinoma	Horne et al. (1976)
Non-specific cross-reacting antigen (NCA)	CML and AML	von Kleist et al. (1972)
Hormones		
Human chorionic gonadotropin (HCG: β-HCG)	Trophoblastic neoplasms, embryonal cell carcinoma of the testis	Vaitukaitis et al. (1972), Vaitukaitis (1979)
Calcitonin	Medullary thyroid cancer (C cells)	Silva et al. (1974), Calmettes et al. (1978)
Ectopic ACTH	Bronchial cancer (oat cell, carcinoid), ectopic syndrome	Gewirtz and Yalow (1974), Podmore et al. (1979)
Insulin	Insulinoma	
Enzymes		
Acid phosphatase	Prostatic cancer, metastases	Schwartz (1975)
Serum prostatic acid phosphatase (PAP)	Prostatic cancer	Foti et al. (1977), Chu et al. (1975), Chu (1978)

Table 1 (continued)

Tumor growth product	Application	References
Placental alkaline phosphatase (Regan isoenzyme)	Adenocarcinoma of the ovaries, testis tumors, pancreatic cancer	Fishman et al. (1968a, b, 1976), Stolbach et al. (1972)
Lactic dehydrogenase (LDH)	Hemoblastic disease, lymphomas	Prochazka et al. (1968), Pfleiderer and Wachsmuth (1961)
γ-Glutamyltranspeptidase (GGTP)	Pancreatic cancer	
Galactosyl-, sialyl-, glycosyl- and fucosyltransferases	Various malignancies	
Immune complexes		
Circulating immune complexes (CIC)	Various malignancies	Gauci et al. (1981), Day et al. (1981)
Neurogenic amines and serotonin metabolitis		
Catecholamines	Neuroblastoma	Schwartz (1975)
Vanilmandelic acid		
Metanephrine		
Cystathionine	Pheochromocytoma	
Dopamine		
Dopamine β-hydroxylase		
Homovanillic acid		
Metanephrine		
5-Hydroxyindole acetic acid	Carcinoid	

Therefore, I will try to explain what I mean by the term "tumor antigen." A tumor antigen is understood to be derived from tumor tissue or cells, but also from other sources, just as sugar may come from sugar cane or sugar beet. The term antigen means that the substance can give rise to and be detected by antibodies by various techniques. If released into body fluids, the concentration of the antigen may be correlated to clinical findings. By defining these findings and their statistical relation to the antigen, the latter gradually becomes a marker, provided that the statistics are good enough. The demand for uniqueness is no longer there, and tumor antigens can be dealt with just as other molecules or mixtures in clinical chemistry.

In oncology, it is essential to determine the activity of tumor disease. The biological basis for activity is cellular proliferation.

Some markers, e.g., TPA, are produced and released by cancer cells in vitro in relation to certain proliferative phases of the cell cycle. The dividing cells contain high concentrations of TPA. Figure 2 shows two dividing HeLa cells and some nondividing cells of the same type. The marker, visualized by anti-TPA antibody and peroxidase, is seen in the cytoplasm of the two cells in prophase and metaphase.

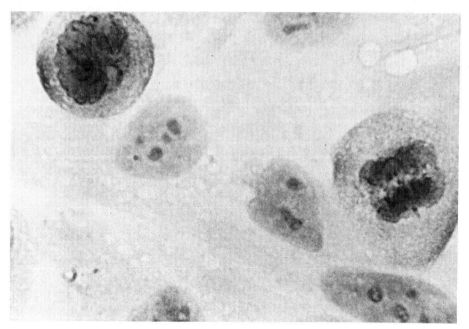

Fig. 2. TPA-stained cytoplasm of two HeLa cells in prophase and metaphase, respectively (PAP technique). The nondividing HeLa cells do not exhibit staining of their cytoplasm

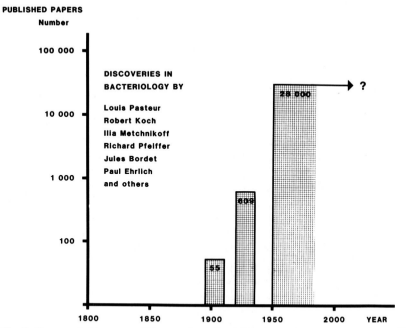

Fig. 3. Exponential increase of the number of published papers on tumor antigens. The years 1895−1911, 1920−1935, 1950−1980 were compared. Between these periods, little activity was seen

Certain necrobiotic or lytic processes may also contribute to the release of marker in vivo. Other factors, which could influence marker concentration in patients' sera, are infections, e.g., hepatitis, and liver damage by alcohol. These conditions can be recognized by the physician. Therefore, in cases of known cancer, the progressive rise of marker may be interpreted as a sign of increased proliferative activity. Adequate therapy should cause the marker to drop.

For various markers which are now available, different schemes have been worked out. There are differences in specificity and sensitivity versus different types of tumors. Table 1 lists a variety of tumor antigens, some of which are markers. Known, but not present in this list, are CA 19.9 [67] and CA 125 [68].

As illustrated by Fig. 3, there has been an exponential increase of interest in tumor antigens. Three waves of enthusiasm followed the great discoveries of the "microbe hunters" of the nineteenth century. It appears as if the interest in antigenicity of tumors is here to stay. Perhaps we will see links from studies of antigen join links from molecular biology, nuclear medicine, oncology, and other fields to give a chain of events to explain the phenomenon of activated proliferation which we call cancer.

Or, to put it otherwise: The elephantness of the problem will lead us to see not just parts, but one day, the whole elephant.

References

1. Richet C, Hericourt J (1895) C R Acad Sc (Paris) 121:567
2. Ehrlich P (1908) Verh Dtsch Pathol Ges 12:13
3. Loeb L (1903) Virchows Arch Pathol Anat 172:345
4. Schöne G (1906) MMW 53:2517
5. Bashford EJ, Murray JA, Cramer W (1908) 3rd Scientific Report of the Imperial Cancer Research Fund, p 315
6. Bridré J (1907) Ann Pasteur 21:760
7. Lambert RA, Hanes FM (1911) J Exp Med 13:505
8. Lumsden T (1925) Lancet 208:383
9. Lumsden T (1926) Lancet 211:112
10. Lumsden T (1928) Arch Exp Zellforsch 6:206
11. Lumsden T (1931) Am J Cancer 15:563
12. Lumsden T (1931) J Pathol Bacteriol 34:349
13. Woglom WH (1929) Cancer Rev 4:129
14. Lumsden T, Macrae T, Skipper E (1934) Lancet 226:721
15. Heidelberger M, Kendall FE (1929) J Exp Med 50:809
16. Buchner H (1889) Zentralbl Bakteriol I Abt 5:817
17. Osborne TWB (1937) Complement or Alexin. Oxford University Press, London
18. Mayer MM, Osler AG, Bier OG, Heidelberger M (1946) J Exp Med 84:535
19. Müller-Eberhard HJ (1975) Ann Rev Biochem 44:697
20. Landsteiner K (1936) The specificity of serological reactions. Thomas, Springfield
21. Kabat EA (1966) J Immunol 97:1
22. Crumpton MJ (1974) Protein antigens: The molecular bases of antigenicity and immunogenicity. In: Sela M (ed) The antigens, vol II. Academic, New York, pp 1–78
23. Pressman D (1957) Ann NY Acad Sc 69:644
24. Day ED, Barnes GW, Planisek JA, Pressman D (1958) JNCI 20:1123
25. Murray MR, Kopech G (1953) A bibliography of the research in tissue culture, 1884–1950, vol I, II, Academic, New York
26. Björklund B, Hellström L (1951) Acta Med Scand 139:122–132

27. Björklund B (1953) Int Arch Allergy 4:340 – 359
28. Björklund B (1953) Int Arch Allergy 4:379 – 414
29. Greenstein JP (1954) Biochemistry of cancer. 2nd ed. Academic, New York, p 362
30. Boyd W (1947) A text-book of pathology. An introduction to medicine, 5th edn. Lea and Febiger, Philadelphia
31. Boyd W (1957) J Can Assoc Radiol 8:45 – 63
32. Everson TC, Cole WH (1956) Ann Surg 144:366
33. Everson TC, Cole WH (1966) Spontaneous regression of cancer. Saunders, Philadelphia
34. Björklund B (1956) Int Arch Allergy 8:179 – 192
35. Björklund B, Björklund V (1957) Int Arch Allergy 10:153 – 184
36 Björklund B, Lundblad G, Björklund V (1958) Int Arch Allergy 12:241 – 261
37. Björklund B, Paulsson JE (1962) Immunol 89:759 – 766
38. Björklund B (ed) (1973) Techniques for detection of cancer. Proceedings Folksam Symposium 1972. Bonniers, Stockholm
39. Björklund B (1983) Tumor products reflecting growth activity. In: Stoll B (ed) Cancer treatment: end point evaluation. Wiley, Chichester, pp 251 – 278
40. Nathrath WBJ, Heidenkummer P, Björklund V, Björklund B (1985) J Histochem Cytochem 33(2):99 – 109
41. Caselitz J, Seifert G, Björklund B, Björklund V (1983) Appl Pathol 1:115 – 120
42. Southam CM, Moore AE, Rhoads CP (1957) Science 125:158
43. Southam CM (1958) Bull NY Acad Med 34:416
44. Southam CM, Moore AE Ann NY Acad Sci 73:635
45. Zilber LA (1958) Adv Cancer Res 5:291
46. Zilber LA (1962) Ann NY Acad Sci 101:264
47. Vygodchikov GW, Crawford R (eds) (1959) Pathogenesis and immunity of tumors. Pergamon, London
48. Lang N (1963) Med Welt 2538 – 2545
49. Day ED, Planisek JA , Pressman D (1961) JNCI 27:1107 – 1114
50. Buinauskas P, McCredie JA, Brown ER, Cole WH (1959) Arch Surg 79:432 – 439
51. Abramoff P, Saunders JW, Gasseling MT (1961) JNCI 26:585 – 599
52. Aizawa M, Southam CM (1960) Ann NY Acad Sci 87:293 – 307
53. Bashkaev IS, Rosenbaum GI (1963) Vopr Oncol 9:83 – 87
54. Gorodilova VV, Shershul'skaia LV (1959) Specific antigens in malignant tumors of man. In: Vygodchikov GV (ed) Pathogenesis and immunology of tumors. Pergamon, New York, pp 101 – 112
55. Itoh T, Southam CM (1963) J Immunol 91:469 – 483
56. McKenna JM, Sanderson RP, Blakemore WS (1964) Cancer Res 24:754 – 762
57. Perez-Cuadrado S, Haberman S, Race GJ (1964) Dallas Med J 50:77 – 84
58. Hirai H, Taga H, Warabioka K (1964) J Biochem 55:178 – 184
59. Blaney DJ, Rotte TC, Siler VE (1964) Surg Gynecol Obstet 118:341 – 346
60. Abelev GI, Perova SD, Khramkova NI, Postnikova ZA, Irlin IS (1963) Transplant Bull 1:174 – 180
61. Abelev GI (1968) Cancer Res 28:1344 – 1350
62. Talerman A (1981) Alpha-fetoprotein and germ cell tumors. In: von Kleist S, Breuer H (eds) Critical evaluation of tumor markers. Karger, Basel
63. Gold P, Freedman SO (1965) J Exp Med 121:439 – 462
64. Gold P, Freedman SO (1965) J Exp Med 122:467 – 481
65. Zamcheck N (1981) Clinical use of carcinoembryonic antigen. In: von Kleist S, Breuer H (eds) Critical evaluation of tumor markers. Karger, Basel, pp 25 – 38 (Contributions in oncology, vol 7)
66. Day ED (1965) The immunochemistry of cancer. Thomas, Springfield
67. Steinberg N et al. (1984) Am Gaster Assoc May, 1984
68. Bast et al. (1983) N Engl J Med 309(15):883 – 887

The Clinical Value of Tumor-Associated Proteins in Gastrointestinal Cancer

H.-J. STAAB[1]

Introduction

Gastrointestinal cancers were one of the first groups of cancers to be extensively investigated with tumor-associated antigens [1−3]. During the last 20 years, carcinoembryonic antigen (CEA) has been established as the first clinically accepted tumor marker in this cancer group [4−5]. Recently, based on monoclonal antibody techniques, the position of CEA as the leading tumor marker in this cancer group has been seriously challenged by a new tumor-associated antigen, CA 19-9 [5−7]. The determinant group of the CA 19-9 antigen was found to be a modified (Lewis) blood group [8]. The monoclonal antibody originally established after immunization with colonic cancer cells was expected to be of high efficacy for this type of cancers [9]. Yet recent data gave evidence that this antigen might be highly useful in the diagnosis and follow-up of pancreatic carcinomas [10].

During the last three years, we investigated the clinical validity of CEA and CA 19-9 in patients with gastrointestinal cancers on the basis of the sensitivity and specificity of preoperative values and in the follow-up. We also considered the possibility of combining the 2 markers. Special attention was dedicated to procedures for deducing therapeutic modalities, mainly assisted by serial measurement of tumor-associated antigens. We also looked retrospectively for possibilities of using tumor-associated antigens in addition to common prognostic parameters.

Material and Methods

Since 1974, 1142 patients, among them 407 with gastric cancer, 667 with colorectal cancer, and 68 with cancer of the pancreas have been followed clinically and with serial CEA determination. 602 patients with histologically confirmed gastrointestinal cancers have also been followed with CA 19-9 since 1981. Additionally, 150 patients with a tentative diagnosis of malignant abdominal disease prior to surgery but in whom nonmalignant disease was confirmed after operation were included in these studies. Of the 602 patients, 287 had pre- and partly postoperative determination of CEA and CA 19-9. Post-

---

1 Klinge Pharma GmbH, Weihenstephaner Straße 28, D-8000 München 80

Nuclear Medicine in Clinical Oncology
Ed. by C. Winkler
© Springer-Verlag Berlin Heidelberg 1986

operatively, the patients were included in the 5 year surveillance program and underwent sequential tumor marker testing at 2- to 3-month intervals together with clinical investigations as described previously [11]. Extension of disease was classified according to the postoperative TNM classification (UICC). The clinical follow-up was carried out according to a standardised program, all medical data were computerized and electronically processed for evaluation. In case a recurrence was suggested from tumor-marker increases or from clinical findings, we performed diagnostic methods including radiological and scintigraphic methods, sonography, endoscopy, and computerized tomography to localize recurrences.

For the investigation of tumor markers we first used a CA 19-9 test from Centocor (Malvern, USA) and thereafter the ELSA CIS CA 19-9 test kit (Isotopen Diagnostic CIS, Dreieich, FRG). For the CEA investigations we used the CEA-RIA test (Roche) parallel to the enzyme immune test CEA-EIA (Hoffmann-La Roche AG, Basel, Switzerland). The tests were routinely controlled with specific reference materials in four different antigen levels (BIOREF GmbH, Mömbris, FRG). For the CEA-EIA test, a cutoff level of 1.5 µg/l [12], for the CEA-RIA test 2.0 µg/l, and for the CA 19-9 test 37 U/ml was used for specifiying a positive test result in the follow-up.

Results

Preoperative Tumor-Marker Values

The specificity of the CEA (EIA) and CA 19-9 tests was determined with 150 patients with nonmalignant diseases, mostly benign tumors and inflammatory abdominal diseases. The sensitivity of the tests was determined for a group of 77 patients with gastric cancer, 27 patients with pancreatic cancer, and a group of 183 patients with colorectal cancers. The 95% percentile of specificity was found to be 4.9 µg/l for the CEA-EIA test and 41 U/ml for the CA 19-9 test. Using this cutoff level of 95% specificity, we evaluated the sensitivity of the test for pancreatic, gastric, and colorectal cancer patients. In Table 1, these data are summarized together with the sensitivity of the combined use of CEA-EIA and CA 19-9 in patients with various stages of diseases. For both tumor-marker tests, sensitivity increased as the disease advanced. Consistent with this observation, an increasing significance of differences between the distributions of tumor-marker values of patients with nonmalignant disease and patients with cancer was calculated using a rank-sum test [13]. When we combined test results which were positive either in one of both tests, sensitivity was increased by 17% over the CEA test in the group of gastric carcinoma, yet only by 3% in the group of colorectal carcinoma. On the other hand, in pancreatic carcinoma, the increase in sensitivity of the CEA test over the CA 19–9 test was only about 4%. Considering the concomitant loss in diagnostic specificity (95% to 91%), a combination of tumor-marker tests appears to be reasonable only in gastric carcinomas.

Table 1. Sensitivity at 95% specifity of the CEA-EIA-m test and the CA 19-9 test compared with the combined use of both tests in subgroups of patients with various primary tumors of different stages. The significance of differences is given between tumor marker values in patients of these subgroups and in patients with benign diseases (After Staab et al. [19])

	Stage	n	CEA			CA 19-9			CEA and/or CA 19-9	
			Sensitivity		Significant at a level of	Sensitivity		Significant at a level of	Sensitivity	
			%	(n)	%	%	(n)	%	%	(n)
Colorectal cancer	I	47	13	(6)	–	4	(2)	–	15	(7)
	II	58	40	(32)	0.1	19	(11)	5	47	(27)
	III	40	35	(14)	0.1	13	(5)	5	38	(15)
	IV	38	74	(28)	0.1	42	(16)	0.1	74	(28)
Total		183	39	(71)	0.1	19	(34)	0.1	42	(77)
Gastric cancer	I	9	11	(1)	n.c.	0	(0)	n.c.	11	(1)
	II	12	0	(0)	n.c.	17	(2)	n.c.	17	(2)
	III	8	0	(0)	n.c.	25	(2)	n.c.	25	(2)
	IV	48	31	(15)	0.1	31	(15)	0.1	48	(23)
Total		77	21	(16)	5	25	(19)	0.1	38	(29)
Pancreatic cancer	II	2		(2)	n.c.		(2)	n.c.		(2)
	III	1		(0)	n.c.		(1)	n.c.		(1)
	IV	24	33	(8)	0.1	88	(21)	0.1	92	(22)
Total		27	37	(10)	0.1	89	(24)	0.1	93	(25)

n.c., not calculated due to low numbers

Long-term Follow-up of Tumor-Marker Determinations

Both CEA and CA 19–9 patterns could be correlated nicely with the clinical course of disease as has already been described earlier [3]. Tumor-marker development was classified as either "increasing", "decreasing", or "essentially unchanged below or above the cutoff levels or fluctuation." These categories were correlated with recurrent disease or no evidence of disease (Table 2). The correlation between long-term CA 19-9 and CEA time courses and the clinical course of disease was accomplished in 379 patients with resected gastrointestinal cancers. While only 7 of 278 patients with essentially unchanged tumor-marker levels had a recurrent disease (2.5%), a recurrent disease was confirmed by clinical methods in all but 2 patients (99 of 101 cases) with increasing tumor-marker levels; in these 2 patients a recurrent disease has not yet been confirmed, but is expected. Of the 54 cases in whom both markers increased, in

Table 2. Correlation of patterns of long term CA 19-9 and CEA time courses with the clinical course of disease in 379 patients with resected gastrointestinal cancers given as ratio recurrence/NED

	Stomach cancer		Colorectal cancer		Total
	Recurr.	NED	Recurr.	NED	
CEA essentially unchanged CA 19-9 essentially unchanged	1	38	6	233	278
CEA increasing CA 19-9 essentially unchanged	3	0	31	2 [a]	36
CEA essentially unchanged CA 19-9 increasing	6	0	5	0	11
CEA increasing CA 19-9 increasing	9	0	45	0	54
Total	19	38	87	235	379

[a] Relapse expected yet clinically not confirmed
Recurr., recurrent disease; NED, no evidence of disease

Table 3. Sensitivity of single or combined determination of CA 19-9 and CEA in the detection of recurrent disease

Site of primary tumor	n	Sensitivity of					
		CEA		CA 19-9		CEA+/or CA 19-9	
		n	%	n	%	n	%
Gastric cancer	19	12	63	15	79	18	94.7
Colorectal cancer	87	76	87	50	57	81	93.1

9 patients the CA 19-9 preceded the initial CEA increase by 2 – 7 months and in 11 patients the CA 19-9 tracked the CEA increase by 1 – 7 months.

In Table 3 the results of the combined CEA and CA 19-9 test in detection of recurrent disease based on trend analyses of tumor markers are evaluated. In gastric cancers, the combination of both markers was most paying, detecting a total of 94.7% of recurrent diseases, i.e., an increase of more than 30% over the CEA. In colorectal cancers, the detection rate was 93.1% for the combined use of CEA and CA 19-9; however, the increase over the CEA was only 6%. Highest complementarity of both tests was therefore achieved in gastric cancers as demonstrated previously [14, 15].

Tumor Markers as an Aid to Introduce Therapeutic Modalities

The median lead time of initial tumor-marker increase preceding a positive clinical diagnosis for the group of patients in Table 2 was 3 months (range 0 – 16 months). This time can be effectively used to introduce therapeutic modalities, i.e., second-look-operations. Recently, the results of a 7-year study on second-look surgery based on serial CEA determinations gave evidence of a sig-

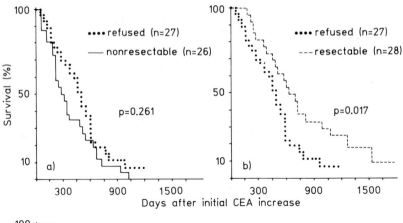

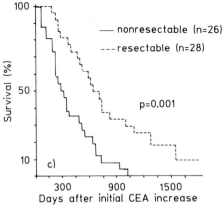

Fig. 1a – c. Survival curves of 81 patients suggested for second-look operations primarily due to increasing carcinoembryonic antigen levels. **a** Patients with nonresectable recurrence compared with patients who refused reoperation. **b** Patients with resectable recurrence compared with patients who refused operation. **c** Patients with resectable recurrence compared with patients with nonresectable recurrence. (After Staab et al. [16])

nificant increase in survival of patients undergoing second-look surgery with radical or palliative resection of their recurrences. Fig. 1 shows the survival curves of 81 patients who were suggested for second-look operations due primarily to increasing CEA levels. Of these patients, 27 refused second-look surgery, 26 patients did not have resectable recurrences, and 28 patients did have resectable recurrences at second-look surgery. It is evident that patients with resectable recurrences fared significantly better than patients who refused second-look surgery ($p = 0.017$) or than patients with nonresectable recurrences ($p = 0.001$). In this study [16] 6 of 54 patients who underwent second-look procedures were cured.

Tumor-Associated Antigens as Prognostic Parameters

The retrospective evaluation of the survival of 563 patients with colorectal carcinomas and 369 patients with gastric carcinoma who underwent no further

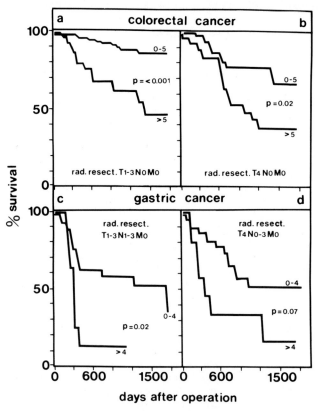

Fig. 2a–d. Correlation of CEA levels with the survival of patients with gastrointestinal carcinomas. Survival curves of patients with radically resected colorectal cancers staged: a T1–3N0M0 ($n=154 + 42$) or b T4N0M0 ($n=50 + 22$) and of patients with radically resected gastric cancer staged c T1–3N1–3M0 ($n=36 + 10$) or d T4N0–3M0 ($n=26 + 10$) according to preoperative CEA ranges of 0–5 vs > 5 (a, b) or 0–4 vs > 4 μg/liter (c, d) (After Staab et al. [21])

therapy after primary operation gave evidence of a high prognostic impact of the preoperative CEA in these cancer groups. It could be demonstrated on a statistically significant basis that a clinically homogenous group of patients with colorectal cancers could, depending on their preoperative values, be split into two subgroups with significantly different survival. In these investigations, those patients with preoperative CEA values under 5 µg/l fared significantly better than patients with values above this level. Likewise, in gastric cancer, a clinically homogenous group of patients did significantly better when their preoperative CEA values were below 5 µg/l in comparison with those patients with CEA values above 4 µg/l [17, 18]. Fig. 2 shows typical survival curves of patients with colorectal cancer and gastric cancer from clinically well-defined groups but belonging to subgroups with different ranges of preoperative CEA values. Prognostic validity of CA 19-9 is not yet established, but studies are currently underway.

Discussion and Conclusion

Though CA 19-9 proved to be of great clinical validity in the follow-up of cancer patients, the tumor marker − similar to CEA − is not useful in the primary diagnosis of cancer of the gastrointestinal tract. There is evidence, however, that CA 19-9 might be helpful for earlier diagnosis of pancreatic carcinomas [10]. In the follow-up of cancer patients, both CA 19-9 and CEA are of high clinical value for the earlier detection of relapse in these patients. While in colorectal cancer the superior role of CEA is still unchallenged [19], in pancreatic carcinoma, CEA certainly has an inferior role in comparison with CA 19-9. In the group of gastric carcinomas, however, both tests are of equal clinical validity. CA 19-9 in colorectal cancers and CEA in pancreatic carcinomas, do not give much additional clinical information of the patient when compared with the leading tumor marker. In gastric carcinomas, however, the highest complementarity of both tests becomes evident since the gain in sensitivity contributed by the CA 19-9 test is about 30% over the CEA test.

Nearly 20 years after the detection of CEA, it has been proven that tumor-associated antigens can be of great help in the management of cancer patients with respect to therapy [16, 20] and prognosis [17, 18]. Since the failure of such serodiagnostic procedures is relatively low, and investigations do not bother patients very much, tumor-associated antigens are to play a predominant role in the follow-up of cancer patients, particularly since they are apt to cut down costs in patient after-care, by selecting those patients with a high probability of relapse for further cost-intensive apparative diagnostic procedures.

References

1. Gold P, Freedman SO (1965) J Exp Med 121:439−462
2. Sugarbaker PH, Skarin AT, Zamscheck N (1976) J Surg Oncol 8:523−527
3. Staab H-J, Anderer FA, Stumpf E, Fischer R (1977) Dtsch Med Wochenschr 102:1082−1086

4. NIH (1981) Tumor Diagn 2:59−61
5. Del Villano BD, Brennan S, Broch P, Bucher C, Liu V, McClure M, Rahe B, Space S, Westrick B, Schoemaker H, Zurawski VR (1983) Clin Chem 29:549−552
6. Herlyn M, Sears HF, Steplenski Z, Koprowski H (1982) J Clin Immunol 2:135−140
7. Del Villano BD, Zurawski·VR (1983) In: Immunodiagnostics. Liss, New York, pp 269−282
8. Magnani JL, Nilsson B, Brockhaus M, Zopf D, Steplewski Z, Koprowski H, Ginsburg V (1982) J Biol Chem 257:14365−14369
9. Koprowski H, Steplewski Z, Mitchell K, Herlyn M, Herlyn D, Führer P (1979) Somatic Cell Genet 5:957−972
10. Klapdor R, Lehmann K, Bahlo M, Greten H, v Ackeren H, Dallek M, Schreiber WH (1983) Tumor Diagn Ther 4:197−201
11. Staab H-J, Anderer FA, Stumpf E, Fischer R (1978) Am J Surg 136:322−327
12. Staab H-J, Glock S, Hornung A (1982) Tumor Diagn Ther 3:183−194
13. Mann HB, Whitney DR (1947) Ann Math Stat 18:50−60
14. Staab H-J, Hornung A, Anderer FA, Kieninger G (1984) Dtsch Med Wochenschr 109:1141−1147
15. Staab H-J, Anderer FA, Hornung A, Kieninger G (1984) In: Protides of the biological fluids. Pergamon, Oxford, pp 617−621
16. Staab H-J, Anderer FA, Stumpf E, Hornung A, Fischer R, Kieninger G (1985) Am Surg 149:198−204
17. Staab H-J, Anderer FA, Brümmendorf T, Stumpf E, Fischer R (1981) Br J Cancer 44:652−662
18. Staab H-J, Anderer FA, Brümmendorf T, Hornung A, Fischer R (1982) Br J Cancer 45:718−727
19. Staab H-J, Brümmendorf T, Hornung A, Anderer FA, Kieninger G (1985) Klin Wochenschr 63:106−115
20. Minton JP, Hoehn JL, Gerber DM, Horsley JS, Connolly DP, Salwan F, Fletcher WS, Cruz AB, Gatchell FG, Oviedo M, Meyer KK, Leffall LD, Berk RS, Stewart PA, Kurucz SE (1985) Cancer 55:1284−1290
21. Staab H-J, Anderer FA, Brümmendorf T, Fischer R (1983) Cancer Detect Prev 6:149−153

The Value of Tumor Markers in the Diagnosis of Urogenital Carcinoma

H. W. Bauer[1] and P. Kühne

In the early diagnosis, course control, and prognostication of urogenital carcinomas, tumor markers may give decisive indications and, at the same time, lead to new findings as to the pathophysiologic mechanisms of tumor genesis.

Prostate Carcinoma

Prostate-Specific Acid Phosphatase = Isoenzyme II (PAP)

Since Foti and co-workers made possible the immunochemical determination of prostate-specific acid phosphatase (PAP) in the early seventies, the value of PAP as a tumor marker in prostate carcinoma has been reassessed.

The list compiled by the most important study groups regarding the sensitivity of immunochemical PAP determination for intracapsular stages shows the very limited value of immunochemical PAP determination for these stages of disease. With a sensitivity rate of 10%–50% in stage A and B, an early diagnosis of prostate carcinomas by immunochemical PAP determination is not possible.

It is not until there are so-called extraprostatic PAP production sites in lymph nodes or other organs, i.e., following formation of metastases, that the sensitivity increases to 80%–95%. A comparative demonstration is given of the results obtained by means of radioimmunoassay, enzyme immunoassay with cloned antibodies, and immunoenzymatic assay. Compared with this, the results obtained by enzymatic and functional means with regard to the recognitive sensitivity to a metastasizing prostate carcinoma are rather poor (36%–68%).

Since the most recent investigations demonstrate the same degree of sensitivity in confirming the presence of metastases using both the PAP method and skeletal scintigraphy with ^{99m}technetium polyphosphate, immunochemical PAP determination may well be regarded as the most important tumor marker used for the course control of metastasizing prostate carcinomas.

---

1 Urologische Universitätsklinik, Klinikum Großhadern der Universität München, Marchioninistraße 15, D-8000 München 70

Nuclear Medicine in Clinical Oncology
Ed. by C. Winkler
© Springer-Verlag Berlin Heidelberg 1986

Table 1. Tumor markers

Prostate carcinoma:	PAP
	PSA
	Hormone receptors
	Hormones
	Unspecific markers
Bladder carcinoma:	Blood-group-antigens
	CEA
	TPA
Kidney carcinoma:	Parameters derived from ectopic formation
Testicular carcinoma:	Alpha-fetoprotein
	HCG
	Unspecific markers

Table 2. Sensitivity of immunochemical PAP determination

		Intracapsular stages:		Clinical staging		
			(%)		(%)	
Foti et al.	1977	A	33	B	79	RIA
Bruce et al.	1979	A/B			10	RIA
Lindholm et al.	1980	A	22	B	29	RIA
Bruce et al.	1981	A/B			22	RIA
Daver et al.	1981	A	15	B	30	RIA
Bauer et al.	1982	A/B			32	EIA
Griffiths et al.	1982	A	24	B	44	EIA
Flüchter et al.	1982	A	22	B	50	RIA/EIA

Table 3. Sensitivity of immunochemical PAP determination

		Extraprostatic metastases			
		n	(%)		E (%)
Foti et al.	1977	25	92	RIA	60
Lee et al.	1980	14	79	IEA	36
Choe et al.	1980	23	78	IEA	
Pontes et al.	1981	10	80	RIA	60
Jacobi et al.	1981	18	87	EIA	53
Wirth et al.	1981	12	83	RIA	39
Flüchter et al.	1982	19	94	RIA	68
Vihko et al.	1982	18	89	RIA	47
Griffiths et al.	1982	25	84	EIA	
Griffiths et al.	1982		76	RIA	
Romas et al.	1982	18	94	IEA	65
Bauer et al.	1982	61	92	EIA	65
Bauer et al.	1982	51	95	IEA	65

Prostate-Specific Antigen (PSA)

Ten years ago, Wang and co-workers were the first to describe the process that confirmed the existence of a prostate-specific antigen in humans, which is relevant for the clinical course control of the prostate carcinoma. In comparison with immunochemically determined PAP, recent investigations did not reveal any higher specificity in the recognition of a prostate carcinoma, since both substances must normally be regarded as exocrine secretion products of the prostate and, in addition, largely reveal identical localization at histological examination. The question as to how far a combined determination of both parameters may lead to an increase in sensitivity and specificity has not yet been answered.

Hormone Receptors and Hormones

The response of a prostate carcinoma to hormone treatment depends on the presence of androgen receptors. Their confirmation in cytosol in part correlates with the response to hormone treatment in prostate carcinoma patients. Although the determination of androgen receptors in prostate carcinoma by means of gel electrophoresis or the carbon dextran method with the more recent specific ligands came to a methodic solution, the problems relating to the initial material, the amount of initial material, the material representation and workup still constitute insurmountable obstacles in diagnosing the prostate carcinoma in contrast to the mamma carcinoma. Thus, the determination of hormone receptors, in particular of androgen receptors, still preserves its clinical experimental characteristics in prostate carcinoma.

Quantitative hormone analyses and unspecific tumor markers − such as, hydroxyproline, lactic dehydrogenase (LDH), complement, transferrin, CK-BB, and cholesterol − may be helpful in the determination of the individual prognostic course; they are, however, inappropriate for the establishment of routine diagnosis or routine course control.

Carcinoma of the Bladder

In 1968, Kovarik and co-workers for the first time demonstrated blood-group antigens of the groups A, B, and 0 on normal urothelium. Their investigations in patients with carcinoma of the bladder showed that lower concentrations of the blood-group antigens on tumor cells indicate an increased invasive tendency of the tumor. It is not clear, however, whether specific defects of biosynthesis or an accelerated decomposition are to be regarded as the cause. The importance of this investigation becomes obvious when the frequency of recidivation of both tumor groups is compared. There is a recidivation rate of approximately 50% in bladder tumors exhibiting blood-group antigens, whereas this rate is 90% for tumors without detectable blood-group antigens. It might thus be concluded from these observations that patients with blood-group-antigen-negative

tumors should undergo early and extensive surgical therapy (radical cystec-
tomy).

CEA and TPA

Determination of carcinoembryonic antigen (CEA) and tissue polypeptide antigen (TPA) in serum of patients with bladder carcinoma may well be useful in
individual cases; they are, however, inadequate for routine course control. The
same holds true for the determination of CEA and TPA in urine. The fluctuations of CEA in the urine of a normal female population are such that an upper threshold value for discrimination between healthy individuals and patients
with bladder carcinoma cannot be given.

Carcinoma of the Kidney

Parameters Derived from Ectopic Formation

Humoral parameters play a role as tumor markers in patients with kidney carcinoma with ectopic formation. In these cases, paraneoplastic syndromes may
occur, which permit a course control and reliable prognosis in selected patients.
These are, for example, the hypersecretion of renin, erythropoietin, and pros-
taglandins A and B as well as the ectopic secretion of parathormone, human
chorionic gonadotropin (HCG), prolactin, and adrenocorticotropic hormone
(ACTH). Otherwise, the diagnosis of kidney tumors remains restricted to imaging procedures, such as sonography, scintigraphy, infusion urography, and
computerized tomography.

Carcinoma of the Testis

AFP and HCG

In the diagnosis and course control of testicular carcinoma, two glycoproteins,
alpha-fetoprotein (AFP) and beta-HCG, have established their clinical relevance.

Of the patients with a tumor other than seminoma 48% had increased alpha-
fetoprotein serum levels, which were not observed in cases of pure seminoma. If
a histologically confirmed seminoma exhibits increased alpha-fetoprotein levels,
a mixed tumor or formation of hepatic metastases has to be assumed.

A combination of both tumor markers with excretory urography and lymphangiography permits a reliable tumor diagnosis in more than 90% of patients
with retroperitoneal metastases from a carcinoma of the testis. This result
underlines the clinical relevance.

Pregnancy-Specific Beta$_1$-Glycoprotein

The presence of a choriocarcinoma or teratoma results in an increased production of a specific beta$_1$-glycoprotein (SP-1) by the involved syncytiotrophoblasts. Its increase in serum is used as an indicator of testicular carcinoma. Furthermore, N-acetyl neuraminic acid (NANA) should be mentioned; its increase in serum allows an earlier identification of therapeutic failure with beginning progression than alpha-fetoprotein and beta-HCG.

Summary

The use if biological tumor markers becomes more and more significant in clinical diagnosis and therapy control of urogenital carcinoma. Tumor markers can be useful in staging most tumors of this type and thus help to decide on an adequate therapeutic procedure. In order to obtain as few false-positive and false-negative results as possible, it is necessary to develop new chemical laboratory procedures and to improve existing methods of examination. The following substances have become clinically relevant: PAP for metastasizing prostate carcinoma, AFP and HCG for testicular tumors, and histochemically demonstrated AB-0 antigenicity loss in the case of bladder tumor.

Tumor Markers for Monitoring Therapy in Lung Cancer

C. GROPP[1], K. HAVEMANN, and R. HOLLE

The ectopic production of several peptide hormones in patients with lung cancer has been described by several authors in recent years. Hormones which are frequently elevated in sera of patients with small cell lung cancer (SCLC) at diagnosis are summarized in Table 1. Only results based on sufficiently large numbers of patients are included. The incidence of elevated levels of a given peptide hormone varies depending on the assay system, the antibodies used, and the upper limits employed in the different studies. For many of the hormones listed in Table 1, increased levels can be detected at diagnosis in up to 70% of patients, and in many cases several hormones are elevated in parallel. Often, however, blood levels are only marginally increased, and evidence of excessive production may be present in only up to 25% [2].

Serum levels of these hormones were evaluated as markers for disease extent and response to therapy. Adrenocorticotropic hormone (ACTH), calcitonin, neurophysins, and other tumor markers, such as carcinoembryonic antigen (CEA), were measured in patients at the diagnosis and then sequentially during therapy [3–5, 7]. The serum levels were correlated with the disease extent and the observed clinical response. While in some studies the presence of increased levels showed a good correlation with disease extent, no such correlation was observed in others.

A close correlation between the tumors' response to cytotoxic therapy and a decrease of hormone levels was shown in some studies [4–6]. This suggests a possibility of treatment monitoring with a subsequent change of therapy according to the serum peptide hormone levels. These results, however, were obtained in rather small groups of patients and in retrospective investigations.

In this paper we report the interim results of a multicenter trial on the treatment of SCLC by chemotherapy and radiation. Patients from 14 participating institutions were randomized between the therapeutic protocols A and B. Under protocol A, patients received a sequential chemotherapy, while the patients in group B were treated with an alternating chemotherapy of different combinations as described in Fig. 1. Responding patients under each protocol received prophylactic cranial irradiation after 3 cycles and chest irradiation after 8 cycles. No maintenance therapy was given to patients in complete remission.

Before each cycle and in monthly intervals during the follow-up period, deep-frozen serum samples were sent to the central marker laboratory in Mar-

---

1 Zentrum für Innere Medizin, Klinikum der Philipps-Universität, Mannkopffstraße 1, D-3550 Marburg

Nuclear Medicine in Clinical Oncology
Ed. by C. Winkler
© Springer-Verlag Berlin Heidelberg 1986

Table 1. Peptide hormones and neuronspecific enolase (NSE) in serum or plasma of untreated patients with small cell lung cancer

	No. of patients	Incidence %	Author	
ACTH	75	29	Hansen et al.	[4]
	50	30	Gropp et al.	[3]
	68	38	Krauss et al.	[5]
	63	24	Ratcliffe et al.	[9]
α MSH	43	19	Gropp et al.	[3]
β Endorphin	58	45	Gropp et al.	[3]
LPH	24	54	Odell et al.	[8]
ADH	41	39	Hansen et al.	(4)
	61	48	North et al.	(7)
	54	17	Greco et al.	(2)
	66	30	Gropp et al.	[3]
Oxytocin	61	30	North et al.	[7]
Calcitonin	75	64	Hansen et al.	[4]
	54	48	Gropp et al.	[3]
	49	73	Krauss et al.	[5]
	54	40	Greco et al.	[2]
	135	56	Luster et al.	[6]
PTH	43	27	Gropp et al.	[3]
β HCG	39	33	Gropp et al.	[3]
Gastrin	69	20	Hansen et al.	[4]
Glucagon	46	11	Hansen et al.	[4]
Secretin, Insulin VIP	46–65	≦5	Hansen et al.	[4]
NSE	94	69	Carney et al.	[1]

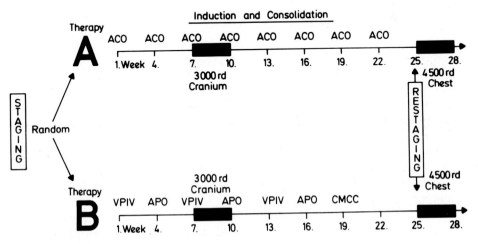

Fig. 1. Treatment plan for the multicentre trial

Table 2. Classification of tumormarker levels

	normal	elevated	pathological
CEA (ng/ml)	$\leq$ 5	5– 20	> 20
Calcitonin (pg/ml)	$\leq$ 100	100–200	>200
ACTH	$\leq$ 80	80–150	>150

burg for determination of calcitonin, ACTH, and CEA. Due to organizational problems, only 60% of the scheduled samples could be tested for these three markers. However, the missing samples mainly belonged to the time period after the end of therapy. About 5% of the samples thawed during transportation. Up to now about 5400 marker analyses of 1816 sera have been performed and the results together with the clinical data are stored in the computer.

For practical reasons, the marker levels were classified as normal, elevated, or clearly pathological, according to Table 2. At the time of this interim analysis, 250 patients were included in the multicenter trial.

Tumor Markers Before Therapy

At diagnosis we observed elevated or clearly pathological levels of calcitonin in 48%, of ACTH in 16%, and of CEA in 41% of patients (Table 3). As expected, the clearly pathological levels were less frequent (viz 9% calcitonin, 19% ACTH, 20% CEA). Thus, the incidence is lower than in retrospective studies, which could be due to the prospective design of our trial or to the transportation of the samples to the central laboratory (especially ACTH is affected by increased temperatures). None of the markers was elevated in 30%, one marker in 39%, two in 26%, and all three markers in only 5% of the patients.

There is a slight positive correlation between any two of the markers, an effect possibly produced by the correlation of the marker levels with the extent of disease. The association between markers and other prognostic variables at diagnosis is given in Fig. 2. The comparisons are based on the percentages of pathological values, because differences between prognostic subgroups are more distinct in the upper ranges of CEA and calcitonin values. There is a direct relationship between the marker levels and the extent of disease. Whereas limited disease and extensive disease without distant metastases show nearly identical marker levels, the serum levels are markedly increased in patients with distant metastases. In addition, patients with multiple distant metastatic sites have higher CEA and calcitonin levels than patients with liver, bone, and bone marrow metastases when compared to patients without metastases in the respective sites. Patients with brain metastases exhibit no significant increase.

As is already known, smoking is strongly correlated with increased levels of CEA and calcitonin. Further positive correlations exist between pathological CEA levels and weight loss and between pathological calcitonin levels and re-

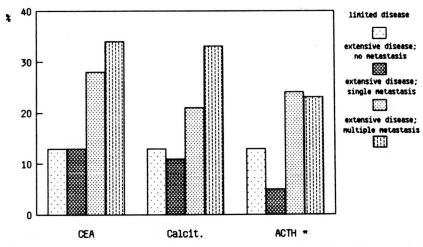

Fig. 2. Percentage of patients with pathological marker levels. * Elevated and pathological values are combined

Table 3. Tumormarker at diagnosis ($n = 172$)

	elevated or pathological (%)	pathological (%)
Calcitonin	48	19
ACTH	16	9
CEA	41	20
No marker	30	65
One marker	39	23
Two marker	26	9
All three markers	5	3
	100	100

duced Karnofsky index, whereas the other variables show less prominent correlations in this analysis.

A relationship between marker levels at diagnosis and survival seems to be indirectly induced by the influence of distant metastases on survival. The results of a stratified analysis show that in patients with limited disease or extensive disease without distant metastases, no influence of the marker levels on survival can be observed. Only in the group of patients with distant metastases do the calcitonin levels seem to be related with survival time. However, further analyses including the number of metastatic sites may explain this correlation.

Tumor Markers in Relation to Tumor Response

For patients with elevated or pathological levels at diagnosis, the change of the markers calcitonin, ACTH, and CEA was compared with the degree of tumor response. In the first analysis, the outcome of treatment was classified as CR (complete remission), PR + MR (partial remission, including minimal response), or NR (no response) and compared with the behavior of the three markers within the first 2 months of chemotherapy (Table 4). A strong correspondence becomes apparent, which is most evident in the cases of complete remission and of no response. Among the CR patients, only two exceptions with continually pathological values of CEA or ACTH at relatively constant levels are found. There was only one patient who had a marker decrease into the normal range without showing any clinical response, but in this case the initial calcitonin level had only just exceeded the normal limit. When marker determinations from the time period after the two months are included in the analysis, patients who achieved a complete remission show a drop of increased values into the normal range in 75% for CEA, 93% for calcitonin, and 63% for ACTH.

To investigate whether a response of the tumor during the first weeks of treatment was accompanied by a change of the marker concentration, a decrease of the marker of at least 10% was compared with the chest X-ray after the first cycle of therapy. With the exception of ACTH, a significant correlation between marker decrease and reduction of tumor size in the chest X-ray can be demonstrated, as shown in Table 5. Corresponding results occur for calcitonin in 78%, for CEA in 73% (not shown), and for CEA and calcitonin combined in 80%. The lack of agreement in the remaining 20% could be due to a delayed marker decrease or could suggest that a decrease in hormone and CEA levels is in some cases a better indicator of tumor reduction than the chest X-ray.

In order to determine the speed of marker decrease, markers which had dropped during the first cycle were studied further during the following cycles. It is evident, as shown in Table 6, that calcitonin decreases much faster than CEA, which does not usually reach normal levels until the end of the second or third cycle or even remains above normal values, especially in the case of initially pathological levels. Although the number of patients with elevated ACTH was rather small, a tendency of response similar to calcitonin could be observed (not shown).

Table 4. Analyses of patients with initially elevated or pathologic marker levels

		Complete remission	Partial or minimal response	No Response
CEA	decrease to normal	7	9	0
	decrease (not normal)	8	18	2
	no decrease of $\geq$ 10%	1	6	5
Calcitonin	decrease to normal	12	32	1
	decrease (not normal)	2	13	5
	no decrease of $\geq$ 10%	0	5	4
ACTH	decrease to normal	4	10	0
	decrease (not normal)	3	0	1
	no decrease of $\geq$ 10%	1	4	1

Table 5. Comparison of marker decrease (at least 10%) and chest x-ray findings after the first cycle of chemotherapy

Decrease of marker ($\geqq$ 10%)		Tumor response in chest x-ray	
		+	$\emptyset$
Calcitonin	+	49	10
	$\emptyset$	5	5
ACTH	+	9	2
	$\emptyset$	5	2
Calcitonin or CEA	+	60	12
	$\emptyset$	5	7

Table 6. Reaching normal values after:

	n	1 cycle	2 cycle	3 cycles or more	never
CEA	23	8 (35%)	3 (13%)	5 (23%)	7 (30%)
Calcitonin	36	24 (67%)	9 (25%)	0	3 (8%)

Table 7. Median survival (days) and the response of tumor markers and of chest x-ray during the first two cycles of chemotherapy

		decrease median (n)	no decrese median (n)	
CEA	1. cycle	319 (35)	230 (19)	$P > 0.1$
	2. cycle	336 (33)	161 (15)	$P < 0.001$
Calcitonin	1. cycle	314 (54)	212 (11)	$P > 0.05$
	2. cycle	319 (50)	154 (8)	$P < 0.001$
All markers	1. cycle	324 (65)	215 (30)	$P < 0.05$
	2. cycle	344 (60)	177 (23)	$P < 0.001$
Chest x-ray	1.–2. cycle	347 (120)	219 (45)	$P < 0.1$

Furthermore, we tested whether the marker levels or the chest X-ray allowed a more reliable prognosis of survival. Table 7 indicates the median survival time of different groups (because of the small sample numbers, ACTH is not included). The decrease of markers was determined 3 and 6 weeks after the start of treatment, i.e., after one or two cycles of chemotherapy.

In order to extend the validity of the results to a larger group, all patients with at least one elevated marker were included in a further analysis. They were only classified as showing a marker decrease if all elevated markers dropped by 10% or more. The mean survival time for patients showing no decrease of CEA, calcitonin, or all elevated markers during the second cycle is significantly shorter than for patients with a decrease of the respective markers. A reduction of the tumor size in the chest X-ray during the first cycle shows nearly the same influence on survival, while the tumor markers appear to have slightly better prognostic value than the chest X-ray, when one compares the respective findings after two cycles of chemotherapy. Nevertheless, the chest X-ray as a monitoring aid cannot be substituted by the tumor markers, since both methods seem to reflect different aspects of tumor response, and since about one third of the patient population shows normal values of all three markers in question.

It has to be mentioned that the results described in this paragraph are dependent on the arbitrary choice of a 10% decrease for the definition of marker response. Further statistical analyses will probably allow the definition of a better suited value.

Tumor Markers During the Further Course of Therapy

To classify the courses of markers during therapy, only those patients could be taken into consideration for whom complete numbers of serum samples were available covering the time from diagnosis up to shortly before the death of the patient. Only 63 patients fulfilled this criterion when the interval between the last serum and the patient's death was restricted to be less than six weeks. Several characteristic types of marker courses can be observed, which may be defined as follows:

Type 1: initially elevated levels decrease to normal and stay normal
Type 2: initially elevated levels decrease to normal and increase again during relapse
Type 3: increased marker levels remain elevated
Type 4: initially normal markers increase to elevated levels
Type 5: markers remain normal over the whole time period

The number of patients with marker courses classified according to this definition are contained in Table 8. It has to be noted that the frequencies of Type 2 and Type 4 have supposedly been unterestimated in favour of Type 1 and Type 5, respectively, because a final rise of the markers could have been missed when the last serum of a patient was collected 4 to 6 weeks before his death. This speculation is supported by the fact that in some of these cases a rise of marker levels into the upper normal range can be observed.

Table 8. Types of marker response during therapy

Type:	1	2	3	4	5	n
	(initially elevated)			(initially normal)		
CEA	3	7	17	10	24	61
Calcitonin	9	10	13	16	15	63
ACTH	1	2	4	4	52	63

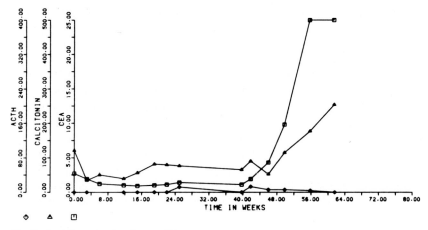

Fig. 3. Serial marker levels, pat. 74

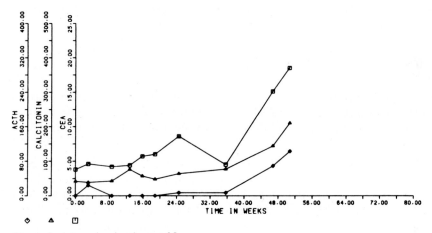

Fig. 4. Serial marker levels, pat. 85

Among patients with increased pretreatment levels, Type 3 is most common. However, this group is heterogenous, because it includes nonresponding patients as well as patients with tumor remission, who do show a marker decrease and fail to fulfil the requirement of normalized levels. Therefore, the generalized type 2, i.e., bathtub-shaped marker courses without reference to normal values, represents an even larger number of patients than indicated by Table 8.

A particularly interesting result of the study is the high percentage of patients with initially normal marker values rising to elevated or even pathological levels during the course of treatment or follow-up (viz 52% of patients with initially normal calcitonin and 29% for CEA). This Type 4 of marker behaviour is demonstrated by two examples (Fig. 3 and Fig. 4) showing an increase of either 2 or 3 markers in parallel, which is obviously related to tumor growth. A further analysis of the CEA courses of Type 4 reveals that nearly all of these patients have pretreatment levels in the upper normal range (i.e., between 3 and 5 ng/ml). In the case of Type 4 calcitonin courses, no similar results could be found, but for some patients the marker rise was only transient and not connected with clinical recurrence.

Combinations of Type 1 for one marker and Type 4 for another occur in some instances. This possibility of a change in the marker profile hints at the necessity of multiple marker determinations for patients with small cell lung cancer. Furthermore, multivariate statistical analyses are required to establish a potential use of tumor markers in the early detection of tumor relapse.

So far, all efforts to use tumor markers as a reliable and clinically useful monitoring aid in patients staying in tumor remission have failed. Although in many cases increasing tumor markers can be observed at the time of recurrence, there are still more exceptions where markers rise too late, indistinctly, or not at all. As in the case of pretreatment marker levels, high levels of one or more markers during relapse can mainly be seen if the recurrence includes distant metastases and not only the primary tumor. Again, the most pronounced increase occurs in patients with liver and bone metastases, while patients with no other than brain metastases show no marker elevation.

Conclusion

In our prospective study, there was a lower incidence of elevated tumor markers as compared with retrospective analyses. Nonetheless, the markers are of some prognostic use and may be helpful in the treatment of patients with small cell lung cancer.

1. A marked increase of ACTH, calcitonin, and CEA indicated the presence of distant metastases. This may allow a better classification of the extent of disease. This finding suggests that there is a direct correlation between tumor burden and the marker levels. Since the tumor burden is negatively correlated with survival, there is also a negative correlation between increased marker levels and survival.

2. There is a positive correlation between the marker values and smoking. In some instances, the multivariate analyses also showed a correlation with weight loss and performance status, whereas a correlation with other variables could not be found.

3. The most important finding of this study is that during the first 2 or 3 cycles of chemotherapy, an immediate control of treatment success by calcitonin and CEA determinations as well as by chest X-ray may allow an early detection of tumor resistance in the individual patient and may suggest a change to another treatment program.

4. So far, monitoring tumor markers during the further course of treatment in order to detect an early relapse is rather disappointing. This is because of the multiple response types observed and the number of cases showing an increase of the marker only during or after clinical relapse. Nevertheless, further research might help to define a more sensitive criterion of marker response.

5. In a considerable number of patients, initially normal values increased during the later course parallel with tumor growth, particularly for calcitonin. This finding may indicate an overgrowth of a resistant hormone-producing tumor cell clone.

References

1. Carney DN, Marangos PJ, Ihde DC (1982) Serum neuron-specific enolase: a marker of disease extent and response to therapy in patients with small cell lung cancer. Lancet 1:583–585
2. Carney DN, Broder L, Edelstein M, Gazdar AF, Hansen M, Havemann K, Matthews MJ, Sorenson GD, Vindelov L (1983) Experimental studies of the biology of human small cell lung cancer. Cancer Treat Rep 67:27–35
3. Gropp C, Luster W, Havemann K, Lehmann FG (1981) ACTH, calcitonin, α-MSH, β-endorphin, parathormone and β-HCG in sera of patients with lung cancer. In: Uhlenbruck G, Wintzer G (eds) CEA und andere Tumormarker. Tumor Diagnostik, Leonberg, pp 358–363
4. Hansen M, Hammer M, Hummer L (1980) ACTH, ADH, and calcitonin concentrations as marker of response and relapse in small cell carcinoma of the lung. Cancer 46:2062–2067
5. Krauss S, Macy S, Ichiki AT (1981) A study of immunoreactive calcitonin, ACTH and CEA in lung cancer and other malignancies. Cancer 47:2485–2492
6. Luster W, Gropp C, Sostmann H, Kalbfleisch H, Havemann K (1982) Demonstration of immunoreactive calcitonin in sera and tissues of lung cancer patients. Eur J Cancer Clin Oncol 18:1275–1283
7. North WG, Maurer H, Valtin H, O'Donell JF (1980) Human neurophysins as potential tumor markers for small cell carcinoma of the lung: Application of specific radioimmunoassays. J Clin Endocrinol Metab 51:892–897
8. Odell WD, Wolfsen AR, Bachelot I, Hirose FM (1979) Ectopic production of lipotropin by cancer. Am J Med 66:631–638
9. Ratcliffe JG, Podmore J, Stack BHR, Spilg WGS, Gropp C (1982) Circulating ACTH and related peptides in lung cancer. Br J Cancer 45:230–238

Tumor Markers for Follow-Up of Thyroid Carcinoma

CHR. REINERS[1]

Malignant epithelial tumors of the thyroid can be characterized oncologically on the basis of some special features (Table 1). For the follow-up, it is very important that most of these tumors secrete hormones or hormone precursors which may serve as very specific tumor markers. Because of the generally good prognosis (the anaplastic type excluded), the number of patients who have to be followed-up increases continuously despite the relative rareness of thyroid malignancies (approx. 40 new cases/year in our department). On the other hand, malignant thyroid tumors not seldom metastasize after several years of uncomplicated course. Therefore, the diagnostic program for follow-up requires sensitive, specific, and cost-effective methods which do not bother the patient. Depending on the histological type of thyroid carcinoma, determinations of different tumor markers can fulfill these criteria.

Table 1. Oncological characteristics of thyroid cancer

Rareness	– incidence $\sim 3/100\,000$
Biological activity	– iodine accumulation, hormone secretion and dependency (hTg, hCT)
Secondaries	– type (N, M) and time of manifestation varying
Prognosis	– extremely variable depending on histological type

Table 2 lists some antigens which may serve as tumor markers. They have to be distinguished – according to the histological type of thyroid cancer – into highly specific and quite unspecific tumor antigens.

Table 2. Specific and unspecific tumor markers for different types of thyroid cancer

Histological type	Specific marker	Unspecific marker
Follicular/papillary	hTg	(TPA)
Oncocytic	hTg	(TPA)
Medullary	hCT	CEA (TPA)

1 Abteilung für Nuklearmedizin der Universität Würzburg, Josef-Schneider-Straße 2, 8700 Würzburg, FRG

Nuclear Medicine in Clinical Oncology
Ed. by C. Winkler
© Springer-Verlag Berlin Heidelberg 1986

First of all, as a glycoprotein of the follicular colloid, thyroglobulin (hTg) serves as a prohormone for the thyroid hormones. It can be used as a specific marker for follicular and papillary carcinoma [39]. These two types of differentiated malignant epithelial thyroid tumors, which often take up radioiodine, are most frequent (37% and 30% respectively in our material). But even malignant oncocytic tumors (Hürthle cell carcinoma), which amount to approx. 12% in our material, mostly produce thyroglobulin in spite of their inability to take up radioiodine [31].

The second specific tumor marker is calcitonin (hCT), a peptide hormone of the parafollicular C cells. hCT is a highly specific and sensitive marker [9, 12] for the rare malignant tumors of those cells (approximately 5% of thyroid malignancies are medullary carcinomas).

On the other hand, some unspecific tumor markers — such as CEA for medullary and TPA for undifferentiated tumors — can be used additionally for follow-up.

Thyroglobulin (hTg) in the Follow-up of Follicular, Papillary and Oncocytic Carcinoma

Figure 1 summarizes the results of hTg determinations in more than 250 patients after thyroidectomy for thyroid cancer. Patients are grouped with regard to the outcome of ablative therapy into patients with nodal (N) or distant (M)

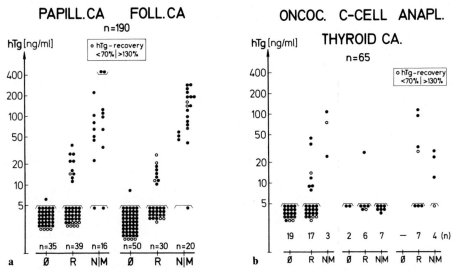

Fig. 1 a, b. Serum thyroglobulin in thyroid cancer **a** 190 patients with papillary and follicular carcinoma. **b** 65 patients with oncocytic, medullary and anaplastic thyroid carcinoma. Ø no thyroid remnant after ablation therapy; R residual tissue in thyroid bed; N/M, nodal/distant metastases. *Open circles* indicate patients with more than ± 30% deviation in the individual recovery test

metastases as well as into patients lacking metastases with residual tissue in thyroid bed (R) or without any thyroid remants (Ø).

It has to be pointed out that determinations of hTg by radioimmunoassay may be interfered with by endogenous autoantibodies against thyroglobulin [2, 3, 11, 19, 24, 25, 28]. For checking the possible interference of such autoantibodies with the hTg RIA, we routinely use individual recovery experiments by adding a defined amount of hTg standard material to each patient sample [24, 25, 28]. Sera with a recovery of less than 70% or more than 130% − which is much less frequent than a diminished recovery in the RIA system we use (hTg RIA Henning Berlin) − are characterized as open symbols in Fig. 1 (approx. 13% of the cases). However in our experience, even recoveries below or above the limits given do not necessarily mean that corresponding hTg results are totally useless for follow-up of thyroid carcinoma. This is in agreement with the observations of other authors [3, 11, 19]. There is no question that hTg values of sera with proven autoantibodies must be interpreted very carefully. Furthermore, sera with hTg autoantibodies detectable by the much less sensitive hemagglutination method (approximately 3% of patients with thyroid cancer) should be excluded from clinical interpretation.

Figure 1 demonstrates that, with few exceptions, patients without thyroid remnants (Ø) have only hTg levels lower than 5 ng/ml. In patients with residual thyroid tissue (R) after incomplete ablative therapy, hTg values are higher: they are measurable in 26 out of 86 cases with papillary, follicular, and oncocytic carcinoma and do not exceed 50 ng/ml. By contrast, hTg is elevated above 30 ng/ml in nearly all cases with nodal (N) or distant (M) metastases of the three types of thyroid tumors mentioned above.

As one should expect, hTg is not very useful as a tumor marker for C cell (or medullary) and anaplastic thyroid carcinoma (Fig. 1 b).

All in all, for papillary, follicular, and oncocytic carcinoma hTg levels higher than 5 ng/ml after *complete* ablation of the thyroid signify progressive tumor disease with a sensitivity of 92% and a specificity of 98%. These probabilities are in agreement with the literature (Table 3). The relatively broad ranges given in this table depend on the fact that some authors evaluated the diagnostic validity of hTg as a tumor marker in patient groups including cases with *incomplete* ablation of the residual thyroid tissue, which impairs the sensitivity [24, 36]. Using a discriminatory level of 30 ng/ml for our patient material, the sensitivity amounts to only 87%, whereas the specificity remains unchanged at 98% [24].

The diagnostic validity of hTg as a tumor marker for differentiated tumors of the thyroid has to be measured against I-131 whole-body scans, which generally serve as sensitive and − above all − specific means for detection and localization of recurrences and metastases. Various evaluations published in recent years clearly showed that hTg determinations are more sensitive than I-131 scans [1, 4, 6−8, 10, 13−15, 17, 21, 23−25, 28, 29, 32−34, 37, 38, 40]. The higher sensitivity of hTg depends mainly on the fact that thyroglobulin synthesis may be maintained even in dedifferentiating tumors or secondaries which often no longer take up radioiodine [14, 34, 38]. This behavior is typical of oncocytic thyroid carcinoma [29, 31] and late metastases of papillary or follicu-

Table 3. Diagnostic validity of thyroglobulin RIA in follow-up of differentiated thyroid cancer. Review from the literature [24]

	Mean	Range
Sensitivity	90%	55%–100%
Specificity	90%	60%–100%

Table 4. Comparison of the sensitivity of thyroglobulin RIA and I-131 scans for detection of early and late metastases of differentiated thyroid cancer [29]

	hTg-RIA		I-131-scan	
	⊕	⊖	⊕	⊖
Primary metastases	30	3	23	10
Late metastases	19	3	9	13
Total	49	6	32	23
Sensitivity	*89%*		*68%*	

lar malignancies [14, 29, 38]. Table 4 proves that the diagnostic sensitivity of hTg in comparison with I-131 scans is highest in patients with late metastases, which may not uncommonly occur after more than 5 years of follow-up [29].

However, there are some restrictions for the use of hTg as a tumor marker in papillary, follicular, and oncocytic carcinoma. The first restriction already mentioned above involves hTg autoantibodies, which may seriously interfere with hTg determinations in about 3% of the cancer patients. Secondly, it has to be pointed out that before surgery only patients with advanced tumor disease (i.e., distant metastases) can be separated from patients with benign goiter [24, 25], in whom hTg is often elevated up to more than 200 ng/ml. The third important restriction depends on the observation that hTg can be suppressed by thyroxine replacement therapy [1, 7, 8, 10, 11, 23–25, 28, 29, 31, 35, 37].

Last but not least, it has to be mentioned that results of different hTg RIA kits may vary widely due to lack of methodological standardization [2, 25].

Figure 2a shows the individual courses of hTg in 10 patients with metastatic disease; endogenous TSH stimulation after withdrawal of thyroxine substitution is characterized by the upright arrows. These data are summarized in Fig. 2b, giving the median differences of hTg on or off thyroxine. It is clear that hTg levels are approximately 60 ng/ml lower under thyroxine substitution. Most important is the observation that hTg is *completely* suppressed by thyroxine in three of the 10 patients with metastases (Fig. 2a). This effect is seen repeatedly over a period of 30 months in one case. In our now extended experience, a total suppression of hTg in spite of metastases has to be considered in approximately 10% of patients with papillary, follicular, and oncocytic cancer [29].

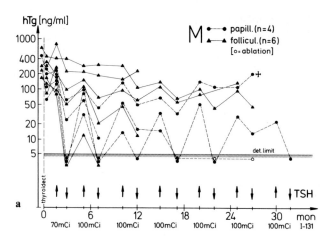

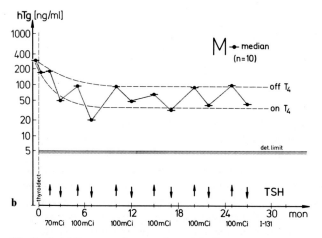

Fig. 2a, b. Follow-up of serum thyroglobulin in relation to endogenous TSH stimulation in 10 patients with metastases of differentiated thyroid carcinoma treated with fractionated high dose I-131 therapy. **a** Individual courses of hTg; **b** medians and mean difference of hTg without or with thyroxine medication. *Upright arrows* indicate endogenous TSH stimulation after withdrawal of thyroxine before I-131 therapy

Table 5. Advantages and problems of thyroglobulin RIA for follow-up of differentiated thyroid cancer

Advantages	– easy to perform, costs moderate
	– sensitivity higher than that of I-131-scans
	– no discomfort for the patient
Problems	– interference of hTg-Ab ($\sim$ 3% of patients with malignancies)
	– suppression of hTg by thyroid hormone replacement ($\sim$ 10% of cases)

In conclusion, hTg has several advantages over I-131 scans (Table 5). However, in our follow-up program [27], we do not replace I-131 scans totally with hTg determinations. Measurements of hTg, which are much easier to perform than I-131 scans, are used as a screening test. If hTg becomes measurable again after total ablation of the thyroid, we immediatedly use I-131 scans to localize suspected recurrences or secondaries.

Calcitonin (hCT) and Carcinoembryonic Antigen (CEA) in Follow-up of Medullary Carcinoma

Figure 3 shows the distribution of hCT and CEA levels in 16 of our patients with medullarly thyroid cancer. Calcitonin is clearly elevated in all of the five cases with proven metastases or recurrences (T+/M+), whereas CEA is normal in one of those patients. On the other hand, both tumor markers are elevated in four out of 11 patients without any clinical evidence of extended tumor disease (T0N0M0). This may be interpreted as a low specificity of hCT and CEA for diagnosis of recurrences or metastases. But it cannot be precluded that these tumor markers precede the clinical detectability of tumor progression.

Some authors prefer CEA determinations for follow-up because immunohistochemical investigations [18] and individual follow-up studies [5] have provided evidence that CEA might be a parameter for dedifferentiation of medullary thyroid carcinoma. Possibly because of this behavior, CEA is supposed to correlate closer than hCT in serum with clinical progression. Indeed, in one of

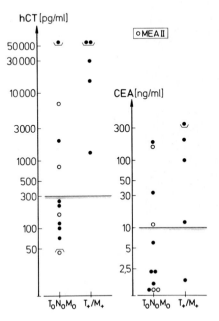

Fig. 3. Calcitonin (*hCT*) and carcinoembryonic antigen (*CEA*) in 11 patients free of disease (*T0N0M0*) and 5 patients with tumor or metastases (*T+/M+*) of medullary thyroid carcinoma

our patients, CEA was unequivocally elevated only shortly before clinical detectability of a local recurrence, whereas hCT was already increased approximately 2 years earlier. After surgical ablation of the local recurrence, CEA
returned to normal again, whereas hCT decreased, but did not normalize.
After two years of additional follow-up, the patient developed a skeletal metastasis although the CEA levels still remained normal. By this observation, we
cannot agree with the opinion that CEA should be more useful than hCT for
predicting the clinical course.

Furthermore, there are two conditions where CEA is unsuited for special diagnostics in medullary thyroid cancer. First at all, hCT determinations can only
be used to screen the relatives of patients with the inheritable form of medullary thyroid carcinoma [12], which is often combined with neoplasias of other
endocrine organs (multiple endocrine neoplasia = MEA II). Figure 4 shows the
results of hCT screening after pentagastrin stimulation in two sons of a patient
with proven medullary carcinoma. Because of the pathological rises of hCT after stimulation, the two young men were operated on despite normal clinical
and scintigraphic findings. Histological examination of the thyroid glands,
which were removed totally, revealed the suspected bilateral small medullary
cancers. The other situation where hCT is clearly superior to CEA is localization of tumor or secondaries by selective venous sampling [30].

Table 6 summarizes the advantages and disadvantages of hCT and CEA
measurements for follow-up of medullary thyroid carcinoma. In our opinion,
both tumor markers should be determined regularly in patients with this rare
type of thyroid malignancy.

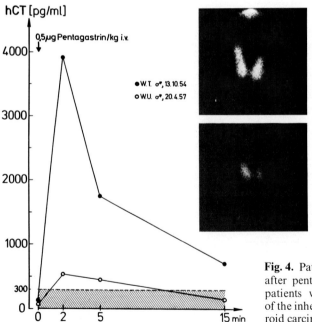

Fig. 4. Pathological rises of calcitonin
after pentagastrin stimulation in two
patients with clinical occult tumors
of the inherited form of medullary thyroid carcinoma

Table 6. Superiority of calcitonin over carcinoembryonic antigen for follow-up of medullary thyroid carcinoma

hCT	– higher specificity for medullary carcinoma
	– localization of tumor tissue by selective venous sampling possible
	– suitable for family screening (pentagastrin stimulation)
CEA	– closer correlation with clinical tumor progression?

Tissue Polypeptide Antigen (TPA) and Carcinoembryonic Antigen (CEA) as Unspecific Tumor Markers in Various Types of Thyroidal Malignancies

Some years ago, we first presented results of TPA and CEA determinations in various types of thyroid cancers [22]. Tissue polypeptide antigen was sometimes elevated in cases of metastasizing papillary, follicular, and medullary carcinoma. This observation has been confirmed by recent immunohistochemical and follow-up studies [16, 20]. Especially the interesting publication of Martino et al. [16] indicates that TPA may be a marker of dedifferentiation of thyroid tumors.

Cases with dedifferentiated metastases could be distinguished better by TPA than by hTg from patients with differentiated metastasizing papillary and follicular carcinoma. Moreover, TPA was elevated in nearly all cases with anaplastic carcinoma or malignant thyroid lymphoma in Martino's study. Additionally, the Italian group proposes TPA as a second-order tumor marker – comparable to CEA – for patients with medullary carcinoma of the thyroid. However, it has to be mentioned that TPA is elevated not only in progressive malignancies but also in inflammatory or infectious diseases [16].

Malignant Thyroid Tumors: An Interesting Challenge for the Application of Tumor Markers

Different tumor markers are of particular importance for follow-up of thyroid carcinoma (Table 7). First of all, they provide valuable information about the

Table 7. Application and interpretation of tumor markers in follow-up of thyroid carcinoma

Information about biological activity and type of the tumor
Early indicators of recurrences and metastases
Control of therapy response in patients with known metastases
Family screening for the inheritable form of medullary thyroid carcinoma

biological activity of tumors which can be used to support histological typing and grading. Secondly, tumor markers are indicators of the aggressiveness of a special tumor.

Thirdly, follow-up determinations can be used for the control of the response to therapy in patients with extended tumor disease. Last but not least, hCT determinations after pentagastrin stimulation represent the only method for early detection and cure of the heritable form of medullary thyroid carcinoma.

References

1. Ashcraft MW, Van Herle AJ (1981) The comparative value of serum thyroglobulin measurements and Iodine-131 total body scans in the follow-up study of patients with treated thyroid cancer. Am J Med 71:806–814
2. Bayer M, McDougall R (1984) Differences in radioimmunoassay results for thyroglobulin that affect management of patients with thyroid cancer. Clin Chem 30:81–86
3. Black EG, Hoffenberg R (1983) Should one measure serum thyroglobulin in the presence of anti-thyroglobulin antibodies? Clin Endocrinol (Oxf) 19:597–601
4. Botsch H (1982) Radioimmunoassay für die Serum-Thyreoglobulinbestimmung. Klinische Anwendung als Tumormarker bei der Verlaufskontrolle des differenzierten Schilddrüsenkarzinoms. Thieme, Stuttgart
5. Busnardo B, Girelli ME, Simioni N, Nacamulli D, Busetto E (1984) Nonparallel patterns of calcitonin and carcinoembryonic antigen levels in the follow-up of medullary thyroid carcinoma. Cancer 53:278–285
6. Castagnoli A, Cappelli G, D'Agata A, Forni S, Milani S, Pupi A (1982) Can thyroglobulin assay really supplant radioiodine scans in patients with differentiated thyroid cancer? Lancet 573
7. Charles MA, Dodson LE, Waldeck N, Hofeldt F, Ghaed N, Telepak R, Ownbey J, Burstein PH (1980) Serum thyroglobulin levels predict total body iodine scan findings in patients with treated well-differentiated thyroid carcinoma. Am J Med 69:401–407
8. Colacchio THA, Lo Gerfo P, Colacchio DA, Feind C (1982) Radioiodine total body scan versus serum thyroglobulin levels in follow-up of patients with thyroid cancer. Surgery 91:42–45
9. Deftos LJ (1974) Radioimmunoassay for calcitonin in medullary thyroid carcinoma. JAMA 227:403–406
10. Echenique RL, Kasi L, Haynie TP, Glenn HJ, Samaan NA, Stratton Hill C (1982) Critical evaluation of serum thyroglobulin levels and I-131 scans in post-therapy patients with differentiated thyroid carcinoma: Concise communication. J Nucl Med 23:235–240
11. Feldt-Rasmussen U, Holten I, Sand Hansen A (1983) Influence of thyroid substitution therapy and thyroid autoantibodies on the value of serum thyroglobulin in recurring thyroid cancer. Cancer 51:2240–2243
12. Hennesy JF, Wells SA, Ontjes DA, Cooper GW (1974) A comparison of pentagastrin injection and calcium infusion as provocative agents for the detection of medullary carcinoma of the thyroid. J Clin Endocrinol 39:487–495
13. Hüfner M, Stumpf HP, Grussendorf M, Hermann HJ, Kimmig B (1982) The significance of whole body scanning and plasma thyroglobulin measurements in the follow-up of metastatic thyroid cancer. Acta Endocrinol (Copenh) [Suppl] 246:59–60
14. Hüfner M, Stumpf HP, Hermann HJ, Kimmig B (1983) Diagnostischer Wert des J-131-Ganzkörperszintigramms in der Nachsorge des differenzierten Schilddrüsenkarzinoms. Dtsch Med Wochenschr 108:1234–1238
15. Jänsch A, Heinze HG, Hast B (1981) Serum-Thyreoglobulin (S-hTg). Ein Tumormarker bei Patienten mit differenziertem Schilddrüsenkarzinom. Strahlentherapie 157:381–392
16. Martino E, Bambini G, Aghini-Lombardi F, Motz E, Pacini F, Lari R, Baschier L, Pinchera A (1984) Serum tissue polypeptide antigen (TPA) in thyroid cancer. J Endocrinol Invest 7:249–252

17. McDougall IR, Bayer MF (1980) Follow-up of patients with differentiated thyroid cancer using serum thyroglobulin measured by an immunoradiometric assay. Comparison with I-131 total body scans. J Nucl Med 21:741−744

18. Mendelsohn G, Wells SA, Baylin SB (1984) Relationship of tissue carcinoembryonic antigen and calcitonin to tumor virulence in medullary thyroid carcinoma. An immunohistochemical study in early, localized and virulent disseminated stages of disease. Cancer 54:657−662

19. Moser E, Braun S, Kirsch CM, Kleinhans E, Buell U (1984) Time course of thyroglobulin autoantibodies in patients with differentiated thyroid carcinoma after radioiodine therapy. Nucl Med Commun 5:317−321

20. Oehr P, Vogel J, Lichius A, Selbach B, Biersack HJ, Winkler C, Gedigk P (1984) Vorkommen und Bedeutung von Thyreoglobulin, Tissue Polypeptide Antigen, Carcinoembryonalem Antigen und Calcitonin in Geweben und im Plasma von Schilddrüsenkarzinom-Patienten. Tumor Diagn 5:129−138

21. Pacini F, Pinchera A, Giani C, Grasso L, Baschieri L (1980) Serum thyroglobulin concentrations and ¹³¹I whole body scans in the diagnosis of metastases from differentiated thyroid carcinoma (after thyroidectomy). Clin Endocrinol (Oxf) 13:107−110

22. Reiners CHR (1981) Spezifische und unspezifische Tumormarker beim Schilddrüsenkarzinom. Simultane Bestimmung von Thyreoglobulin, Kalzitonin, Carcinoembryonalem Antigen, Alpha-Foetoprotein, Beta-Choriongonadotropin, Tissue Polypeptide Antigen, Immunoglobulin E, Ferritin und Tennessee Antigen. Tumor Diagn 2:199−208

23. Reiners CHR (1983) Serum thyroglobulin as a substitution of I-131-scans in follow-up of differentiated thyroid cancer? Act Endocrinol (Copenh) [Suppl]252:66−67

24. Reiners CHR (1983) Serum-Thyreoglobulin und Thyreoglobulin-Antikörper. Ergebnisse beim Schilddrüsenkarzinom und anderen Schilddrüsenerkrankungen. Thieme, Stuttgart

25. Reiners CHR (1984) Klinische Wertigkeit der Thyreoglobulin-Bestimmung im Serum. Akt Endokrinol 5:76−82

26. Reiners CHR, Baum K, Wiedemann W, Schick F, Becker W, Spiegel W, Eilles CHR, Gerhards W, Börner W (1983) Special diagnostics in follow-up of C-cell (medullary)-carcinoma of the thyroid. Act Endocrinol (Copenh) [Suppl]252:61−62

27. Reiners Chr, Börner W (1982) Ein differenziertes Nachsorgeprogramm für das Schilddrüsenkarzinom. Med Klin 77:34−41

28. Reiners Chr, Börner W, Wiedemann W, Becker W, Schick F, Spiegel W, Eilles CHR, Gerhards W (1982) Kritische Betrachtungen zur diagnostischen Wertigkeit der Thyreoglobulin-Bestimmung beim differenzierten Schilddrüsenkarzinom. In: Höfer R, Bergmann H (eds) Radioaktive Isotope in Klinik und Forschung, vol 15/I. Egermann, Vienna, p 417

29. Reiners CHR, Reimann J, Schäffer R, Baum K, Becker W, Eilles CHR, Gerhards W, Schick F, Spiegel W, Wiedemann W, Börner W (1984) Das metastasierende differenzierte Schilddrüsenkarzinom. Diagnostische Treffsicherheit des Thyreoglobulin-RIA im Vergleich zur J-131-Ganzkörperszintigraphie. Fortschr Röntgenstr 191:306−313

30. Reiners CHR, Schramm A (1981) Nachsorge des C-Zell-Karzinoms der Schilddrüse. Ergebnisse der Kalzitoninbestimmung nach selektiver Venenkatheterisierung. MMW 123:1708−1710

31. Schäffer R, Reiners CHR, Reimann J, Börner W (1983) Das onkozytäre Schilddrüsenkarzinom: Klinisch-pathologische Renaissance einer Tumorform? Tumor Diagn 4:161−168

32. Schatz H, Horn W, Grebe SF, Müller H (1983) Thyreoglobulinmessung oder ¹³¹Jod-Szintigraphie in der Nachsorge von Patienten mit differenziertem Schilddrüsenkarzinom? Dtsch Med Wochenschr 45:1737−1738

33. Schatz H, Grebe SF, Horn W, Müller H (1984) Nachsorge bei differenziertem Schilddrüsenkarzinom: Serumthyreoglobulinbestimmung statt routinemäßigem J-131-Szintigramm? Wien Klin Wochenschr 96:389−393

34. Schatz H, Grebe S, Mäser E, Teuber J, Horn W, Schröder O, Schatz Ch (1982) Serum-Thyreoglobulinspiegel als Tumormarker bei Schilddrüsenkarzinom. Klin Wochenschr 60:457−464

35. Schlumberger M, Charbord P, Fragu P, Lumbroso J, Parmentier C, Tubiana M (1980) Circulating thyroglobulin and thyroid hormones in patients with metastases of differentiated thyroid carcinoma: relationship to serum thyrotropin levels. J Clin Endocrinol 51:513−518

36. Schlumberger M, Fragu P, Parmentier C, Tubiana M (1981) Thyroglobulin assay in the follow-up of patients with differentiated thyroid carcinomas: comparison of its value in patients with or without normal residual thyroid tissue. Act Endocrinol 98:215−221
37. Schneider AB, Line BR, Goldman JM, Robbins J (1981) Sequential serum thyroglobulin determinations, ^{131}I scans, and ^{131}I uptake after triodothyronine withdrawal in patients with thyroid cancer. J Clin Endocrinol 53:1199−1206
38. Stumpf HP, Hüfner M, Hermann HJ, Kimmig B (1984) Langzeitbeobachtung bei 15 Patienten mit differenziertem Schilddrüsenkarzinom und unklar erhöhten Plasmathyreoglobulinspiegeln (Tg). Klin Wochenschr 62:417−422
39. Van Herle AJ, Uller RP (1975) Elevated serum thyroglobulin. A marker of metastases in differentiated thyroid carcinoma. J Clin Invest 56:272−277
40. Weissel M, Bergmann H, Höfer R (1980) Klinische Wertigkeit von Serumthyreoglobulin- und J-131-Ganzkörperretentionsmessungen bei der Metastasensuche von differenzierten Schilddrüsenkarzinomen. Act Med Austriaca 7:114−119

Use of Tumor Markers for Patient Monitoring in Breast Cancer

M. Lüthgens[1], G. Schlegel, and H. D. Schoen

Monitoring of patients with breast cancer under therapy is based on the results of our previous studies on the surveillance of approximately 1000 patients in clinical routine since 1979. As we have shown before, tissue polypeptide antigen (TPA) and carcinoembryonic antigen (CEA) are highly potential markers in the follow-up of various malignancies. In breast cancer, statistical analysis demonstrated that both markers, each separately, had more discriminatory power than 18 other common laboratory parameters taken together. In combination, TPA and CEA were able to discriminate at 95% probability between patients with progressive disease and those without evidence of disease. On this basis, the two markers can well serve as an aid in diagnosing early recurrence and in monitoring therapy. In the follow-up of breast cancer cases undergoing cytotoxic chemotherapy and/or hormone therapy, we have found that the concordance with the clinical status amounted to 91% in TPA, 77% in CEA, and 71% in TPA + CEA. The lower concordance of CEA in comparison with TPA is due to differences in cellular development and secretion of the markers into the peripheral blood stream. Our findings are in general agreement with those of other clinicians. The importance of marker analysis is accentuated by the fact that in 11% of patients, a recurrence was indicated by TPA or CEA marker analysis only, whereas the usual diagnostic means including clinical findings failed.

Furthermore, the relevance of prolactin determination in monitoring therapy is discussed. In refractory cases hyperprolactinemia is eliminated by bromocriptine under continuation of applied therapy.

---

1 Katharinenhospital, D-7000 Stuttgart

Nuclear Medicine in Clinical Oncology
Ed. by C. Winkler
© Springer-Verlag Berlin Heidelberg 1986

Tumormarkers for Monitoring Breast Cancer Patients

P. Oehr[1] and B. Hünermann[1]

In the framework of our investigations on the significance of TPA and CEA determinations as well as their combined application, we examined the sensitivity and specificity of the markers in patients with breast cancer. The concentration in the plasma was determined simultaneously for TPA (RIA Sangtec Medical) and CEA (RIA Abbott). The group examined comprised patients with recidivations and/or metastases ($n = 59$). Plasma of blood donors served as control.

To determine sensitivity and specificity the inverse distribution function [1] and ROC curves [2] were used. Combined analysis was reached by calculating product values [3] or by variation of cut-off levels for sensitivity optimization [4], respectively. The sensitivities of the different findings were compared at specificity values of 95% or 98%. The results are presented in the table below:

Specificities (%)	Sensitivities (%)				
	TPA	CEA	TPA × CEA	TPA and CEA	TPA or CEA
95	91	94	99	93	100
98	84	91	98	93	100

The analysis shows that the constellation "increased TPA or CEA" leads to the highest sensitivities and thus has the greatest accuracy in follow-up studies and particularly early recognition of recidivation. – No comparable results have hitherto been reported in the literature, as far as we know. With regard to other localisations of tumors we have likewise established that the "TPA or CEA-method" leads to the most favourable sensitivity results when monitoring cancer patients [5].

References

1. Oehr P, Wustrow A, Derigs G, Bormann R (1981) Evaluation and inverse distribution function. Tumor Diagnostik 2:195–198
2. Oehr P, Derigs G, Altmann R (1981) Evaluation and characterization of tumorassociated antigens by conversion of inverse distribution function values into specificity-sensitivity diagrams. Tumor Diagnostik 2:283–290
3. Oehr P, Fischer L, Kersjes W, Kunath U, Biersack H-J, Sipeer U, Winkler C (1982) Verteilung, Sensitivität und Spezifität von TPA, CEA und CEA × TPA Marker Produktwerten bei Patienten mit gastrointestinalem Carcinom. Tumor Diagnostik und Therapie 3:195–198
4. Oehr P, Fischer L, Kersjes W, Biersack H-J, Winkler C (1984) Ermittlung der optimalen Sensitivität multipler Marker durch kombinierte Grenzwertvariationen bei festgelegter Spezifität für Patienten mit kolorektalen Karzinomen. Tumor Diagnostik und Therapie 5:189–195
5. Oehr P (1984) Tumormarker-Untersuchungen zum diagnostischen und prognostischen Wert. medwelt 35:1504–1512

1 Institut für klin. und exp. Nuklearmedizin der Universität Bonn, D-5300 Bonn-Venusberg

Nuclear Medicine in Clinical Oncology
Ed. by C. Winkler
© Springer-Verlag Berlin Heidelberg 1986

VIII. Therapeutic Use of Radiopharmaceuticals Including Labelled Antibodies

Radioiodine Treatment of Thyroid Carcinomas

H. Rösler[1]

The well-differentiated thyroid carcinoma is the only tumor which can be treated with radioiodine. But this very tumor is not highly aggressive: even without therapy, long survival is possible [8, 15]. The total thyroidectomy plays the most important role in the successful treatment. From the data of Mazzaferri et al. it is clear that the 15-year survival rates in patients with papillary thyroid carcinoma increase from 78% after lobectomy to 92% after bilateral thyroidectomy, and to 98% after additional radioiodine treatment [22]. It is because of this 6% improvement in the survival rate that practically all patients must be referred to the nuclear medicine department [see also 20, 21]. Here the lifelong follow-up is coordinated, even though the majority of patients require no additional radioiodine treatment after ablation of their thyroid remnants.

Serial determinations of hTG (human thyroglobulin as the tumor marker) and whole-body tumor scintigraphy with thallium-201 have replaced the more complicated and time-consuming examinations with radioiodine in the routine. Interruptions in the substitution with thyroid hormone are no longer necessary for every control. This also helps to break the circle between diagnostics and therapy; for example, residual radioiodine uptake in the tumor leads to a therapeutic radioiodine application, after which another diagnostic control with radioiodine is necessary, the result of which justifies the next treatment. Today, it should no longer be necessary to submit these patients to a diagnostic procedure which by the nature of its extent can be justified only with tumors of much higher aggressivity.

Additional treatment with reasonable doses of radioiodine have few immediate side effects and no apparent late complications. This may have inspired some authors to generously apply higher amounts of radioiodine. However, ^{131}I therapy must follow clinically defined guidelines:

- Cure of a malignant tumor which without radioiodine therapy would lead to death
- Prolongation of life and
- Improvement in the quality of life in patients in whom other treatments are more invasive and less effective

Bearing these points in mind, a therapist must also avoid an underdosage in patients in whom only the highest possible amounts of ^{131}I are effective.

---

1 Nuklearmedizin des Inselspitals, CH-3010 Bern

Nuclear Medicine in Clinical Oncology
Ed. by C. Winkler
© Springer-Verlag Berlin Heidelberg 1986

Long-term results should be measured individually in terms of clinical improvement and tumor involution. Special nuclear medicine techniques are of
use in the follow-up of these patients.

Basic Physical Requirements

It is the absorption of ionizing energy in the tumor which leads to therapeutic
effects. With doses lower than 2000 rads (20 Gy), tissue alterations are not
clearly seen. With doses higher than the tenfold, the therapeutic effects no
longer increase in proportion to the dose increase.

After radioiodine, which is measured in millicuries or Becquerels, is given to
the patient, a certain amount is accumulated and retained in the tissue. The
mean absorbed dose is not only proportional to this amount, but also to a complex factor which summarizes the dose constant of iodine-131, the size of the
target, and an additional factor Φ. Phi represents the fraction of emitted energy
which is absorbed in the target and thus takes the microdosimetry into account
[24]. Phi depends on the three-dimensional dose grid spread between the points
of disintegration and thus depends on the ^{131}I tissue concentration. Phi is
smaller than 1 when the distance between the points is greater than the average
range of the beta particles. With targets smaller than this, the conditions for a
quantitative dose absorption are even worse: the smaller the target, the larger
the dose which is deposited outside of the target. In order to compensate for
these losses, one must increase the concentration of iodide-131 in the tumor by
a factor of 3 in structures measuring 0.5 mm, and by a factor of 13 in structures
measuring 0.1 mm in diameter [27].

Typically, for thyroid remnants after operation, the parameters which are
needed for dose calculation are well known (phi is $\sim$ 1.0). The ablation dose,
therefore, can be calculated in units of absorbed dose. In order to deliver 50,000
rads (500 Gy) to the thyroid remnants, we needed an average of 45.5 mCi
(1,7 MBq) [131]I [31].

In contrast, the variables for the later treatment doses cannot be determined
as exactly: values approximated from diagnostic doses are representative, but
not reliable [25].

There is always a large amount of radioiodine which is distributed throughout the body. This amount is largely diluted by the body, and the retention time
is shorter than in actively retaining tissue. But still a significant whole-body
radiation burden results. This dose is proportional to the blood dose, which can
be determined from the iodine-131 concentration over time [after 18].

It is the organically bound radioiodine which has the longer retention time
in blood (in contrast to the virtually constant 50 rad/100 mCi contribution resulting from the iodide phase). This leads to a higher radiation exposure when
gross thyroid remnants or large tumors with effective hormone synthesis and secretion are present. Authors who have calculated the radiation exposure individually from the blood levels have found varying results: 100 mCi can give
less than 50 or more than 200 rads [18, 27].

On the other hand, one tends to overestimate the dose that is absorbed in the
tumor.

Example [after 10]. A tumor of approximately 20 g (its diameter would be somewhat larger than 3 cm) has taken up 5% of the 150 mCi radioiodine applied to the patient. With an effective half-life of 2 days, 10,000 rads are absorbed. Thus, for the subsequent scintigraphy the 7.5 mCi retained in the tumor are utilized − a gigantic diagnostic dose.

Even with 7.5 μCi (i.e., 1/1000th of that amount) one would see good contrast in the scintigram. But in this realistic situation, one would achieve an absorbed dose of only 10 rads/tumor using the given calculations. This ^{131}I accumulation can identify a nodule or tumor as being derived from the thyroid, but it has no therapeutic effect.

Tumors Suited for Treatment with Radioiodine

Only papillary and follicular thyroid carcinomas have an effective hormone synthesis, i.e., more than mere uptake of radioiodine.

A scale which subdivides the tumors suitable for ^{131}I therapy parallels their histopathologic classification [17]. Among the *highly differentiated follicular carcinomas* are potentially and even overtly toxic carcinomas [32]. They are as autonomous in function as "toxic adenomas" but have a less efficient hormone synthesis per unit of volume. We have observed 29 similar patients (in addition to more than 70 related cases in the literature) in whom the malignant tumor itself caused hyperthyroidism [32]. As a group, these carcinomas have the best radioiodine uptake and the longest effective retention times.

Example. The 81-year-old patient was seen after her doctor and her family had given up on her. She had been operated upon 5 times because of recurrent hyperthyroidism with goiter growth. Two surgeons now refused to perform even a palliative goiter resection, since it was technically impossible. The patient had become increasingly hard of hearing due to a displacement of the auditory canal by the tumor and had multiple lung metastases. 100 mCi and, 3 months later, another 200 mCi radioiodine were tolerated without any side effects. The neck tumor has decreased markedly in size, the lung metastases are no longer detectable on chest X-ray.

The normal thyroid tissue, initially suppressed with a RIA-T$_3$ value higher than 5 ng/ml, was reactivated after the tumor destruction. Today, substitution therapy with thyroid hormone is necessary.

In comparison, the hormone production rate is lower with the *well-differentiated follicular carcinoma;* hyperthyroidism is seen only with monstrous tumor growth: Cunningham et al. extrapolated that a tumor weight of more than 3 kg would be necessary to cause thyrotoxicosis [10]. In addition, the effective halftime of radioiodine is shorter. The well-differentiated papillary carcinomas and mixed papillary-follicular tumors have, as a rule, similar behavior.

A pathognomonic peculiarity of these tumors is their tendency to progressive dedifferentiation. The *moderately or less well-differentiated follicular or papillary carcinoma* is a tumor which often takes up no, or only an insufficient, amount of radioiodine.

Example. The 38-year-old patient with a solitary cold nodule in her recurrent goiter correctly underwent bilateral thyroidectomy after the frozen section had revealed a moderately well-differentiated follicular carcinoma. While under treatment with radioiodine, residual tumor tissue was imaged and successfully eliminated. Several years later bone, lung, and brain metastases appeared, none of which accumulated radioiodine.

Next in this sequence are the *poorly differentiated follicular or papillary tumors.* They may take up radioiodine, even in the metastases. But the accumulation alone is insufficient to achieve adequate absorbed doses. This is understandable when serial scintigraphic examinations are performed.

Example. In another patient, 2 h after radioiodine application there is a tumor mass on the left side of the neck which has taken up radioiodine homogeneously and in about the same amount as the normal lobe on the right. This tumor is cold 48 h later, but the thyroid lobe on the right has continuously accumulated radioiodine. A similar but accelerated sequence can be seen before and after giving perchlorate (= acquired peroxydase defect).

Such a tumor has lost its ability for an effective hormone synthesis. Additional doses of TSH (thyroid stimulating hormone) are unable to increase the uptake or prolong the retention time [29].

One must continue this scale with another important group of tumors, those which do not take up any radioiodine but which can be followed with hTG levels and thallium-201 scintigrams: the *large cell or eosinophilic cell thyroid carcinomas*, i.e., the former Hürthle cell carcinomas.

With *undifferentiated and anaplastic tumors*, even hTG determinations are worthless for follow-up. In patients with these tumors, radioiodine has no indication [5, 6, 30].

Treatment Plan

Ablation of the Thyroid Remnants: "Elimination"

Only in those exceptional cases in which radioiodine can be seen simultaneously in the tumor and in the thyroid remnants is the first therapeutic radioiodine application identical with the first treatment of the tumor itself [32]. As a rule, however, the first application of radioiodine has to prepare for the following tumor treatments, i.e., to enable later tumor residues or recurrences to be efficiently treated with radioiodine [5, 6, 14, 15, 18, 22, 23, 25, 31, 35]. At least the ablation should enable the reliable follow-up with hTG determinations and ^{201}Tl scintigrams. We think it highly important to distinguish between the later tumor treatments and this *ablation or "elimination" of the thyroid remnants*, which aims at the thyroid, not at the tumor itself.

Surgeons try to avoid mutilating the patient and, therefore, always leave some thyroid remnants after thyroidectomy. These remnants can be eradicated without complications using radioiodine [31]. The residual thyroid tissue should be stimulated as much as possible: additional TSH injections are obligatory, even though there is already an overproduction of endogenous TSH.

As a rule, radioiodine is given in an amount which results in an absorbed dose of at least 30 krad, more typically and better $50-60$ krad $(500-600$ Gy) [5, 6, 10, 11, 12, 15, 26, 31, 39]. An "overkill" of the thyroid remnants with more than 100 mCi (3.7 MBq) makes no sense, even though propagated by some highly prominent therapists [2, 3, 33]. These high doses result in painful irradiation thyroiditis and increase the whole body radiation exposure. If necessary, a second elimination dose with 80 mCi (3 MBq) radioiodine can be given, which is less painful and gives less radiation exposure. This amount of radioiodine can also be given primarily in those patients in whom the calculation of a correct dose is impossible because of too little thyroid tissue or because of too low values for the radioiodine uptake.

It is necessary to make a short digression into the criteria for a successful "elimination". The problem of the "unsuccessfully" ablated "remnant" is well-known: after three months half of the patients have residual thyroid tissue *scintigraphically*. If the elimination dose given was too small [19], it must have failed to eliminate all thyroid remnants: then the remaining thyroid tissue may be relevant and compete with later tumor uptake. But after doses of 50,000 rad (or 80 mCi in the special situations discussed) as a standard dose, there is no longer an uptake value higher than 1%, and, therefore, no competition with later ^{131}I tumor treatment doses.

There is one publication which may help to get a more realistic approach to this situation. Scintigrams performed after serial single doses of 150 mCi (5.6 MBq) iodine-131 show, even after having accumulated over 1 Ci, that in more than 70% of these patients some thyroid remnants are seen in the scintigrams [37].

The good intentions of eradicating the thyroid completely — at all costs — need to be corrected [39]. Such an effort is unrealistic from the physical point of view due to the microdosimetry, as shown. More important: the increasing whole body irradiation (for the patient population as a whole) with such a procedure is, at least theoretically, hardly justifiable.

Even with such a cautious regimen, ablation doses less than 100 mCi were sufficient to allow confirmation within the first three months of 80% [23] and 75% [31] of all those metastases which were observed over a much longer follow-up period. And these results were independent of whether the thyroid was eliminated with success (scintigraphically) or not. All those metastases found years later would not necessarily have been found earlier, even with higher amounts for the ablation dose. Even very high amounts of radioiodine are not able to destroy all micrometastases. The insufficiency of a maximizing concept may be illustrated.

Example. A 15-year-old patient, at first treated only with a lobectomy, afterwards because of locoregional recurrent tumor correctly with a bilateral thyroidectomy, presented with regional metastases in the posttreatment scintigraphy after the 80 mCi ablation dose. Between the following treatment doses of 200 mCi, new metastases are appearing. But these very metastases should have been destroyed with the former radioiodine dose because they were present, at least microscopically, at the time of the previous treatments (Fig. 1, A–D).

With an ablation dose of 100 mCi iodine-131, up to 200 rads are applied to the whole body [27]. Larger amounts would increase the exposure proportionally. Bone marrow and ovaries, as the most sensitive tissues, will be altered the most. Thus, because of changes secondary to a too high ablation dose, one may be forced to discontinue a potentially successful treatment series in the further course of the disease.

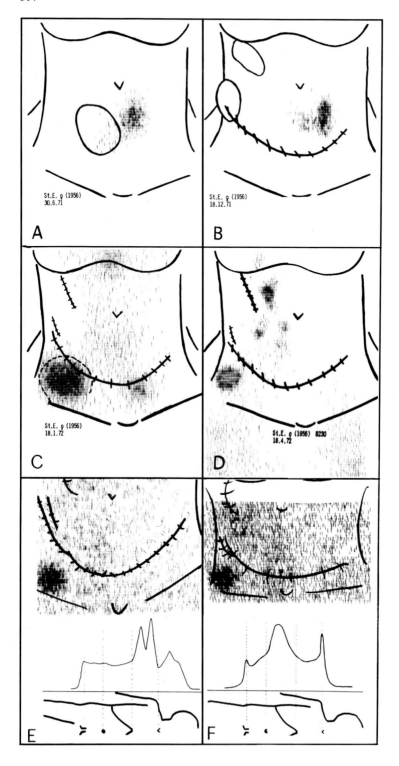

There are more important arguments for an adequate, but not too high, amount of radioiodine in this situation, i.e., to avoid excessive radiation in patients who never will need further radioiodine treatments. These patients cannot be identified initially but represent more than ⅔ of patients referred for ablation. One should be aware that, from an ethical point of view, any radiation side effect (even if merely theoretical) is only justified when it results in a prolonged or improved life for the individual patient.

Criteria which help to reject patients for ablation should be respected [4]. In patients with tumors smaller than 1.5 cm in diameter, the ablation is no longer recommended in some centers in the USA. But in our experience, many occult or nearly nonpalpable tumors have been followed by locoregional and even distant meatstases [31]. A size limit of 1 cm would at least conform with the TNM-staging (pT1 $\leq$ 1 cm). Most of our colleagues can be convinced that the criteria for patient selection should be handled in a flexible way, demonstrating to them the better quality of life resulting from one noninvasive ablation dose, in contrast to repetitive interventions with complications in the case of recurrences, and the more effective follow-up using serial hTG values.

The Tumor Therapy

After ablation of the thyroid remnants, the way is free for beginning the tumor therapy, *if necessary*. Now Beierwaltes' statement, "first dose kills best" [2] must be considered. 200 mCi ^{131}I are well tolerated and, as a rule, the best "dose". Conversion into rads [10, 24, 27] are not done routinely. But the therapist should be able to perform such a calculation in order to be aware of possible side effects. Thus, any dissipation of our therapeutic potential with inadequate single doses can and must be prevented (see Schneider 1982 [35]).

Example. Such a dose calculation is seen in a 60-year-old man who was treated in 1977 for vertebral tumor residues after laminectomy because of an incomplete paraplegia. The 200 mCi ^{131}I resulted in an absorbed dose of 62,500 rads from both β- and γ-emission. After an additional 200 mCi ^{131}I and percutaneous irradiation, the patient has so far been free of symptoms.

One can try to increase the tumor uptake by giving exogenous TSH. But this is only justified because well-tolerated products are available today; anaphylactic reactions were a problem previously. The endogeneous stimulation seen in athyroidism is considered sufficient by most authors [12, 15, 31].

Surely, the increase of endogenous TSH after cessation of the T_4 for 6 weeks and the T_3 medications for 2 weeks as seen in almost every case [1, 11] is a correct observation; but one cannot assume that good therapeutic results are due to increased TSH stimulation [14, 32]. Tumor autonomy was one of the earliest findings in scientific medicine and holds true in thyroid carcinomas.

Fig. 1 A−F. St. E. ♀ 19. 4. 56. Papillary SD-Ca with a small follicular part. **E** One year after the third (last) radioiodine application; **F** four years after the third (last) radioiodine application

More important for the increasing tumor uptake after stopping the thyroid hormone substitution is the continuously decreasing inactive iodine level. Even the most well-differentiated thyroid tumor has a very small iodine pool. The binding of iodide-131 by the tumor is blocked by the smallest amount of inactive iodide. Every measure which decreases the level of "cold" iodide makes sense [11]. Diuretics do increase the tumor uptake [16], but they also accelerate turnover in the tumor. Lithium increases the iodine-131 uptake in the tumor and delays its release. It deserves to be evaluated further [7, 13, 28, 36, 38].

The Practice of Radioiodine Treatment

The first radioiodine treatment is indicated only when scintigraphy with a diagnostic dose or the scintigrams done subsequent to the ablation dose show tumor uptake and retention. For the very first treatment, the effectiveness need not always be guaranteed in advance. From an ethical point of view, one cannot deny such a trial therapy in any patient with ^{131}I-accumulating metastases. But in patients with poor uptake, no uptake in some of the metastases, or with a predominance of less differentiated elements histologically, the timing of the first treatment can be critical since the hormone substitution must be interrupted. During these long waiting periods, one must consider tumor reduction by surgery or an additional percutaneous irradiation.

A late first treatment, i.e., when the treatment begins several years after "elimination" in patients with tumor recurrence, can be indicated on the basis of a positive thallium-201 scintigraphy alone, if the tumor is known histologically to be sufficiently differentiated.

A second treatment dose should not be given earlier than 3 months after the preceding one, again with a 200 mCi "standard-dose", after discontinuing T_3 and T_4 treatments for 2 and 6 weeks. Now, and for all the following treatments, the functional properties of the individual tumor, its size, and its behavior under the preceding radioiodine doses, are well known. One can follow a *series of scintigrams each done after application of a treatment dose* which shows the potential of tumor and metastases to further take up radioiodine and to retain it long enough to be of therapeutic value. With constant or only slightly decreasing uptake values but with continuous tumor regression, further ^{131}I therapies may be discussed. But with decreasing tumor uptake, one should try to interrupt the sequence of treatments and await an overt tumor recurrence, when even a smaller absorbed dose may hit the tumor in a more sensitive state.

Ending the Radioiodine Treatment

Successful tumor eradication, stabilization with residual tumor which does not threaten the patient's life, and failure: these three situations mark the end of all ^{131}I treatments.

A tumor which was just barely seen after the last treatment dose and a tumor which has absolutely no more ^{131}I uptake: both are outside the realm of further

[131]I treatment. Now we have to admit that we have not met our therapeutic goal. Perhaps the tumor was functionally too poorly differentiated to respond to [131]I. Or a tumor reduction has been achieved, but the remaining tumor residues or a new tumor growth initiated by less differentiated cells oblige us to discontinue ^{131}I treatment.

Such a tumor may grow very slowly, slowly enough that an older patient may never experience painful bone lesions or pulmonary failure due to metastases.

Example. In a 70-year-old patient the tumor seemed to regress after ablation and the first tumor dose; this was confirmed by decreasing hTG values. Newly increasing lung metastases gave rise to another treatment with 200 mCi iodide-131. But this time the tumor uptake was insufficient, no further treatment effects were observed. The patient is now 78 years old. She knows that she has a tumor and knows that when necessary a palliative radiation can help. There is no use wasting the patient's time with further radiodine treatments or even performing follow-up examinations and thus interrupting her substitution regimen.

Following a favorable course one should once again consider the observations made with the ablation: one may have reached an optimum before the tumor or its metastases are eradiated scintigraphically. Once more our scintigraphic criteria may be too sensitive and mislead us to an undue overtreatment. One should discontinue the series of treatments, even with positive scintigraphic findings, when the tumor is no longer palpable or seen in the X-ray, and when primarily high hTG values tend to decrease.

Example. With the 15-year-old patient (Fig. 1 E, F) residual radioiodine uptake in the initially largest metastases can be seen today, more than 10 years after the first contact with nuclear medicine. But from the sequence of the absolute uptake values, one can see an ongoing reduction of the radioiodine retention in the tumor: what was initiated by the treatment with radioiodine has been completed by the healthy organism itself.

In these patients, young as well as older ones, we primarily wanted to reserve the last therapeutic doses for a later tumor recurrence, but in none of our patients have we yet observed a recurrence, mostly more than 10 years after ablation. The spontaneous and progressive tumor regression continues. The tumor residues which are scintigraphically visible because of their specific function seem to have lost their capacity to proliferate. Whether or not this "clonogenic death" [6] is identical with clinical healing must be affirmed by further observations. One can not be sure of cure. But fertility is preserved and the best quality of life is assured, both of which seem to be more important than a normal scintigraphy with radioiodine. (Thallium-201 scintigrams showed no pathological accumulation in these patients.)

Conclusion

The treatment with radioiodine is a supplement to the total thyroidectomy. The surgeon has the main responsibility for the patient's further life without complications and without the necessity for late reinterventions. In his decision to perform a more radical operation, he will find help with the very worthwhile

list of postulates given by Clark, a surgeon himself, in 1982 [9]. There is one
most important point which stresses the special behavior of the differentiated
thyroid carcinoma: its ability to grow older and develop into more and more
malignant forms. This tumor transformation can only be prevented by an early,
radical surgery and radioiodine ablation of the thyroid remnants together with
any residual tumor. This is the more important, the younger the patient is. Every small residue of a follicular or papillary carcinoma can be the source of a
more malignant and finally fatal anaplastic tumor.

Example. A 71-year-old patient had had a lobectomy 15 years previously because of a papillary carcinoma and was irradiated percutaneously. Now she is referred with a local recurrence
which does not take up radioiodine. Cytologically, one finds not only elements of the old
papillary tumor but also osteoclast-like giant cells. The patient died 2 months after a new attempt at percutaneous radiation therapy.

There are some successes with individuals even in advanced stages, which
seem to justify all the efforts which are necessary with the radioiodine treatment of thyroid carcinomas. More often, the merits of this treatment remain
unknown. But large studies make it clear that there are many more individuals
who must have been cured by a "prophylactic" treatment [2, 21, 22, 34]. Dis-
astrous late results, such as shown with the last patient, enable us to appreciate
this additional beneficial side of our profession.

References

1. Allweiss P, Braunstein GD, Katz A, Waxman A (1984) Sialadenitis following I-131 therapy for thyroid carcinoma: concise communication. J Nucl Med 25:755–758
2. Beierwaltes W, Haynie T (1978) A discussion of the presentations. In: Spencer RP (ed)
Therapy in nuclear medicine. Grune and Stratton, New York, pp 375–376
3. Beierwaltes W, Rabbani R, Dmuchowsk C, Lloyd V, Eyre P, Mallette S (1984) An analysis
of "ablation of thyroid remnants" with I-131 in 511 patients from 1947–1984: experience
at University of Michigan. J Nucl Med 25:1287–1293
4. Berchtold R, Rösler H, Büll U, Leisner B, Emrich D, Becker HD, Droese M, Pichlmaier
H, Reinwein D, Röher HD (1984) Differenzierte Schilddrüsenkarzinome. Dtsch Med Wochenschr 109:626–634
5. Biersack HJ, Helpap B, Koch U, Janson R, Baumgarten C, Winkler C (1983) Should treatment of highly differentiated thyroid carcinoma be conservative? Nucl Med 12:20–23
6. Bloomer WD, Adelstein SJ (1982) The mammalian radiation survival curve. J Nucl Med
23:259–265
7. Brière J, Pousset G, Darsy P, Guinet (1974) Intérêt de l'association lithium-iode 131 dans
le traitement des métastases captantes du cancer thyroïdien. Ann Endocrinol (Paris)
35:281–282
8. Byar DP, Green SB, Dor P, Williams ED, Colon J, van Gilse HA, Mayer M, Sylvester RJ,
van Glabbeke M (1979) A prognostic index for thyroid carcinoma. A study of the
EORTC-thyroid cancer cooperative group. Eur J Cancer Clin Oncol 15:1033–1041
9. Clark OH (1982) The treatment of choice for patients with differentiated thyroid cancer.
Am Surg 196:361–370
10. Cunningham RM, Hilton G, Pochin EE (1955) Radioiodine uptake in thyroid car-
cinomata. Radiology 18:252–256
11. Edmonds CJ (1978) Radioiodine. In: Werner SC, Ingbar H (eds) The thyroid. Harper and
Row, Hagerstown, Maryland, pp 569–575
12. Edmonds CJ, Smith T (1984) Long term hazards of 131-I treatment of thyroid cancer. Ann
Endocrinol (Paris) 45:83

13. Gershengorn MC, Izumi M, Robbins J (1976) Use of lithium as an adjunct to radioiodine therapy of thyroid carcinoma. J Clin Endocrinol 42:105−111
14. Halnan KE (1975) The non-surgical treatment of thyroid cancer. Br J Surg 62:769−771
15. Halnan KE (1980) Perspectives and prospects. In: Duncan W (ed) Thyroid cancer. Springer, Berlin Heidelberg New York, pp 129−137
16. Hamburger JK (1969) Diuretic augmentation of 131-I uptake in inoperable thyroid cancer. N Engl J Med 280:1091−1094
17. Hedinger Chr (1975) Klassifizierung der Schilddrüsentumoren. Schweiz Med Wochenschr 105:997−1000
18. Hüfner M, Stumpf HP, Grussendorf M, Hermann HJ, Kimmig B (1983) Comparison of the effectiveness of 131-I whole body scans and plasma Tg determinations in diagnosis of metastatic differentiated carcinoma of the thyroid: Retrospective study. Acta Endocrinol 104:327−332
19. Kuni CC, Klingensmith WC (1980) Failure of low doses of 131-I to ablate residual thyroid tissue following surgery for thyroid cancer. Radiology 137:773−774
20. Maheshwari YK, Hill CS, Haynie TP, Hickey RC, Samaan NC (1981) 131-I therapy in differentiated thyroid carcinoma: M.D. Anderson Hospital experience. Cancer 15:664−671
21. Massin J-P, Savoie J-C, Garnier H, Guiraudon G, Leger FA, Bacourt F (1984) Pulmonary metastases in differentiated thyroid carcinoma: Study of 58 cases with implications for primary tumor treatment. Cancer 53:982−992
22. Mazzaferri EL, Young RL (1981) Papillary thyroid carcinoma: a 10 year follow-up report of the impact of therapy in 576 patients. Am J Med 70:511−518
23. Moser E, Braun S, Buell U, Kirsch CM, Tosch U, Wendt T (1984) Thyroglobulin levels to follow-up patients with treated differentiated thyroid carcinoma. Cancer Detect Prev 7:79−86
24. NCRP Report Nr. 70 (1982) Nuclear Medicine − Factors influencing the choice and use of radionuclides in diagnostics and therapy. Bethesda, pp 51−60
25. Nemec J, Röhling S, Zamrazil V, Pohunkova D (1979) Comparison of the distribution of diagnostic and thyroablative I-131 in the evaluation of differentiated thyroid cancers. J Nucl Med 20:92−97
26. Pfannenstiel P, Hoffmann G (1967) Szintigraphische Kontrolle der Radiojodtherapie bei Struma maligna. In: Hoffmann G, Scheer KE (eds) Radioisotope in der Lokalisationsdiagnostik. Schattauer, Stuttgart, pp 471−476
27. Quimby EH, Feitelberg S (1963) Radioactive isotopes in medicine and biology. Lea and Febiger, Philadelphia
28. Rassmusson B, Olsen K, Rygard J (1983) Lithium as adjunct to 131-I therapy of thyroid carcinoma. 3rd International Thyroid Symposium, Innsbruck, Austria. Acta Endocrinol [Suppl] (Copenh) 252:74
29. Rösler H, Kinser J (1973) The leakage phenomenon in thyroid nodules. Acta Endocrinol [Suppl] (Copenh) 179:80−81
30. Rösler H (1982) Restriktive Indikationsstellung zur Radiojodtherapie beim undifferenzierten Schilddrüsenkarzinom. In: Biersack HJ, Winkler C, Beyset D (eds) Neue Aspekte in Diagnostik und Therapie des Schilddrüsen-Karzinoms. Schattauer, Stuttgart, pp 75−79
31. Rösler H (1982) Das papilläre Schilddrüsenkarzinom in Bern heute. Schweiz Rundsch Med (Praxis) 71:541−554
32. Rösler H, Wimpfheimer C, Ruchti Ch, Kinser J, Teuscher J (1984) Hyperthyreose bei maligner Struma. Nucl Med 23:293−300
33. Sarkar SD, Beierwaltes WH, Gill SP, Cowley BJ (1976) Subsequent fertility and birth histories of children and adolescents treated with 131-I for thyroid cancer. J Nucl Med 17:460−464
34. Samaan NA, Schultz PN, Haynie TP, Ordonez NG (1985) Pulmonary metastasis of differentiated thyroid carcinoma: treatment results in 101 patients. J Clin Endocrinol Metab 60:376−380
35. Schneider C (1982) Prinzipien der Radiojodbehandlung. In: Biersack HJ, Winkler C (eds) Neue Aspekte in Diagnostik und Therapie des Schilddrüsenkarzinoms. Schattauer, Stuttgart, pp 65−74

36. Schraube P, Kimmig B, zum Winkel K (1984) Lithium als Adjuvans in der Radiojodtherapie des Schilddrüsenkarzinoms. Nucl Med 23:151–154
37. Schümichen C, Bulczak-Schmidt M, Blattmann H, Pauli-Harnasch C (1984) Wirksamkeit der hochdosierten Radiojodtherapie zur Ausschaltung von Restgewebe nach totaler Thyreoidektomie. Nucl Med 23:265–269
38. Sedvall G, Jönsson B, Petterson U, Levin K (1968) Effects of lithium salts on plasma protein-bound iodine and uptake of 131-I in thyroid gland of man and rat. Life Sci 7:1257
39. Sisson JC (1983) Applying the radioactive eraser: I-131 to ablate normal thyroid tissue in patients from whom thyroid cancer has been resected. J Nucl Med 24:743–745

Therapy of the Neuroblastoma with ^{131}I-MIBG

U. FEINE[1], T. KLINGEBIEL, and J. TREUNER

The neuroblastoma is the second most prevalent malignant tumor type in children. One third of the children over 1 year of age demonstrate the disseminated form already at the initial diagnosis of the tumor. Despite intensive therapy, chance of survival is extremely low: no therapy including immune stimulation, differentiation factors or interferons, has yet proved effective in considerably improving the chance of survival. Allogenic and autologous bone marrow transplantations after complete body irradiation still seem to achieve a certain level of success. However, bone marrow transplantation therapy is limited by the necessity of finding suitable donors.

For this reason, the investigation of new therapy possibilities seems to be justified.

With the at times amazingly high and specific enrichment of ^{131}I-metaiodobenzylguanidine (^{131}I-MIBG) in the cells of the neuroblastoma, this substance, which was used for the first time in 1983/84 by Kimmig and colleagues [5] and our working group in Tübingen [2], presented itself for application in therapeutic doses. A corresponding therapy had already been tried with the malignant pheochromocytoma with metastases [1, 4].

In our first report at the Nuclear Medicine Congress in Helsinki in 1984 on the therapeutic application of ^{131}I-MIBG on neuroblastoma, we reported on 5 children and a total of 8 treatment cycles [3].

In the intervening period, this therapy has been used at various clinics in Europe and the U.S.A.

By May 1985 we ourselves had treated 8 children with stage IV neuroblastomas with ^{131}I-MIBG in 21 therapy cycles. 6 other children were treated in Frankfurt by Hör, Maul, Kornhuber, Schwabe. One treatment was conducted by Fischer and Wehinger in Münster/Kassel, and another in Hannover by Weinel (Table 1). I have been graciously permitted to give a short summary of the results (Table 2).

Seven of the children have suffered a relapse of the neuroblastoma. The children were being chemotherapeutically, radiologically and surgically treated in stage IV without complete remission.

The average radioactivity used per cycle was 130 (50–240) mCi in Frankfurt, 130 in Hannover, 123 in Kassel, and 92 (35–212) in Tübingen (see Table 3). The radioactivity per patient, administered in several cycles, was between

---

1 Nuklearmedizinische Abteilung, Med. Strahleninstitut der Universität Tübingen, Röntgenweg 11, D-7400 Tübingen

Nuclear Medicine in Clinical Oncology
Ed. by C. Winkler
© Springer-Verlag Berlin Heidelberg 1986

Table 1. ^{131}I-MIBG therapy of neuroblastomas

Center	Patients	Therapy Cycle
Frankfurt	6	13 (1–4)
Hannover	1	1
Kassel	1	3
Tübingen	8	21 (1–5)
	16	38

Table 2. ^{131}I-MIBG therapy of neuroblastomas

Patients	Free of fever	Free of pain	Local tumor size	BM Infiltration	Catechol-amine	LDH	Remiss. Status 6/85	
1. C. E.	+	+	stop-progression	temp. reduct. ↑		↓	†	(120 days)
2. T. T.	+	+	stop-progression	temp. reduct. ↑		↓	†	(55 days)
3. H. S.	+	+	consolidat. of path. fractures	temp. free of tumor ↓			†	(249 days)
4. I. H.			local without tumor (+RT)	temp. free of tumor ↓			CR	(BMT)
5. J. C.	+	+	local without tumor (+RT)		↓	↓	†	
6. C. A.			progression (+RT)	–	–		†	(129 days)
7. S. A.			–	–	–		†	(188 days)
8. A. K.			–	–	–		CR	(122 days)
9. A. T.			consolidat. of path. fractures				CR	(BMT)
							PR	(115 days)
10. J. S.	+		tumor progress.				†	
11. L.			–	temp. free of tumor			CR	(BMT)
12. D. O.	+	+	diminishing				†	(118 days)
13. A. S.			no MIBG-uptake				†	(40 days)
14. G.	+	+	progression				†	(20 days)
15. K. H.			incert. reduction				PR	(45 days)
16. A. W.			diminishing				PR	(40 days)

BMT, bone marrow transplant; CR, complete remission; PR, partial remission

Table 3. ^{131}I-MIBG therapy of neuroblastomas

Center	Activity per cycle	Activity per patient
Frankurt	130 mCi (50–450)	346 mCi (125–650)
Hannover	130 mCi	130 mCi
Kassel	123 mCi	370 mCi
Tübingen	92 mCi (35–212)	241 mCi (85–596)
	119	282

Table 4. ^{131}I-MIBG therapy of neuroblastomas

Center	Time between two therapy cycles	Observation time after first ^{131}I-MIBG cycle
Frankfurt	19–56 days (M: 31 days)	20–181 days (M: 74 days)
Kassel	29 days	115 days
Tübingen	15–48 days (M: 37 days)	54–249 days (M: 142 days)

Table 5. ^{131}I-MIBG therapy of neuroblastomas

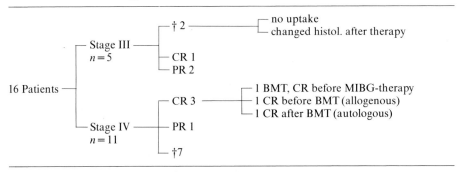

BMT, bone marrow transplant; CR, complete-remission; PR, partial remission

346 and 385 mCi. In most of the cases doses totaling 350 mCi were administered in 3–4 series (Table 3, 4). For the last six patients we administered the dose as a continuous infusion over 24–30 h. The other departments did similarly, however, usually in a shorter time of 2–12 h.

So far, an essential difference in storage for the various infusion times not been determined with any significance. Our decision to employ a long-term infusion was based on examinations of cell cultures which showed that in various cell cycle segments the absorption of the ^{131}I-MIBG can be quite variable.

In accordance with our instructions the firms Henning in Berlin and later Amersham Buchler in Brunswick kept the specific activity as high as possible, between 25 and 35 mCi per mg MIBG.

Table 5 gives the results from 16 patients. So far 7 of 16 children have survived (as of 5/85). Seven children died in stage IV, and 2 in stage III as a result of the bone marrow infiltration. Three children were given bone marrow transplants after undergoing whole-body irradiation: in one child the transplant was autogenous, in one child syngeneic, and in the third child autologous. All three children are still living.

The most important side effect is a reversible bone marrow depression corresponding to the bone marrow radiation dosage in the tumor-free bone marrow of approximately 50–150 rad with radioactivity between 80 and 150 mCi

Table 6. ^{131}I-MIBG-therapy in neuroblastoma (Tübingen)

Patient	Course	^{131}I-MIBG	Radiation dose (rad/cGy)	
			Major lesion	Whole body
E. C.	1	35 mCi	1450	57
	2	80 mCi	2000	70
	3	108 mCi	2950	140
T. T.	1	92 mCi	3000	120
	2	60 mCi	1670	70
Sh. H.	1	50 mCi	–	–
	2	100 mCi	2470	57

^{131}I-MIBG. The determination of whole-body, bone marrow, and tumor dosages can be established by whole-body scintigraphy. Table 6 shows the calculated tumor and bone marrow doses of the 3 children (see also Fig. 1).

The results of the treatment are difficult to analyze as a unit.

Emphasis should be placed on the rather rapid clinical improvement which occurs in the first few days after injection of ^{131}I-MIBG. Fever and, most importantly, the occasionally very severe pain in the bones disappeared rapidly, as was also the case with the opiate-dependent patients. In almost all cases, a clear to very good regression of the tumor metastases and bone marrow infiltration could be detected (Fig. 2) and the catecholamine secretion was reduced. Most of the children, however, suffered relapses, so that a longer lasting success cannot yet be achieved.

How are the results to be judged?

With the doses of ^{131}I-MIBG used to date, despite occasionally higher doses, no final success has been achieved, except for the 3 children who were given bone marrow transplants following whole-body irradiation of short duration. Although there was in each case a clear effect on the tumor, most of the children have suffered relapses.

In most of the children, the storage of MIBG in the tumors was, compared with the first examination, negatively affected by simultaneously administered cytostatic therapy, so that the specific concentration was, in part, clearly lower than in the primary diagnosis before the start of therapy. In the ongoing national multicenter study, MIBG is being administered only during stage IV following a 4 block cytostatic treatment when tumor absorption is still good.

A pilot study should now attempt to introduce MIBG therapy at the beginning during stage IV with high radiation doses in order to apply the highest possible dose to the tumor.

The second possibility which chould be discussed is the combination of ^{131}I-MIBG therapy in high doses with a bone marrow transplant. Because of the specific concentration of MIBG in the tumor cells, with the radiological effect primarily on the tumor nests, the infiltrated bone marrow and solid tumors may absorb a significantly higher dose than the bone marrow with little or no infiltration.

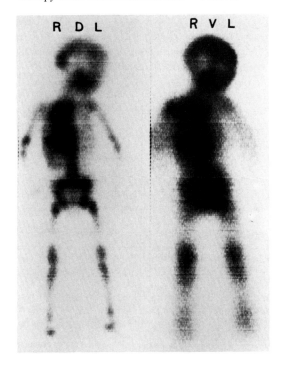

Fig. 1. Whole-body scan dorsal and ventral during therapy for tumor bone marrow with ^{131}I-MIBG

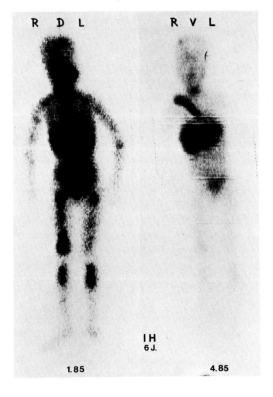

Fig. 2. 6-year-old boy, neuroblastoma stage IV. Whole-body scan during ^{131}I-MIBG therapy. Multiple bone marrow infiltration (**left**). Second therapy 3 months later. Bone marrow infiltration has disappeared. Resting tumor in the left pelvis. Radioactivity in the thorax region is due to uptake in a vena cava superior catheter

In summary, it be can said that with the currently very bad prognosis for neuroblastomas in stage IV, further study into the therapeutic use of ^{131}I-MIBG appears to be thoroughly justified. Due to the low number of cases in the individual centers, a jointly evaluated multicenter study offers the only possibility of rating the value this therapy in the near future.

References

1. Beyerwaltes WH (1981) New horizons for therapeutic nuclear medicine in 1981. J Nucl Med 22:549−554
2. Feine U, Treuner J, Niethammer D, Borchelt G, Dopfer R, Eibach E, Grünbach S, Kaiser W, Klingebiel T, Meinke J, Müller-Schauenburg W (1984) Erste Untersuchungen zur szintigraphischen Darstellung von Neuroblastomen mit ^{131}J-metajodbenzylguanidin. Nuc Compact 15:23−26
3. Feine U et al. (1984) Scintigraphic imaging of neuroblastoma with ^{131}I-MIBG and first attempts of its therapeutic use. 22nd Int. Annual Meeting Soc. Nuclear Medicine Europe, Helsinki, 1984. In: Nuklear-Medizin, Schattauer, Stuttgart
4. Fischer M, Winterberg B, Müller-Rensing R, Zidek W, Vetter H (1983) Nuklearmedizinische Therapie des Phaeochromozytoms. Nuc Compact 14:172−176
5. Kimmig B, Brandeis WE, Eisenhut M, Bubeck B, Herrmann HJ, Zum Winkel K (1983) Szintigraphische Darstellung eines Neuroblastoms. Nuc Compact 14:320−326
6. Treuner J, Feine U, Niethammer D, Müller-Schauenburg W, Meinke J, Eibach E, Dopfer R, Klingebiel T, Grünbach S (1984) Lancet I:333−334

Treatment of Pheochromocytomas with ^{131}I-Metaiodobenzylguanidine

M. Fischer[1] and H. Vetter

[131]I-metaiodobenzylguanidine (^{131}I-MIBG) is used for the scintigraphic localization of catecholamine-producing tissue in patients with pheochromocytomas, neuroblastomas, and apudomas. In high concentrations and doses, the same radiopharmaceutical agent can be used for the treatment of tumors showing a high tracer uptake.

Between October 1981 and May 1985, 43 patients with pheochromocytomas were studied with ^{131}I-MIBG scintigraphy in our department. The final diagnosis and/or localization were confirmed by surgery in 41 of 43 patients. Six of the 43 patients suffered from malignant pheochromocytoma, one of them from a pheochromocytoma of the organ of Zuckerkandl with a single metastasis of a neighboring lymph node. Five of these 6 patients had multilocular metastases. Five patients with multilocular metastases and one female patient with an intraadrenal, probably benign, pheochromocytoma, who could not be operated because of a catecholamine-induced myocarditis, were treated with ^{131}I-MIBG.

Multiple treatments were administered with intervals of 3−5 months (Table 2). Single doses of 65−210 mCi with a specific activity of 10−35 mCi/mg benzylguanidine in a volume of 50 ml were infused intravenously in 45−90 minutes. In all patients, the thyroid was blocked with 600 mg perchlorate/day and 150 μg L-T_4 for 4 weeks, starting 1 day before tracer administration. The therapeutic effect was controlled by clinical follow-up, catecholamine secretion, and in four of six patients by determination of tumor volume by computed tomography.

All patients with multilocular metastases were operated before ^{131}I-MIBG therapy, four of them were also treated with chemotherapy and external radiation treatment.

In all patients we observed a clinical improvement after the first therapeutic doses of ^{131}I-MIBG, leading to a significant reduction of antihypertensive drugs. In two patients (patients No. 1 and No. 2), a reduction of tumor volume of about 61% and 10% was measured by computed tomography (see Table 3). In patient No. 4, who had extensive liver metastases, increasing tumor necrosis in the liver could be visualized by CT during treatment. In this patient, a single-photon-emission computed tomography (SPECT) was performed after administration of 5 mCi ^{123}I-MIBG after his third treatment in an interval. SPECT

---

1 Westfälische Wilhelms-Universität, Medizinische Klinik und Poliklinik, Nuklearmedizinische Abteilung, Albert-Schweizer-Straße, D-4400 Münster

Nuclear Medicine in Clinical Oncology
Ed. by C. Winkler
© Springer-Verlag Berlin Heidelberg 1986

Table 1. Patients with pheochromocytoma, treated with ^{131}I-MIBG: age at the beginning of therapy and location of the lesion(s)

Patient	Sex	Age	Location of lesion
1. K. A.	f	16y	multilocular metastases (bone and soft tissue)
2. W. M.	f	16y	multilocular metastases (bone and lung)
3. J. H.	f	73y	intra-adrenal tumor
4. T. H.	m	43y	multilocular metastases (bone and liver)
5. G. B.	m	43y	multilocular metastases (bone)
6. D. G.	f	29y	multilocular metastases (bone and soft tissue)

Table 2. Number of treatments, total doses and time of follow-up

Patient	No. of treatment	Total doses	Time of follow-up
1. K. A.	8×	1055 mCi ^{131}I-MIBG	36 months
2. W. M.	6×	890 mCi ^{131}I-MIBG	29 months
3. J. H.	3×	435 mCi ^{131}I-MIBG	14 months
4. T. H.	4×	520 mCi ^{131}I-MIBG	15 months
5. G. B.	3×	405 mCi ^{131}I-MIBG	11 months
6. D. G.	4×	480 mCi ^{131}I-MIBG	13 months

Table 3. Results of treatment with ^{131}I-MIBG in patients with pheochromocytoma

1. K. A.	61% tumor reduction (after 435 mCi ^{131}I-MIBG); no tumor progression until now.
2. W. M.	10% tumor reduction (365 mCi), then tumor progression (new lung and bone metastases)
3. J. H.	local tumor growth (435 mCi)
4. T. H.	local tumor reduction (liver), but new bone metastases (405 mCi)
5. G. B.	progression of bone metastases under treatment
6. D. G.	stop of tumor growth

showed high tracer accumulation in the marginal zone of the lesions in the liver with decreased uptake in the central zone, taking a characteristic ring-form appearance.

In patient No. 2 new lung metastases and bone metastases could meanwhile be imaged by control scintigraphies and X-ray films after further treatment. Some of these new lung metastases did not show a tracer uptake. The female patient with the intra-adrenal pheochromocytoma (patient No. 3) died after a total dose of 435 mCi because of an obstruction of the large intra-abdominal vessels by the growing tumor. Patient No. 4 died from a tumor anemia. In patient No. 5 we stopped treatment because his bone metastases were growing under therapy. Approximately one half of his metastases did not show a tracer uptake during diagnostic scintigraphy before starting treatment and during posttherapeutic scintigraphies. He had to be operated 3 times because of tumor destruction of cervic and lumbar vertebras and of his right femoral head. In our last patient (patient No. 6) tumor growth has so far been stopped by treatment with ^{131}I-MIBG. During tracer infusion and in the intervals, no severe side effects were observed.

About 10% of pheochromocytomas are malignant. They may cause serious symptoms either by secretion of catecholamines or by metastatic or invasive growth of the tumor. In general, malignant pheochromocytomas do not respond to chemotherapy or external radiation therapy [1, 5]. For a therapeutic effect of radiation therapy, a minimum of 15,000 rad to the tumor should be the goal [3].

Our results in six patients with pheochromocytomas show that the selection of patients for treatment with ^{131}I-MIBG still remains problematic. It was discussed by Sisson et al. [6] that tumors with rapid progression are more responsive to therapy. This may be evident in our female patient with the intraadrenal, probably benign, pheochromocytoma with a high intratumoral tracer uptake, but no response to a total dose of 435 mCi ^{131}I-MIBG. Similar observations were reported in 3 patients who had very slowly progressive malignancy [4].

Nevertheless, in patient No. 1 a tumor reduction of about 61% was measured by CT after a dose of 415 mCi ^{131}I-MIBG although in this patient the malignant pheochromocytoma was diagnosed 8 years before we started treatment with this new radiopharmaceutical agent.

Whereas the mean biologic half-life of ^{131}I-MIBG in adrenergic tissue during diagnostic or therapeutic procedures is about $2.7-3$ days, in one of our patients treated with ^{131}I-MIBG (patient No. 4) a delayed biological half-life was observed, but the patient developed an increasing number of new bone metastases during treatment with a poor tracer uptake and died from tumor anemia. Therefore, we would like to add a further point for discussion to those mentioned by McEwan et al. [4]: whether or not shorter intervals between treatments would be more effective.

Although the early results in four therapeutic centers (Ann Arbor, U.S.A.; Southampton and St. Bartholomew's, London, U.K.; Münster, Germany) first seemed encouraging, we are now less optimistic. In our experience, we may improve clinical symptoms in patients with malignant pheochromocytomas and multilocular metastases for a period of weeks to years [2, 7], but this treatment is probably not curative.

References

1. Drasin H (1978) Treatment of malignant pheochromocytoma. West J Med 128:106−111
2. Fischer M, Winterberg B, Müller-Rensing R, Friemann J, Zidek W, Vetter H (1983) Nuklearmedizinische Therapie des Phäochromocytoms. Nuc Compact 14:172−176
3. McDougall IR (1984) Malignant pheochromocytoma treated by ^{131}I-MIBG − Teaching editorial. J Nucl Med 25:249−251
4. McEwan AJ, Shapiro B, Sisson JC, Beierwaltes WH, Ackery DM (1985) Radioiodobenzylguanidine for the scintigraphic location and therapy of adrenergic tumors. Semin Nucl Med 15:132−152

5. Scott HW, Reynolds V, Green N (1982) Clinical experience with malignant pheochromocytomas. Surg Gynecol Obstet 154:801–818
6. Sisson JC, Shapiro B, Beierwaltes WH, Glowniak JV, Nakajo M, Mangner TJ, Carey JE,
   Swanson DP, Copp JE, Satterlee WG, Wieland DM (1984) Radiopharmaceutical treatment
   of malignant pheochromocytoma. J Nucl Med 25:197–206
7. Vetter H, Fischer M, Müller-Rensing R, Vetter W, Winterberg B (1983) ^{131}I-MIBG in treatment of malignant pheochromocytomas. Lancet II:107

Treatment of Neuroblastoma by ^{131}I-Meta-iodobenzylguanidine (^{131}I-MIBG): Qualitative and Quantitative Scintigraphic Evaluation of the Treatment Effect

J. Happ[1], J. Griese, F. D. Maul, R. P. Baum, K. H. Manegold, V. Gerein, D. Schwabe, D. Klinter, S. Szepesi, B. Kornhuber, and G. Hör

Introduction

[131]I-meta-iodobenzylguanidine (^{131}I-MIBG), a newly synthesized radiopharmaceutical probably taken up by adrenergic neurotransmitter vesicles and thus concentrated in neuroadrenergic tissue [1, 2], has successfully been used for imaging of benign or malignant neuroectodermal tumors such as pheochromocytoma [3], paraganglioma [4], and neuroblastoma [5]. ^{131}I-MIBG has also been applied in treatment of malignant pheochromocytoma [6]. Several groups of investigators recently started ^{131}I-MIBG treatment in patients with neuroblastoma; this paper is one of the first publications on the results of such treatment. The report is restricted to the scintigraphic evaluation of the effects of seven treatments in two patients out of a total of 20 treatments in eight patients performed in our division between December 1984 and August 1985.

Methods

Two patients with neuroblastoma stage IV (Table 1) were chosen for treatment with ^{131}I-MIBG (Henning Berlin GmbH, Berlin, FRG and Amersham Buchler, Braunschweig, FRG). The tumors were diagnosed and classified histologically (biopsy of the tumor and/or iliac crest), biochemically (catecholamines, metanephrines, vanillylmandelic acid in blood and urine, respectively) and by diagnostic ^{131}I-MIBG scans showing disseminated bone marrow infiltration. A more detailed description of the clinical data on the patients will be given in succeeding papers of our group. Repeat diagnostic ^{131}I-MIBG scintigrams (whole body scintigraphy by multiple views) were produced at intervals of 1 to 4 days up to 7 days after the administration of the radiopharmaceutical [0.38 and 0.36 mCi intravenously (i.v.)].

Cytostatic treatment was stopped about 10 or 11 months prior to the beginning of ^{131}I-MIBG therapy. Before ^{131}I-MIBG therapy, written consent was obtained from the parents of the children. Thyroidal uptake was blocked by Endojodin, 1/3 ampoule per day, for 9 days, beginning 2 days before ^{131}I-MIBG administration and thereafter, by oral administration of 0.1 g potassium iodide

---

1 Zentrum der Radiologie, Klinikum der Johann-Wolfgang-Goethe-Universität, Abt. für Allg. Nuklearmedizin, Theodor-Stern-Kai 7, D-6000 Frankfurt am Main 70

Nuclear Medicine in Clinical Oncology
Ed. by C. Winkler
© Springer-Verlag Berlin Heidelberg 1986

Table 1. Clinical data on patients with neuroblastoma stage IV

Patient	Sex	Age (yrs; mths)	Height (cm)	Weight (kg)	Location of primary or solid tumor	Previous treatment
1	male	4; 4	96	14	upper mediastinum[a]	cytostatics
2	female	8; 6	134	35	unknown	cytostatics

[a] Primary tumor removed by surgery from right abdomen, solid metastasis in the left supra- and infraclavicular region.

Table 2. ^{131}I-MIBG treatment schedules used in 2 patients with neuroblastoma stage IV

	Treatment course			
	I	II	III	IV
Patient 1				
Activity (mCi)	185	80	85	
Specific activity (mCi/mg)	35	42	35	
Infusion time (h)	24	24	16	
Time after previous ^{131}I-MIBG treatment (d)		27	21	
Patient 2				
Activity (mCi)	158	270	100	48
Specific activity (mCi/mg)	15	20	28	9
Infusion time (h)	30	30	12	4
Time after previous ^{131}I-MIBG treatment (d)		32	57	48

tablets, 3 times daily, up to 3 weeks after ^{131}I-MIBG administration. The exact ^{131}I-MIBG treatment schedule is given in Table 2. The therapeutic doses were infused (i.v.) at a constant rate by an automatic pump. High doses of ^{131}I-MIBG were split into two fractions. After a first dose of $50-100$ mCi, ^{131}I-MIBG uptake by the tumor was approximated and radiation doses were calculated for the tumor as well as for the liver and the whole body. Depending on these calculations, a second dose of ^{131}I-MIBG was administered within 24 h. A detailed description of dosimetry will be given in a separate paper of our group.

After a residual whole body activity of less than 2 mCi was recorded serial post-treatment scintigrams were produced (whole body scintigraphy by multiple anterior and posterior views) at intervals of about 1 week. Scintigraphy was performed using a gamma camera (Searle, LFOV, Desplaines, Illinois, USA) with a parallel-hole collimator. The images were documented on X-ray films as well as acquired on a computer system (Philips, Processing and Display System, Appeldoorn, Netherlands).

Quantitative evaluation of the scintigrams was restricted to the pelvic region (Tu) and the liver (L). The serial scintigrams acquired (matrix 128×128) were evaluated by measuring background activity in the left mid abdomen (posterior view), activity of the hottest region of the tumor located in the pelvic bone marrow (posterior view), and of the one found in the liver (posterior view in patient 1, anterior view in patient 2) by determination of counts per minute (cpm) recorded within standardized regions of interest (ROI). If necessary in single cases, views of the opposite side were taken for evaluation; in this case, the data were corrected for the difference of about 7% between the cpm obtained from the anterior or posterior view (for the activity of the pelvic region, higher values by posterior views; for the liver activity, higher values by anterior view). For evaluation of background, a ROI of 64 pixels was placed on the mid abdomen half way from the spine to the waist, corresponding to 16 pixels from mid spine in patient 1 or 18 pixels in patient 2, respectively. At this distance from the spine, the site of minimum activity was chosen for placing the ROI which usually was at the height of lumbar vertebra III to IV. In patient 1, a ROI of 200 pixels included a part of the sacrum and the ilium, i.e., the region of spinae iliacae posteriores of both sides and the upper part of the sacrum; the same anatomic region was included in a ROI of 296 pixels in patient 2. A ROI of 64 pixels included the hottest region of the right lobe of the liver. Count rates of the pelvic region and the liver were corrected for ROI area and for background. ^{131}I-MIBG uptake ratios (UR) were calculated for the tumor in the pelvic bone marrow (Tu) and the liver (L) as follows: $(\mathrm{cpm_{Tu,\,L}} - \mathrm{cpm_{BG}})/\mathrm{cpm_{BG}}$, where cpm were normalized for a ROI of 64 pixels.

Results

Diagnostic scintigrams as well as scintigrams after the first treatment showed high ^{131}I-MIBG uptake in the mediastinal solid metastasis in patient 1 and in nearly all regions of the skeleton in both patients: skull, spine, ribs, scapulae, pelvis, and long bones, especially the metaphyses. The liver was visualized optimally on the earliest diagnostic scintigram in patient 2, on the latest one in patient 1 and on the post-treatment scintigrams of both patients. By visual evaluation of the scintigrams, regression of skeletal ^{131}I-MIBG uptake during treatment was noted as a reduction or loss of activity contrast. Quantification of these changes, however, was difficult, especially if liver or parts of this organ were included in the field of view. Changes in distribution pattern of ^{131}I-MIBG-accumulating tissue could be observed during the treatment: while regression of ^{131}I-MIBG uptake was observed in most parts of the skeleton, additional sites of ^{131}I-MIBG accumulation could be found. This applies to patient 1 whose right tibia primarily was not visualized and presented ^{131}I-MIBG accumulation during treatment II and III.

Changes in ^{131}I-MIBG uptake by the tumor or the liver were quantified by determination of UR. Tumor uptake ratios (TuUR) increased in the series of diagnostic scintigrams during the 1st week after administration of ^{131}I-MIBG (Fig. 1). One day after the administration, the UR was about 1 in patient 1 and

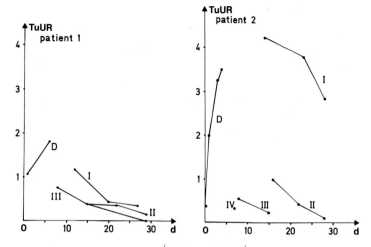

Fig. 1. Tumor uptake ratios $\left(\dfrac{cpm_{Tu} - cpm_{BG}}{cpm_{BG}}\right)$ for ^{131}I-MIBG as functions of time after administration of diagnostic (D) or therapeutic doses of ^{131}I-MIBG in two patients with neuroblastoma who underwent 3 to 4 courses of treatment ($I-IV$)

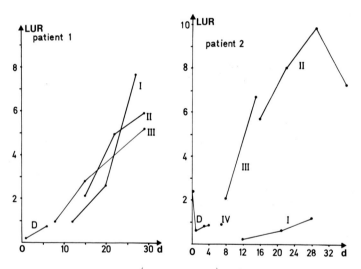

Fig. 2. Liver uptake ratios $\left(\dfrac{cpm_{L} - cpm_{BG}}{cpm_{BG}}\right)$ for ^{131}I-MIBG as functions of time after administration of diagnostic (D) or therapeutic doses of ^{131}I-MIBG in two patients with neuroblastoma who underwent 3 to 4 courses of treatment ($I-IV$)

about 2 in patient 2. During the following days a further increase was observed and a value of 1.8 was reached after 6 days in patient 1 whereas patient 2 presented a value of 3.5 on day 4. In both patients, especially in patient 2, similar or even higher values were obtained about 2 weeks after the administration of the first therapeutic dose of ^{131}I-MIBG. Four weeks after tracer administration, the values had fallen towards 0 in patient 1 whereas a very high value of 3 remained in patient 2. In patient 1, UR were generally lower throughout treatment II than during treatment I. No significant further decrease was found in this patient comparing treatments II and III. In patient 2, UR decreased progressively with every treatment; this was most marked during treatment course II, since it can be assumed that the initial UR during treatment II was about as high as the last value obtained during treatment I.

Liver uptake ratios (LUR) varied between 2.4 and 0.7 during the week (2.5 h to 6 days) after the administration of the diagnostic dose of ^{131}I-MIBG (Fig. 2). Markedly higher values were observed during treatment with ^{131}I-MIBG where LUR increased after about 1 or 2 weeks after administration of the therapeutic doses and reached values ranging between 5.2 and 9.8 about 4 weeks after the administration. No significant increase, however, was found in patient 2 during treatment I. LUR determined during treatment were inversely related to the TuUR.

The clinical results of the treatment (iliac crest biopsy, bone and bone marrow scintigrams, tumor markers, blood cell counts, kidney and liver laboratory tests) will be published separately.

Conclusions

^{131}I-MIBG uptake ratio is a useful parameter by which the avidity of an adrenergic tumor may be expressed. The avidity determined by repeat diagnostic scintigrams may serve to predict the uptake of a therapeutic dose of ^{131}I-MIBG and possibly also to calculate roughly the radiation dose to be expected after administration of a given ^{131}I-MIBG dose. The two patients with neuroblastoma stage IV studied during ^{131}I-MIBG therapy presented marked differences in the avidity of their tumors. The patient with the tumor of high ^{131}I-MIBG avidity showed the best treatment effect, finally was submitted to bone marrow transplantation and is still alive (i.e., survival time of 4 months after treatment). The patient with low ^{131}I-MIBG avidity of the tumor died about 1 month after the last ^{131}I-MIBG treatment. Thus, prognosis of a patient treated with ^{131}I-MIBG seems to depend on the avidity of the tumor for this agent.

Loss of ^{131}I-MIBG avidity during ^{131}I-MIBG therapy may result from destruction of the tumor, at least of the ^{131}I-MIBG accumulating clones of tumor cells, as well as from a loss of adrenergic function of the tumor. It is rather likely that the decrease in ^{131}I-MIBG avidity of the tumor observed during treatment in patient 1 is due to selection of dedifferentiated tumor cells with reduced or lost adrenergic function. The changing pattern of ^{131}I-MIBG uptake found in this patient during ^{131}I-MIBG therapy supports this hypothesis. In the other patient, high ^{131}I-MIBG avidity of the tumor persisted during the first course of treatment and complete loss of ^{131}I-MIBG uptake occurred during treatment II, the treatment with the highest ^{131}I-MIBG dose. In patient 1, the greatest change in ^{131}I-MIBG uptake was also observed during the treatment with the highest dose of ^{131}I-MIBG, which was treatment I.

The role of the liver after application of ^{131}I-MIBG can also be studied by determination of uptake ratios. Changes recorded during the first few days after the administration of a diagnostic dose may be helpful for characterization of the tumor with respect to its adrenergic activity [7]. The changes occurring during the weeks following administration of a therapeutic dose probably reflect uptake of ^{131}I-MIBG released by the tumor being damaged by radiation. This is suggested by the inverse relationship of uptake ratio of the tumor as compared with the uptake ratio of the liver.

Our observations favor the concept of primary ^{131}I-MIBG therapy in patients with neuroblastoma stage IV or inoperable cases of earlier stage. The treatment would then be given at a time when the tumor is well differentiated. The most efficient reduction of tumor mass might within the safety limits of radiation doses be achieved by few courses of treatment with high doses of ^{131}I-MIBG rather than with multiple courses of treatment with lower doses. By this procedure, selection of dedifferentiated cells and further tumor growth might be prevented which possibly could be the basis for a curative cytostatic treatment or conditioning for bone marrow transplantation.

References

1. Wieland M, Wu JI, Brown LE, Mangner TJ, Swanson DP, Beierwaltes WH (1980) Radiolabeled adrenergic neuron-blocking agents: adrenomedullary imaging with [131]I Iodobenzylguanidine. J Nucl Med 21:349−353
2. Wieland M, Brown LE, Tobes MC, Rogers WL, Marsh DD, Mangner TJ, Swanson DP, Beierwaltes WH (1981) Imaging the primate adrenal medulla with (^{123}I) and (^{131}I) Meta-Iodobenzylguanidine: concise communication. J Nucl Med 22:358−364
3. Sisson JC, Frager MS, Valk TW, Gross MD, Swanson DP, Wieland DM, Tobes MC, Beierwaltes WH, Thompson TW (1981) Scintigraphic localization of Pheochromocytoma. N Engl J Med 305:12−17
4. Cordes U, Hahn K, Eißner D, Weigand H, Günther R, Braun B, Hey O, Rothmund M, Lenner V, Lorenz J, Bohl J, Strohbach H, Beyer J (1982) Szintigraphie adrenerger Tumoren mit ^{131}I-meta-Benzylguanidin. Dtsch Med Wochenschr 107:1349−1352
5. Kimmig B, Brandeis WE, Eisenhut M, Bubeck B, Hermann HJ, zum Winkel K (1983) Szintigraphische Darstellung eines Neuroblastoms. Nuc Compact 14:347−348
6. Fischer M, Winterberg B, Müller-Frensing R, Friemann J, Zideck W, Vetter H (1983) Nuklearmedizinische Therapie des Phaeochromocytoms. Nuc Compact 14:172−176
7. Nakajo M, Shimabukuro K, Miyaji N, Shimada J, Shirono K, Sakata H, Yoshimura H, Yonekura R, Shinohara S (1985) Rapid clearance of Iodine-131-MIBG from the heart and liver of patients with adrenergic dysfunction and pheochromocytoma. J Nucl Med 26:357−365

Endolymphatic Radionuclide Therapy (ELRT) in Malignant Melanoma of the Lower Extremities

P. Pfannenstiel[1], R.-P. Müller, and P. E. Peters

Metastatic malignant melanoma of the lower extremities is known to spread early via the lymphatic route. Lymph node metastases are considered to be rather resistant to ionizing radiation, thus requiring high radiation doses, which can only be applied by endolymphatic radiotherapy.

Any attempt to determine the value of a new therapeutic approach in malignant melanoma requires a large number of patients, since there are many factors of prognostic importance to be considered, such as localization of the primary tumor, clinical staging, histological classification, including the level of invasive growth.

Therefore, in 1972, four German medical centers in Berlin, Essen, Münster, and Wiesbaden decided to pool their experience in a joint study group. In these institutions ELRT is performed in a standardized manner [8 – 11].

The main indication for endolymphatic radiotherapy (ELRT) is stage I disease of malignant melanoma with the primary tumor located in the lower extremities (Table 1). In the great majority of cases the intralymphatic application was performed within 4 – 6 weeks of a wide surgical excision of the primary tumor.

A relative indication is given in stage II disease as seen in patients with clinically positive regional lymph nodes. In these cases the surgeon would like to have information about the possible extent of the metastatic involvement of lymph nodes. In these patients ELRT is performed prior to lymph node dissection, mainly to obtain sufficient diagnostic information because of the radiopaque contrast medium lipiodol UF, in which the $^{32}P/^{131}$iodine is dissolved [4], but not for definitive treatment of the lymph nodes.

By restricting ourselves to melanoma of the lower extremities, we were able to accumulate a well-defined group of patients in stage I. The number of patients [4, 6, 7, 9, 10, 12, 15] in this stage is now 290 (Table 2).

ELRT was performed in two different ways of application technique (Table 3):

- The diseased extremity is treated by unilateral application of 5 mCi phosphorus-32 (^{32}P in the form of tri-*n*-octylphosphate). 0.5 mCi ^{131}I-labelled triolein is added for dosimetric purposes only. Both radionuclides are dissolved in 3.5 ml lipiodol UF, an oily contrast medium for lymphography.
- Bilateral application of the radioactive substances, administering 2.0 mCi ^{32}P combined with 0.5 mCi 131-I-lipiodol UF on each side.

---

1 Fachbereich Nuklearmedizin, Deutsche Klinik für Diagnostik, Aukammallee 33, D-6200 Wiesbaden 1

Nuclear Medicine in Clinical Oncology
Ed. by C. Winkler
© Springer-Verlag Berlin Heidelberg 1986

Table 1. Indications for endolymphatic radiotherapy in malignant melanoma (only as an adjunct to competent surgical therapy)

1. Stage I – disease of the lower extremities
2. Stage II – disease of the lower extremities *prior* to lymphadenectomy
3. Other locations of malignant melanoma (e g., upper extremities, trunk) if technically possible

Table 2. Endolymphatic radiotherapy in malignant melanoma – level of invasive growth – stage I

II	Tumor infiltrates into upper portion of papillary dermis	10
III	Tumor is layered on the interface of the papillary and reticular dermis	53
IV	Tumor involves reticular dermis	153
V	Tumor involves subcutaneous tissue	17
	Undetermined	57
		290

Table 3. Endolymphatic radiotherapy (ELRT) – volume and radiation dose compound: ^{32}P/^{131}I tri-n-octylphosphate (LIPIODOL-UF)

Unilateral application (lower extremity):	3.5 ml	5.0 mCi ^{32}P	0.5 mCi ^{131}I
Bilateral application (lower extremities):	3.5 ml	2.0 mCi ^{32}P	0.5 mCi ^{131}I each side
Unilateral application (upper extremity):	2.0 ml	2.0 mCi ^{32}P	0.5 mCi ^{131}I

We completely discontinued ELRT in malignant melanoma of the upper extremities because of the rather high rate of complications and poor clinical results.

Following intralymphatic application of the labelled contrast medium, the distribution of radioactivity is measured by profile scanning. Figure 1 shows the variations of ^{131}I in the region of the abdomen. These variations can be determined by planimetry of the individual sections of the curves.

The radioactivity in the pelvic and para-aortal lymph nodes as well as in the whole body and lungs is measured at set intervals following the administration of the radioactive contrast medium. By plotting radioactivity against time, a curve showing the ^{131}I retention in different parts of the body is obtained [12 – 15].

Figure 2 shows an example of this with high uptake of radioactivity in the retroperitoneal lymph nodes and only small amounts of radioactivity over the thoracic region due to overflow of the ^{131}I-labelled contrast medium from the thoracic duct to the lungs. Usually about 75% of the applied radioactivity is retained by the inguinal, iliac, and retroperitoneal lymph nodes, and about 25% is found in the lungs.

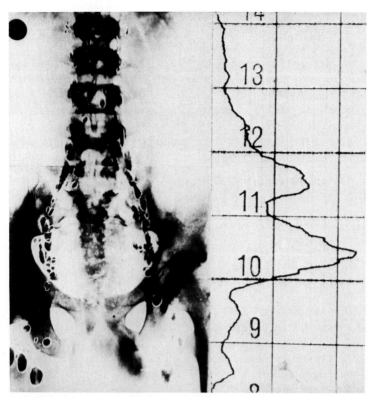

Fig. 1. ^{131}I distribution as measured by a profile scanner on successive days demonstrating the different rates at which ^{131}I is discharged from the abdominal region. In order to calculate the weight of the lymph nodes, the length and breadth of each lymph node as projected on the anterior-posterior X-ray is measured (formula see text)

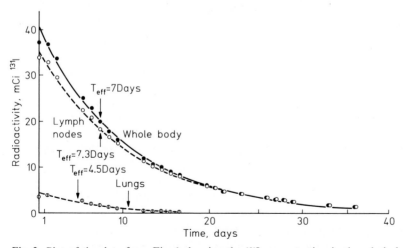

Fig. 2. Plot of the data from Fig. 1 showing the ^{131}I-concentration in the whole body, lymph nodes, and lungs following endolymphatic ^{131}I-therapy. The effective half-life (T_{eff}) of the ^{131}I, as shown on the time scale, is 7.3 days for the lymph nodes and 4.5 days for the lungs

From these curves we derive the rate at which ^{131}I is discharged from certain parts of the body. The effective half-life (T_2) of ^{131}I accumulated in the lymph nodes varies from 5.3 to 8 days with an average of 7.0 days.

For dosimetry an average absorbed energy of 0.203 MeV for ^{131}I was assumed. Since phosphorus-32 was used together with ^{131}I an average absorbed energy of 0.685 MeV was assumed.

For dosage calculations we have attempted to assess the weights of the lymph nodes. Given an ellipsoidal shaped lymph node, the depth can be considered to be the same as the breadth, and the length and the breadth are measured on the anterior-posterior X-ray (Fig. 1).

$$V_{\text{lymph node}} = \frac{4}{3}\pi\frac{\text{length}}{2}\left(\frac{\text{breadth}}{2}\right)^2\left(\frac{110-17}{110}\right)^3$$

$$V_{\text{lymph node}} = 0.312 \times \text{length} \times (\text{breadth})^2$$

This method was proved by estimating the weight of the lymph nodes from their projections on the X-rays of lymph nodes of known weights. The total weight of the retroperitoneal lymph nodes averages 20 g.

The absorbed radiation doses in the region of the pelvic and para-aortal lymph nodes vary according to the $^{131}I/^{32}P$ distribution in the body, the effective half-life (T_2), and the calculated volume of the lymph nodes. They were found to range from 5000 to 700,000 rads. These doses are only approximate, as the calculations presume a homogenous distribution of the contrast medium within the lymph nodes. The mean radiation absorbed dosage to the lymphatic system was found to be 180,000 rad or 180 Gy [12–15].

The radiation dose to the lungs averaged 220 rad (2,2 Gy) [6, 7]. However, only two patients obtained more than 1000 rad (10 Gy) whole lung irradiation. This dosage might cause clinical symptoms, which, in fact, did not appear. Only 22% of the patients had no measurable radioactivity within the lungs.

From 1972 to 1984, 378 patients with malignant melanoma of the lower extremities were treated by uni- or bilateral ELRT. At the time of operation of the primary tumor, 290 patients had no evidence of regional lymph node metastasis and thus belonged to the clinical stage I.

Since ELRT in advanced stages of malignant melanoma is only a palliative step due to the limited range of penetration of ^{32}P-beta irradiation, we concentrated our attention on patients with stage I disease, where ELRT was performed to treat micrometastases, which clinically occur in about 20%–30% of cases.

In the clinical stage I there were 2.6 times more female than male patients. This is due to the fact that the lower extremities are the preferential site of malignant melanoma in women, while men more often show involvement of the trunk. The calf was the preferential location in 62%, followed by the foot in 24%, and the thigh in 14% of the patients.

Histological classification according to MIHM and Clark (Table 4) was available in most cases, revealing a relatively high incidence of nodular-type melanoma – 27% in our material as opposed to 15% in large statistics. This particular subtype of malignant melanoma is known to have a rather poor prognosis.

The treated patients were aged between 14 and 87 years; the mean age was 49 years for both female and male patients.

Concerning treatment-related side effects, our patients suffered from mild, mostly transient lymphedema and radiodermatitis in only 13%. A specific therapy was necessary in only 3% following radioulcera at the site of extravasation of radioactive material (Table 5).

The survival rates were calculated using the actuarial method of UICC (1976). The 5-year survival rate was 70.5% (165/234 patients) and the 10-year survival rate was 65% (98/137).

There was no statistically significant difference between unilateral and bilateral application of the radioactive substances (Table 6). However, there was a difference in the survival rates according to the clinical stage of the disease. Prognosis for patients with stage II disease was distinctly worse than for the group with stage I [4, 6, 7].

Our data compare favourably with earlier reports by Edwards et al. [1] and others [3, 21]. Endolymphatic radiotherapy following wide surgical excision of the primary tumor cannot totally prevent development of lymph node metastasis and/or skin metastases, but ELRT can reduce the incidence of such prognostically significant occurrences. As compared with isolated perfusion and radical lymph node dissection, it is a rather simple procedure with very little morbidity and no mortality.

About 30% of our patients were younger than 40 years at the time of ELRT. The prognosis was better than in the older age group. Localization of the primary tumor apparently had no influence on the prognosis.

From our more than ten years' experience considering the advantages and disadvantages of endolymphatic therapy with radioactive substances, we believe that this type of internal irradiation has definite advantages as opposed to

Table 4. Endolymphatic radiotherapy in malignant melanoma – classification according to MIHM and Clark – stage I

Lentigo maligna melanoma	24
Superficial spreading melanoma	120
Nodular melanoma	78
Equivocal	17
Undetermined	51
	290

Table 5. Endolymphatic radiotherapy (ELRT) – complications

Severe:	Radiation pneumonitis or fibrosis of the lung
	Radiation damage at the site of injection due to extravasation of radioactive material
Moderate:	Transitory edema
	Delayed healing of skin incisions
	Radiation induced lymphangitis

Table 6. Unilateral and bilateral application of endolymphatic radionuclide therapy

Years	ELRT: Unilateral total 205		Bilateral total 85	
	±	%	±	%
0– 1	6	3.0	0	–
1– 2	15	7.0	6	7.0
2– 3	13	6.3	2	5.9
3– 4	9	4.5	5	2.4
4– 5	4	2.0	2	2.4
5– 6	6	3.0	2	2.4
6– 7	3	1.5	0	–
7– 8	1	0.5	2	2.4
8– 9	1	0.5	2	2.4
9–10	0	–	1	1.0
10–11	0	–	0	–
Total	58	28.3	22	25.9

Table 7. Endolymphatic radiotherapy (ELRT) – limiting factors

Anatomic variations:
  – Incomplete filling of lymph nodes
  – Inhomogeneous dose distribution
  – "By passing" of lymph nodes
  – Lympho-venous anastomoses
Metastases larger than range of penetration of beta radiation

external radiation therapy in this particular disease. The limiting factors for endolymphatic radiotherapy are anatomical variations (Table 7).

It is, however, impossible to end this discussion without a comment on the initial treatment of the primary lesion. It is evident that the bad prognosis of many of our patients was significantly influenced by the inadequacy of the initial surgical treatment. Despite almost universal agreement in the literature to the necessity of wide excision and grafting or local amputation concerning different anatomical locations, many patients are sent to our departments in whom the primary tumor has been cut into, partially excised, or excised with little or no margining.

The advantages of ^{32}P endolymphatic radionuclide therapy in stage I patients with malignant melanoma of the lower extremity may be summarized as follows: It prevents a block dissection of inguinal/iliacal lymph nodes by sufficient devitalization of microscopic metastases. The technique is minimally invasive and the patients suffer very little in the way of side effects as compared with surgical intervention or isolated groin perfusion.

References

1. Edwards JM, Kinmonth JB (1968) Endolymphatic therapy for malignant melanoma. Br Med J I:18—22
2. Edwards JM (1981) Treatment of malignant melanoma by endolymphatic therapy. In: Ariel IM (ed) Malignant melanoma. Appleton-Century-Crofts, New York, p 237
3. McBride CM (1982) Treatment analysis of a group of patients with primary malignant melanoma on a limb. Prog Clin Cancer 333
4. Müller R-P, Peters PE, Fischedick A-R, Tilkorn H (1984) Endolymphatic radiotherapy using $^{131}J/^{32}P$-lipiodol in malignant melanomas of the lower extremities — long term results. In: Höfer R, Bergmann H (eds) Radioaktive Isotope in Klinik und Forschung. Internationales Symposium 1984 Gastein, Austria
5. Müller R-P, Peters PE (1985) Die Strahlenbelastung der Lunge nach endolymphatischer Radionuklidtherapie (ELRT) von Melanomen der unteren Extremıtäten. Strahlentherapie 161:23—29
6. Müller R-P, Peters PE, Pfannenstiel P, Pötter R (1985) 10 years follow-up of patients with stage I malignant melanoma of the lower extremities treated by endolymphatic radionuclide therapy. 10th International congress of lymphology, Adelaide, South Australia, 26 Aug—2 Sept, 1985
7. Müller R-P, Peters PE, Pfannenstiel P, Pötter R (1985) Long term results of endolymphatic radionuclide therapy (ELRT) in stage I malignant melanomas of the lower extremities. 2nd Annual scientific meeting of the American Society for Therapeutic Radiology and Oncology, Miami Beach/Florida, USA, 29 Sept—4 Oct, 1985
8. Peters PE, Makoski HB, Pfannenstiel P, Scherer E, Schnepper E, Wannenmacher M, Weissleder H, zum Winkel K (1977) Endolymphatic radiotherapy in malignant melanoma of the lower extremities. Results of a joint study. In: Malek P, Bartos V, Weissleder H, Witte MH (eds) Lymphology. Proceedings of the VIth International Congress, Prague, 1977
9. Peters PE, Weissleder H, Kipper S, Ehring F, Makoski HB, Pfannenstiel P, Schnepper E, zum Winkel K (1979) Intralymphatic isotope therapy, an effective alternative to the wait-and-see policy in the treatment of stage I malignant melanoma of the lower limb. In: Weissleder H, Bartos V, Clodius L, Malek P (eds) Progress in lymphology. Proceedings of the VIIth International Congress, Florence, 1979
10. Peters PE, Makoski HB, Pfannenstiel P, Scherer E, Schnepper E, Wannenmacher M, Weissleder H, zum Winkel K (1979) Endolymphatic radiotherapy in malignant melanoma of the lower extremities. Results of a joint study. In: Malek P, Bartos P, Weissleder H, Witte MW (eds) Lymphology. Thieme, Stuttgart, pp 460—462
11. Peters PE, Weissleder H, Kipper S, Ehring F, Makoski HB, Pfannenstiel P, Schnepper E, zum Winkel K (1981) Intralymphatic isotope therapy — an effective alternative to the wait-and-see policy in the treatment of stage I malignant melanoma of the lower limb. Avi Cenun Verlag, Prague, pp 373—376
12. Pfannenstiel P, Wetzig E, Kleine N (1967) Strahlendosimetrie bei der endolymphatischen Therapie mit ^{131}J. In: Hoffmann G, Höfer R (eds) Radionuklide in Kreislaufforschung und Kreislaufdiagnostik. pp 440—448
13. Pfannenstiel P, Wetzig E, Weissleder H, Strickstock KH, Kleine N, Hoffmann G (1969) Probleme der Strahlendosimetrie bei endolymphatischer Therapie mit Radionukliden. In: Maligne Melanome. Urban and Schwarzenberg, München, pp 186—196
14. Pfannenstiel P, Weissleder H, Hoffmann G (1969) Problems of radiation dosimetry in endolymphatic therapy with radioactive isotopes. Lymphology 2:160—166
15. Pfannenstiel P, Weissleder H, Peters PE (1979) Endolymphatische Behandlung mit P-32-J-131. Nuklearmediziner 4:300—313
16. Weissleder H, Pfannenstiel P, Strickstock KH, Hoffmann G (1967) Die endolymphatische Therapie mit radioaktiven Substanzen (Technik und Radiometrie). Fortschr Röntgenstr 107:758—764
17. Weissleder H, Pfannenstiel P, Strickstock KH, Hoffmann G (1968) Principles of endolymphatic therapy with radioactive substances. In: Viamonte M, Koehler PR, Witte M, Witte

C (eds) Progress in lymphology II, 2nd International congress of lymphology, Miami, USA, 1968
18. Weissleder H, Pfannenstiel P (1972) Endolymphatische Metastasentherapie mit Radioisotopen bei malignem Melanom. Arch Dermatol Forsch 244:403–405
19. Weissleder H, Pfannenstiel P (1973) Radionuklidbehandlung von Lymphknotenmetastasen bei malignem Melanom. Hautarzt 24:21–24
20. Weissleder H, Pfannenstiel P (1979) Endolymphatische Radionuklidbehandlung. In: Emrich D (ed) Nuklearmedizin, Funktionsdiagnostik und Therapie, 2nd edn. Thieme, Stuttgart
21. Zum Winkel K (1981) Intralymphatische Strahlentherapie. In: Frommhold W, Gerhardt P (eds) Erkrankungen des Lymphsystems (ohne Lymphogranulomatose). Klinisch-radiologisches Seminar, vol 11. Thieme, Stuttgart, pp 135–148

On the Efficacy of Strontium-89 Therapy.
Preliminary Evaluation of a Double-blind Study

H.-J. Correns[1], K. Buchali, D. Schnorr, Hildegard Lips, Karin Sydow, M. Schürer, and B. Johannsen

In 1970 and 1982, we reported on the results of Sr-89 treatment of pain caused by bone metastases in 81 patients with prostate carcinoma [1, 2]. Due to uncertainty inherent in the evaluation of this treatment within the manifold therapy of such patients, we decided, in agreement with the therapy commission of our Faculty of Medicine, to start a double-blind investigation in order to differentiate the Sr-89 effect from effects of simultaneously applied drugs (hormones, cytostatics etc.)

Patients were selected as previously reported. One prerequisite was a positive Sr-85 scintigram indicating an accumulation of strontium in the multiple bone lesions. The outpatient therapy consisted of a sequence of 3 intravenous injections of 75 MBq Sr-89 chloride (Amersham) each at monthly intervals. The placebo group received physiological saline. The patients were classified into the two groups according to a random parameter. Follow-up examination involved subjective evidence of the skeletal associated pain and blood count both at the time of injection and 3 months later. Further investigations including Tc-99m EHDP skeletal scintigraphy were made 6−12 months after the start of therapy (Table 1).

Results

Which preparation (Sr-89 or NaCl) was given to 24 patients of the double-blind study has been disclosed for evaluation. Thirteen were treated with Sr-89 chloride (Sr group) and 11 patients with placebo (Pl group).

In 5 patients, the therapeutic procedure could not be completed. Due to the severity of the underlying disease, they died after the first ($n = 1$) or second ($n = 4$) injection. Four other patients died within 6 months of the third therapeutic application. The dead comprised 6 (55%) out of the Pl group and only 3 (23%) of the Sr group (Table 2).

Five patients with only slight pain showed no clear change. Thus, the efficacy of their treatment is not definitely assessable.

There were 10 cases with pain relief, 3 (38%) from the Sr group and 7 (64%) from the Pl group (Table 3). Table 4 shows the outcome in dependence of the duration of the disease: of the 7 patients whose disease was diagnosed early

1 Direktor der Nuklearmedizinischen Klinik, Bereich Medizin (Charité), Humboldt-Universität zu Berlin, Schumannstr. 20−21, X-1040 Berlin (DDR)

Table 1. Steps of the procedure applied

Tc-99m diphosphonate scintigraphy
↓
Sr-85 chloride scintigraphy
↓
Sr-89 chloride therapy
(3 × 75 MBq)
1 injection/month
↓
Tc-99m diphosphonate scintigraphy

Table 4. Comparison of patients diagnosed early and late

Patients	Relief of pain	
	+	0
Diagnosed early (< 1 year)	6	1
Diagnosed late (> 1 year)	4	8

Table 2. Comparison of survival rate between Sr group and Pl group

Group	Survival	
	No	Yes
Sr	3	10
Pl	6	5

Table 5. Result of follow-up scintigraphy

Group	Uptake	
	Regressive	Progressive
Sr	4	–
Pl	–	2

Table 3. Result of treatment obtained with patients of Sr and Pl group

Group	Relief of pain	
	+	0
Sr	3	5
Pl	7	4

Table 6. Side effect on thrombocytes

Group	Thrombocytes count	
	↓	=
Sr	7	6
Pl	2	9

(< 1 year), 6 were treated successfully; among them 4 from the placebo group. Pain relief could be observed in 4 out of 12 patients with a late diagnosed disease (> 1 year).

While 4 (Sr group) of the 6 patients who were followed up scintigraphically showed reduced radioactivity accumulation, 2 (Pl group) had a more intense uptake (Table 5).

A transient thrombocytopenia was observed in 7 cases (54%) from the Sr group and 2 (18%) from the placebo group (Table 6).

Discussion

Pain is a subjective sensation and thus the effectiveness of analgesic treatment cannot yet be evaluated with objective methods. Therefore, subjective assessment has been further recommended, partly with a graduation registered by the patient himself [3].

When evaluating the Sr-89 effect on skeletal metastases, certain subjective influences on the patients have to be taken into account (circumstance of injection, instructions on the radiotherapeutical agent, etc.). Secondary cures, which we also observed, can be explained along this line.

As for the underlying mechanism of Sr-89 therapy, the interval prior to the response, which often occurs within a week of injection, is to a certain extent informative. Considering the effective half-life of approximately 25 days in the region of metastases (Firusian, Buchali), the radiation dose absorbed during 1 week amounts to 18% of the total dose (approx. 0.22 Gy/MBq), i.e., about 3 Gy/75 MBq/week and is thus in the range of doses used for irradiation of inflammations.

Though not yet proved and contradicting earlier results, a total dose of approximately 50 Gy seems to influence the metastatic process as demonstrated by the follow-up scintigrams made until now. The observed distribution of the dead between the Sr and the Pl groups is congruent with this suggestion.

On the other hand, the beneficial effect in respect of pain appears to be less than earlier reported.

In agreement with previous results, there is a better effect in patients diagnosed early, but it is a point of discussion whether this is a merit of the basic therapy, since 4 cases with placebo injections are included.

We want to emphasize that side effects concerning haematopoiesis, especially thrombocytes, appear in about half the cases. The placebo group shows that the radioactivity is not the only reason for haematological complications in these patients under complex treatment.

In conclusion, at this stage of our double-blind study, we cannot derive a final assessment. In order to obtain as soon as possible a conclusive evaluation of the therapeutic efficacy we intend to extend our investigation to a multicentre study.

References

1. Correns H-J, Mebel M, Buchali K, Schnorr D, Seidel C, Mitterlechner E (1979) 89-Strontium therapy of bone metastases of carcinoma of the prostatic gland. Eur J Nucl Med 4:33
2. Correns H-J, Buchali K, Sydow K, Schürer M, Schnorr D, Richter K (1982) Nuklearmedizinische Therapie von Metastasen des Skelettsystems. 19th Symp Nuklearmedizin, Reinhardsbrunn 1982
3. Cziske R (1983) Faktoren des Schmerzerlebens und ihre Messung: Revidierte mehrdimensionale Schmerzskala. Diagnostica 29:61

Cancer Treatment with Radioactive Labeled Antibodies

G. L. DeNardo[1], S. J. DeNardo, and D. J. Macey

Introduction

The potential of radioimmunotherapy based upon monoclonal antibodies has elicited considerable excitement within the scientific community. This type of disease targeting has been a long-standing goal of medicine. Bale [1] explored the use of polyclonal antibodies produced against fibrin and labeled with I-131 to deliver radiation therapy to tumors more than 20 years ago. The potential usefulness of this approach has been demonstrated [2], but success was limited by inadequate specificity of these polyclonal antibodies. The superiority of monoclonal antibodies over conventional polyclonal antisera has been demonstrated [3]. Monoclonal antibodies are uniquely attractive targeting molecules. Two other technological developments have occurred at precisely the same time as the hybridization technology for producing monoclonal antibody so that the simultaneous collision of these three technologies provides a unique opportunity for provision of radionuclide therapy based upon not only the specificity of monoclonal antibodies, but also treatment planning techniques of the type which have proved necessary in external beam and radionuclide sealed source radiation therapy. Contrary to common misconception, radionuclide therapy does not necessarily require more favorable target to nontarget relationships than radionuclide imaging. The critical element for radionuclide therapy is the nature of the nontarget or critical organ and its radiosensitivity. For example, bone marrow is a particularly vulnerable critical organ, whereas the spleen does not represent an essential organ. Furthermore, time is an ally to successful therapy using monoclonal antibodies as targeting molecules, because the latter usually have a prolonged residence time on the cancerous tissue, particularly when compared to other tissues. The situation is analogous to that of treatment of differentiated thyroid cancer with ^{131}I-iodide, wherein this radionuclide is incorporated into thyroid hormone and resides in the thyroid cancer for a prolonged interval of time. A variety of systemically infused monoclonal and polyclonal radiolabeled antibodies have been demonstrated to target both primary malignancies and metastatic cancers [4]. The science of determining the dose distribution, toxicity, and tumor response following the administration of systemic radioactive agents for therapeutic purposes is in the process of being developed [5, 6]. Significant results have been reported in melanoma [7],

---

1 University of California, Davis, School of Medicine, Division of Nuclear Medicine, 4301 X Street, Folb II/E, Sacramento, CA 95817, USA

Nuclear Medicine in Clinical Oncology
Ed. by C. Winkler
© Springer-Verlag Berlin Heidelberg 1986

hepatoma, and lymphoma [8]. The current clinical experience in radiolabeled antibody therapy has been accomplished through ongoing multi-institutional protocols in the treatment of hepatoma and lymphoma, and through individual institutional protocols in the treatment of melanoma and cancerous effusions.

In some situations of very avid tumor localization, it is clear that radio-therapy with antitumor antibody is feasible. Using these antibodies as carriers, preliminary results indicate that it is possible to deliver several thousand rads to a tumor without inflicting excessive damage to bone marrow. However, it is too early to comment on the absolute clinical utility of these methods.

Theoretical Basis for Radioimmunotherapy

In order for radioimmunotherapy to be effective, certain minimal requirements must be met. The antibodies must retain acceptable biological activity after coupling with the radionuclide. The radioantibody preparation must possess sufficiently high specific radioactivity to deliver a lethal dose of radiation after attaching to the cell, the required level of activity depending on the number of antibodies which can be bound by the cell. The relative selectivity of tumor cells as compared with normal cells for the antibody must be high enough that destruction of normal cells remains at a tolerable level. A fundamental question is whether enough radionuclide can be localized on the tumor cell to deliver a lethal dose of radiation to the tumor cells while maintaining the dose to normal tissues at tolerable levels. The number of specific antigenic sites on tumor cells is many times greater than the number of radioantibodies required to deliver the dose. A number of antigen-antibody systems have now been defined where-in there are $10^4 - 10^6$ antigenic sites per cell [9]. This number represents the number of antigenic sites potentially available on the cell membrane for target-ing by an antibody against a discrete epitope of that antigen. There are 10^9 cells in each gram or cubic centimeter of cancer tissue so that $10^{13} - 10^{15}$ antibody molecules can be accumulated in 1 g cancer tissue. Additional antigen-antibody systems within the same cancer cell line, as well as the possibility that more than one epitope of a particular type may exist on a single antigen, provide the possibility of targeting more antibody. Analogous calculations suggest that use of monoclonal antibodies against fibrin present in cancer tissue provides at least as many potential targeting sites [5].

Antibodies can be labeled with at least one atom of radionuclide per mol-ecule of protein without altering their immunogenicity. As an example, 1 μCi ^{131}I in the carrier-free state has 3.6×10^{10} atoms of iodine. If we restrict ra-diochemical labeling to one atom of iodine introduced to each molecule of anti-body, then 2.7×10^2 to 2.7×10^4 μCi ^{131}I represent the maximum amount of this radionuclide that can be introduced in 1 g cancer tissue using a single antigen-antibody system. One μCi of ^{131}I distributed in 1 g tissue results in ap-proximately 120 rad of absorbed radiation in that tissue through its physical lifetime (physical half-life: 8 days). Thus, 32,400 to 3,240,000 rads can theoreti-cally be delivered to cancer tissue in the absence of biologic turnover of the antigen-antibody complex. Other radionuclides provide somewhat greater dose.

The actual situation in a patient is more complicated. An antibody protein will distribute in the intravascular and interstitial spaces to all tissues of the body. A characteristic of importance to successful radioimmunotherapy, that is, that the biologic lifetime in the cancer of radiolabeled immunospecific antibody must be, and is, longer than that in other tissues adds to the therapeutic ratio.

Theoretical calculations and published data have suggested to McGaughey [10] that it is possible to deliver a highly therapeutic dose of β-radiation to individual free floating tumor cells solely by means of ^{131}I- or ^{133}I-antibodies attached to tumor-specific antigens on the cell membrane over one half-life of either isotope. He concluded that such an approach would be useful for destroying circulating cancer or leukemia cells or early metastases, and might also be used for the therapy of disseminated tumors. Such an approach would be analogous to the technique of extracorporeal irradiation of the blood which has proven beneficial in some cases, especially in conjunction with chemotherapy.

Using a theoretical model of biodistribution and clearance with target to nontarget localization indices based on current estimates, Wessels [11] assessed the potential of several radionuclides for radioimmunotherapy. By assuming a standard geometry and tumor location in humans and applying available biodistribution data for radiolabeled tumor-associated antibodies or their fragments, a generalized comparison of nuclide radiolabeling potential for these applications was obtained. It was assumed that for these modeling calculations a therapy dose of 100 mCi of immunologically active and purified labeled tumor-associated antibody was administered to a 70-kg patient with a 500-g solid tumor target (T) located heterogeneously in a normal size (1833-g) liver. If T/NT ratios in excess of 10 are reached after a few days for tumor-associated antibodies or their fragments, the calculations indicate that useful radioimmunotherapy is feasible. Without additional consideration to any other specific critical organ, and assuming a T/NT dose ratio in excess of 10, it is possible to deliver fractionally 100–150 rads to tumor without excessive whole body radiation doses. If the bone marrow is taken to be the critical organ, up to 300 rads may be delivered to the tumor for several radionuclides under current consideration. Dose values described in this work for large heterogeneous tumors are probably less than doses delivered to small tumors or micrometastases. A review of particle LET and dose deposition per track length for a variety of radionuclides has been presented by DeNardo [12].

Antiferritin and Related Antibodies

While not the first use of radiolabeled antibodies to treat cancer, the work of the pioneering group at Johns Hopkins has certainly been the most prolonged and extensive. More than 100 patients have now been treated with more than 300 doses of radiolabeled polyclonal antibody (P. Leichner, pers. communication 1985). This work initially encompassed several polyclonal antibodies, but is now focused primarily on the use of polyclonal antiferritin antibody in patients with hepatoma.

Ferritin is a tumor-associated protein found in experimental and human hepatoma and other cancers [13, 14]. Normal tissues secrete ferritin in response to physiologic mechanisms. Much of the ferritin in normal tissues is intracellular and may not be available for initial binding. Binding of polyclonal antiferritin antibody in the H-4 II-E rat hepatoma model could be inhibited by unlabeled antiferritin but not by unlabeled normal rabbit IgG. Normal tissues did not target with antiferritin. The maximum tumor targeting was dependent on the amount of injected IgG. At very low amounts of injected antibody, optimal tumor targeting did not occur (Table 1), perhaps due to nonspecific absorbtion in normal tissues of the limited amount of specific antibody available for binding. The antiferritin preparation contains 80% normal IgG [13]. Many normal tissues have capacity to bind IgG nonspecifically [15]. An optimum therapeutic window of injected antiferritin exists for maximal tumor targeting over concomitant nonspecific normal tissue accumulation. The injection of large amounts of antiferritin resulted in decreased specific targeting of tumor in this model system. The physiologic reasons for such selective localization is not known, but the term "biologic window" has been used to describe the differential availability of tumor ferritin for binding [13].

Following successful use and lack of appreciable toxicity in pilot studies, Phase I–II studies were initiated in patients with advanced primary liver malignancies using ^{131}I-labeled anti-CEA antibody (biliary carcinoma) or antiferritin (hepatoma). These patients were studied in an integrated program combining external irradiation and chemotherapy, followed by radioimmunotherapy. Initial patients treated with 50–100 mCi demonstrated retention of radiolabeled antibody in the tumor target for up to 8 days.

Several factors became obvious in the Phase I study. Significant toxicity with doses up to 100 mCi of radiolabeled polyclonal antibody did not occur, while total tumor dose of 1000–2000 rads was provided. Secondly, the dose rate to the tumor was between 5 and 10 rads per hour and, therefore, this "biologic radioactive implant" was in the low dose (Table 2) range unlike standard implantation where the dose rate is 40 rads per hour or more. The effective half-life in the body of isotopic labeled antibody was approximately 3 days and delivered 1 rad of total body radiation per mCi administered.

Studies included liver and tumor volume computations based on computerized axial tomographic scan analysis, in vivo quantitation of the activity deposited in hepatic tumors and normal liver tissue, and effective half-life

Table 1. Illustration of effect of amount of *polyclonal* antiferritin antibody on effective half-life. (Estimated from data by Leichner et al. [16])

Number of patients	Estimated antiferritin amount (mg)	Effective T-1/2 (days)	
		Tumor and liver	Body
4	250	7.4	3.6
5	10	2.9	2.7

Table 2. Total radiation absorbed dose (rads) and maximum dose rate (rads/hr) from administration of polyclonal antiferritin antibody to patients with hepatoma. (Modified from Leichner et al. [16])

Range of doses (rads)			Range of maximum dose rates (rads/h)		
Tumor	Liver	Body	Tumor	Liver	Body
360–610	50–150	25–130	3.1–4.2	0.5–1.3	0.3–1.1

Table 3. Specific activities (μCi/g) in tumor and liver tissues and tumor-to-liver ratios (Leichner et al. [16])

No. of patients	Tumor volumes (cm^3)	Mean (range)		Tumor-to-liver ratios
		Specific activity		
		Tumor	Liver	
18	220–1700	8.4 (6.2–12)	1.8 (1.1–3.4)	4.8 (1.9–7.0)
4	2290–3020	2.6 (1.7– 3.6)	1.6 (1.1–2.3)	1.6 (1.1–2.2)

measurements of the activity in the tumor, liver and total body. The ^{131}I activity in the tumor and liver was quantitated by the method of conjugate gamma-camera views [16].

For tumor volumes ranging from 220 to 1700 cm^3, the maximum tumor activity was linearly proportional to tumor volume. In this range of tumor volumes, the mean value of the tumor-to-liver ratios of specific activities was 4.8 (Table 3). Hepatomas ranging from 2290 to 3020 cm^3 had reduced tumor uptake of radiolabeled antiferritin antibody. There was a linear relationship between the volume of normal liver tissue and the maximum activity deposited. However, the percent of administered radioactivity deposited in tumor decreased from 30% in the lower range (approximately 30 mCi) of administered dose to 3% at 157 mCi of administered dose. These data, in conjunction with toxicity studies and tumor effective half-life measurements, led to the present treatment regimen of administering 30 mCi on day 0 and 20 mCi on day 5 following the first injection. This has resulted in the same range of absorbed dose to the tumor as was achieved with larger administered activities, but with a significant reduction of total-body irradiation to the patient.

Despite combination with radiation and chemotherapy, the singular additional toxicity from the ^{131}I-antibody was marrow hypoplasia reflected by transient thrombocytopenia. This study has demonstrated lack of serious toxicity from radiolabeled antibody, the biological characteristics of the agent, and its potential effectiveness. Their extensive experience has led to the conclusion that this therapy, while not adequate in itself, represented a promising adjunct to the conventional radiation and chemotherapy. While complete remission from combined therapy occurred in only a few patients with small tumors, tumor regression greater than 30% and lasting more than 8 weeks occurred in approximately one-half of the patients [3]. Antiferritin antibody labeled with ^{90}Y is under exploration with the expectation of substantial increase in dose rate delivery.

Antimelanoma Antibodies

Hellstrom and Larson's group at the University of Washington and the National Cancer Institute have studied human melanoma using monoclonal antibodies or Fab fragments that recognize the human melanoma-associated antigens p97 and "high-molecular-weight antigen" [7, 17].

The antigen best characterized is p97, a 97,000 molecular weight glycoprotein on the cell surface, which is present in concentrations of up to 400,000 molecules per cell. It is expressed at very low concentrations in most normal adult tissues but at high levels in more than 50% of melanomas and in fetal colon, thus characterizing it as an oncofetal antigen [18]. Sequencing of the amino acid structure showed 60% homology with serum transferrin and lactotransferrin [19]. The second antigen system targeted is a proteoglycan on the cell surface, with weights of 250 and 400 kd described as high-molecular-weight antigen [20].

Hellstrom and Larson's group at the University of Washington and the National Cancer Institute have now treated 15 patients with ^{131}I on 5–10 mg of Fab fragment on three occasions over 3–4 weeks. The largest cumulative dose has been 861 mCi. The results can be described as encouraging as occasional transient objective responses have occurred [7].

Three patients were particularly evaluable because of their length of follow-up and delivered dose (374–861 mCi), with an estimated 3800–8500 rads to tumor. One patient developed progressive disease and died 90 days after the first treatment dose. One patient received three doses totaling 519 mCi. There was stabilization of his previously rapid-growing liver metastasis for 3 months, which subsequently continued to increase in volume as determined by transmission CT measurements. A fourth dose with 342 mCi of ^{131}I anti-p97 was administered, and stabilization for 2 months was seen with subsequent rapid tumor growth. The third evaluable patient had metastatic disease to inguinal and pelvic nodes. He received 2 treatments totaling 374 mCi within a 2-week interval. A comparison of pre- and 6-week post-treatment transmission CT images showed a greater than 50% reduction of disease and disappearance of some nodes with no new lesions visualized. Tumor growth was again noted 3 months later, with new lung lesions and enlargement of pelvic nodes.

Eight patients had biopsies of subcutaneous nodules at 48 and 72 h post-injection in order to assess whether localization of radioactivity was antigen specific. Antigen-specific localization was observed with average ratios of specific to nonspecific uptake of 3.7 (48 h) and 3.4 (72 h); uptake was strongly correlated with tumor p97 concentration. Imaging studies of the biodistribution of ^{131}I-labeled anti-p97 Fab in patients selected for high p97 tumor concentration showed avid tumor uptake and more prolonged retention of labeled Fab in tumor than in normal tissues. In addition to tumor, ^{131}I-Fab uptake was also seen in liver and kidney.

Dosimetry estimates were performed based on the biodistribution of ^{131}I-Fab in these patients, and for every 100 mCi of ^{131}I-Fab given, tumor received 1040 rads; liver 325 rads; and bone marrow, 30 rads. Marrow would be expected to be the critical organ, if doses greater than 500 mCi ^{131}I-Fab are given.

Toxicity has been limited. No significant changes in pre- and posttreatment liver function or renal function tests were observed. Patients receiving therapy with greater than 500 mCi ^{131}I-Fab showed a drop in neutrophil and platelet counts, with nadirs at 3−4 weeks and gradual improvement thereafter. Four acute reactions were observed: one episode each of transient chills and fever; flushing and hypotension; and two skin rashes. All of these reactions responded promptly to symptomatic therapy. Marrow toxicity led to the conclusion that cumulative doses of up to 800 mCi ^{131}I anti p97 antibody could be administered [7].

Tumor Models

Our group's experience began 6 years ago with the production of polyclonal and monoclonal antibodies against P51 cells from the B16 syngeneic mouse melanoma. Polyclonal antibodies were produced by immunizing rabbits with irradiated melanoma cells. Monoclonal anti-bodies were produced by hybridizing spleen cells from C-57 black mice previously immunized with irradiated melanoma cells and NS-1 myeloma cells [21−24]. Equivalent amounts of ^{131}I-labeled monoclonal antibody produced 10 times greater kill in cell culture than ^{131}I-labeled polyclonal antibody.

Tissue biodistribution in mice bearing melanomas revealed 3−4 times more uptake of the ^{131}I monoclonal immunospecific antibody in the tumor than that or ^{131}I-labeled nonspecific gamma globulin. Tumor to muscle ratio was 20:1 and the mean percent of injected dose per gram of tumor was 15% at 72 h. All mice given calculated tumoricidal radiation doses (10,000 rads) by the ^{131}I monoclonal antibodies survived and the tumors regressed within 5 days. The mice survived 6 months without evidence of recurrence, and then were sacrificed.

More recently, we have cured the Raji human B cell lymphoma implanted in athymic mice with doses of ^{131}I-lym-1 monoclonal antibody [25, 26]. The doses of ^{131}I-lym-1 were estimated to have delivered approximately 5000 rads to the tumor and 1500 rads to the liver based upon biodistribution data. Mice injected with lym-1 labeled with [67]Cu using a bifunctional chelate had somewhat greater concentrations of radioactivity in the tumors [27]. These results suggested that curative radiation could be delivered with tumor-specific radiolabeled antibodies.

Patients with Cancer

Our group has successfully imaged patients with cancer using a variety of specific monoclonal antibodies and radionuclides. Lymphoma and breast cancer

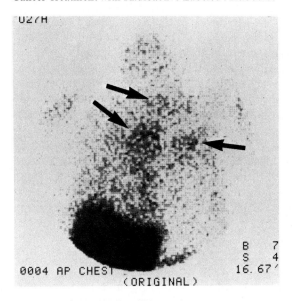

Fig. 1. 58-year-old female with breast cancer. Image of chest 3 days after injection of 1.6 mCi ^{111}In-IgM anti-breast cancer monoclonal antibody (19 mg) produced from human lymphocytes revealed several sites of uptake by cancer

have been visualized with ^{123}I-labeled anti-B-cell lymphoma and anti-breast cancer antibodies, respectively. Melanoma has been visualized with either anti-p97 or anti-HMW antibodies labeled with [111]In. Prostate cancer has been visualized with prostate-specific antibodies. All these antibodies were produced by mouse clones. However, we have recently imaged breast cancer strikingly well with an ^{111}In-labeled antibody produced from the fusion of human lymphocytes (Fig. 1). This experience is even more unique because this human antibody is of the IgM type, which has been presumed to be unsuitable for clinical application. These studies with IgM human monoclonal antibodies have raised many questions, but do point to one of the many options for eliminating foreign protein reactions (HAMA) and nonspecific receptor uptake of antibody.

Unfortunately, the obstacles to successful treatment of a patient with cancer are more formidable. Only a small fraction of the cardiac output is delivered to the tumor because the tumor is a relatively smaller fraction of the body weight of a patient when compared with a mouse. Mouse monoclonal antibody is a foreign protein for the patient. While monoclonal antibodies have been tolerated remarkably well by patients, they are treated differently than the patients' immunoglobulins. Small amounts of mouse immunoglobulin are cleared from the blood very rapidly by receptor sites, requiring administration of larger amounts of antibody in order to enhance accumulation in the tumor [28]. Many other choices, such as choices of antigen-antibody system, choices of radionuclides, of amounts, of timing, and so forth, must be made.

Radionuclide Selection

The work of Adelstein [29] has shown the lethality of Auger and low-energy electrons on microorganisms and mammalian cells. Of course, α-emitters give off high linear energy transfer (LET) particles. We have examined the micro-dosimetry of [211]At and several low-energy Auger-electron-emitting radio-nuclides [12]. One of the more attractive of these is [197]Hg. The path length of ionization from this class of emitters is suitable for therapy where circum-stances permit uniform or relatively uniform targeting of all the cancer cells. Emissions of short range are desirable when the antigen and thus the antibody are uniformly distributed throughout the cancer, because short-range emissions reduce the radiation dose to surrounding tissue and have the potential for en-hanced relative biological effectiveness. Possible examples include circulating cancer cells, small metastases, postoperative prevention of metastases, and selective irradiation of diffuse, infiltrating cancer cells in the marrow. These agents may permit sparing of the marrow in the latter circumstance.

Beta particles are less densely ionizing and thus deposit energy over more cell diameters. Even so, they too may be effective tumorcidal agents as they im-part more uniform irradiation of the cells in solid tumors.

The optimum radionuclide to deliver radioimmunotherapy should have a physical half-life consistent with the residence time of the monoclonal anti-bodies or their fragments on the tumor cell. Iodine-131 has a rather long physi-cal half-time for radioimmunotherapy. Thus, there is need for radionuclide op-tions within these physical parameters and for the evaluation of detailed micro-dosimetry. We believe [67]Cu is an attractive candidate because of its physical half-life, beta energy, and gamma emission suitable for tracing distribution of the dose in vivo. [123]I and ^{131}I represent a tracer-treatment radionuclide combi-nation suitable for tracing the distribution of the radiation from the treatment dose (Table 4). [111]In and ^{90}Y have been proposed as a similar tracer-treatment combination. Like [67]Cu, ^{90}Y, a pure beta emitter, theoretically has better properties for therapy than [131]I. The lack of gamma radiation associated with disintegration of ^{90}Y reduces the "innocent bystander" exposure to radiation-sensitive organs such as marrow.

Table 4. Radionuclides for radioimmunotherapy

Nuclide	T-1/2 (h)	Electron energies (%)	Primary gamma energies (%)
[67]Cu	62	577 keV (20) 484 keV (35) 395 keV (45)	184 keV (47)
[90]Y	64	2.29 meV (100)	none
[197]Hg	64	64 keV (71) 52 keV (5) 7 keV (50)	77 keV (97)
[186]Re	90	1.07 meV (77) 0.93 meV (23)	137 keV (9)
[131]I	193	807 keV (1) 606 keV (86) 336 keV (13)	364 keV (81)

Treatment Planner

The athymic mouse tumor model is not a satisfactory source of information upon which to make the choices required for optimal radioimmunotherapy. These decisions need to be made from studies in patients of a type comparable to the biodistribution studies which are obtained in animal tumor models. Fortunately, tracer techniques can now be implemented by advanced equipment for quantitative radionuclide imaging and strengthened by dynamic modeling of the physiological parameters which govern radionuclide distribution, and hence radiation dose distribution [5].

We have pursued an ultimate goal of development of a treatment planner based upon radiation absorbed dose distribution [5] as a basis for not only making the choices defined earlier, but also the following decisions: (1) whether to treat the patient or not; (2) how to treat the patient; and (3) comparison of results of treatment with radiation absorbed dose distribution. The success or failure of radiation therapy can depend upon the accuracy with which a dose prescription is fulfilled. The establishment of tumor-cure probabilities, optimized time-dose schedules, and radiobiological efficiencies requires that the systematic uncertainties in dosimetry be made as small as possible. The mainstay of therapy decision should be quantitative radionuclide tracer studies performed on the individual patient before therapy and with each therapy dose. The general approach to radioimmunotherapy that we propose is applicable to various radionuclides or combination of radionuclides for which the signal source and the ionization source (e.g., ^{67}Cu or the combination of ^{123}I with ^{131}I or ^{111}In with ^{90}Y) are documented to have identical biologic behavior.

Single photon emission computed tomography represents a powerful technological advance in quantitative clinical radionuclide studies. It eliminates most of the cross-contamination from one source to another in imaging the body. The validity of this technique has been documented in phantom simulations. Some of the difficulties of determining absolute radionuclide uptake in patients remain to be resolved. An accurate boundary for each transverse section is important for areas of the body where an ellipse is a poor approximation for shape. Transmission methods can define organs, while in general other methods define only the body boundary. This may prove especially important in the transitional zones between chest and abdomen, or through the heart. The accuracy of attenuation correction, by any method, depends upon knowledge of the tissue composition in each transverse section. The use of mean linear attenuation coefficient values corresponding to identifiable areas of different tissue type in a section, such as bone, muscle, and lung, as suggested by Gullberg [30], may prove to be an adequate solution, but requires further investigation. The use of an average linear attenuation coefficient is not sufficiently accurate. The choice of attenuation correction method is not clear.

It is relatively straightforward to determine volumes of radioactively labeled tissue down to about 10 cm³ using commercially available emission computed tomographic systems. The lower limits of accuracy of determination of volume are related to the inherent spatial resolution of the detection system, and, unfortunately, impose a limitation on the definition of small metastases. In such cir-

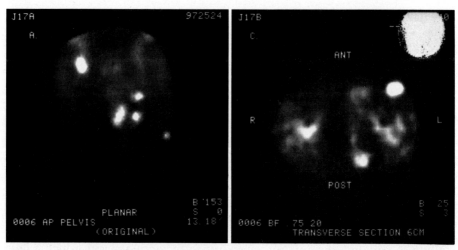

Fig. 2. Planar (*left*) and SPECT tomographic (*right*) images of lower pelvis and upper legs of male with metastases from melanoma were obtained 24 h after administration of ^{111}In-HMW melanoma monoclonal antibody. Radioactivity in melanoma exceeds that in the marrow

cumstances, the concentration of radioactivity cannot be obtained, and therefore absorbed radiation doses can only be approximated by assuming a volume which conforms to known anatomic structures. Fortunately, most structures of these small dimensions tend to be spheroidal or ellipsoidal in configuration.

Planar imaging techniques for in vivo quantitation are simpler and more straightforward [31]. They are satisfactory for many circumstances (Fig. 2), but cannot entirely avoid the problem of superimposition of tissues which accumulate radioactivity. The problem of defining a suitable body background is unmanageable except when background is a relatively insignificant fraction of target radioactivity.

Kinetic modeling is not essential to the estimation of absorbed radiation doses by the proposed methods. However, it should improve the accuracy of these estimates by better interpolation between the serial computed tomographic studies.

Other Routes of Administration

If the antibody is administered into a restricted space, such as a pleural, pericardial, or peritoneal cavity, it is possible to achieve higher uptake by the tumor target and lower uptake by normal organs, and in particular, the organs, such as liver, lymphatics, and blood, that are involved in immunoglobulin catabolism. Mouse monoclonal antibody HMFG2, an IgGl [32], detects a differentiation antigen expressed by carcinoma as well as by some normal epithelia. It is not tumor specific but it is epithelium specific. A tumor-associated monoclonal antibody was given intrapleurally to a patient with malignant pleural effusion, intrapericardially to a patient with pericardial effusion and a tumor mass invading the pericardium, and intraperitoneally to a patient with stage III ovarian carcinoma resistant to chemotherapy [32]. The dose of radiation delivered was 500–700 rads to the malignant sites, 2–20 rads to normal organs, and 1–2.5 rads to whole body. Cytological examination after antibody-guided therapy showed no neoplastic cells in the residual fluid from the patients. In one patient, computerized tomography of the pericardium showed that the tumor had diminished and the pericardial effusion had resolved. No side effects were observed or reported by the patients. There were no hematological, biochemical, or other signs of toxicity.

This work is not only important because of the frequency and troublesomeness of malignant fluid accumulations, but also because it points the way toward methods for reducing the obstacles to selective delivery of the radiolabeled antibodies to their target. We believe problems in delivery of the radiolabeled antibody to the antigenic targets on the cancer cell will prove to be the major factor limiting radioimmunotherapy [3]. Therefore, all creative approaches to selective delivery of the antibodies to their targets are worthy of exploration. Several other methods have been considered or explored and include delivery via the lymphatics or use of antibodies to deliver boron-10 to tumor cells [33]. The combination of thermal neutrons with ^{10}B produces a fission reaction yielding locally destructive ionizing alpha particles.

Summary

Tumor targeting radiolabeled antibodies are capable of achieving experimental and clinical results. The concern that foreign immunoglobulin would not be tolerated or that other complications would be excessive have proved unfounded. The results from treatment of patients with cancer have been modest but encouraging. New areas of research require technical advancement to allow further development of this potential modality for cancer therapy. Many of the major restrictions have been overcome, but improvements can be anticipated for many years. Monoclonal antibodies from human clones, better radionuclides, and radiochemistry, and methods for preventing nonspecific receptor uptake are but a few of a great many avenues for improving the results of therapy. Careful quantitative evaluation will allow integration of these new agents and methods into the management of patients with cancer. Our goal is a comprehensive treatment planning system for clinical cancer therapy with radiolabeled monoclonal antibodies against cancer-associated antigens. We expect the system to provide estimates of the radiation dose distributions associated with various choices of radionuclide and targeting molecule. These approaches are now possible because of technological advances in quantitative radionuclide imaging.

References

1. Bale WF, Spar IL, Goodland RL (1960) Experimental radiation therapy of tumors with ^{131}I-carrying antibodies to fibrin. Cancer Res 20:1488–1494

2. Spar IL, Bale WF, Marrack D, Dewey WC, McCardle RJ, Harper PV (1967) ^{131}I-labeled antibodies to human fibrinogen: diagnostic studies and therapeutic trials. Cancer 20:865−870

3. DeNardo GL, DeNardo SJ (1983) Perspectives on the future of radioimmunodiagnosis and radioimmunotherapy of cancer. In: Burchiel SW, Rhodes BA (eds) Radio-immunoimaging and radioimmunotherapy. Elsevier, New York, pp 41−60

4. Brady LW, Order SE, Leigel SA, Markoe AM (1984) Radionuclides for systemic on-cotherapy. Cancer Treat Symp 1:127−134

5. DeNardo GL, Raventos A, Hines HH, Scheibe PO, Macey DJ, Hays MT, DeNardo SJ (1985) Requirements for a treatment planning system for radioimmunotherapy. Int J Radiat Oncol Biol Phys 11:335−348

6. Leichner PK, Klein JL, Garrison JB, Jenkins RE, Nickoloff EL, Ettinger DS, Order SE (1981) Dosimetry of ^{131}I-labeled antiferritin in hepatoma: A model for radio-immunoglobulin dosimetry. Int J Rad Oncol Biol Phys 7:323−333

7. Carrasquillo JA, Krohn KA, Beaumier P, McGuffin RW, Brown JP, Hellstrom KE, Hell-strom I, Larson SM (1984) Diagnosis of and therapy for solid tumors with radiolabeled antibodies and immune fragments. Cancer Treat Rep 68:317−328

8. Order SE (1982) Monoclonal antibodies: potential role in radiation therapy and oncology. Int J Rad Oncol Biol Phys 8:1193−1201

9. Boone CW, Brandchaft PR, Irving DN, Gilden R (1972) Quantitative studies on the bind-ing of syngeneic antibody to the surface antigens of AKR virus-induced rat lymphoma cells. Int J Cancer 9:685−692

10. McGaughey C (1974) Feasibility of tumor immunoradiotherapy using radioiodinated antibodies to tumor-specific cell membrane antigens with emphasis on leukemias and ear-ly metastases. Oncology 29:302−319

11. Wessels BW, Rogus RD (1984) Radionuclide selection and model absorbed dose calcu-lations for radiolabeled tumor associated antibodies. Med Phys 11:638−645

12. DeNardo SJ, Jungerman JA, DeNardo GL, Lagunas-Solar MC, Cole WC, Meares CF (1984) The choice of radionuclides for radioimmunotherapy. In: The developing role of short-lived radionuclides in nuclear medicine practice. Oak Ridge, Tennessee, De-partment of Energy Technical Information Center, CONF-82-523, NTIS, pp 396−409

13. Rostock RA, Klein JL, Kopher KA, Order SE (1984) Variables affecting the tumor locali-zation of ^{131}I-antiferritin in experimental hepatoma. Am J Clin Oncol (CCT) 6:9−18

14. Rostock RA, Klein JL, Leichner P, Kopher KA, Order SE (1983) Selective tumor locali-zation in experimental hepatoma by radiolabeled antiferritin antibody. Int J Radiat Oncol Biol Phys 9:1345−1350

15. Noltenius HW (1981) Fc and complement receptors on malignant tumor cells. Cancer 48:1761−1767

16. Leichner PK, Koein JL, Siegelman SS, Ettinger DS, Order SE (1983) Dosimetry of ^{131}I-labeled antiferritin in hepatoma: specific activities in the tumor and liver. Cancer Treat Rep 67:647−658

17. Larson SM, Carrasquillo JA, Krohn KA et al. (1983) Localization of ^{131}I-labeled p97-spe-cific Fab fragments in human melanoma as a basis for radiotherapy. J Clin Invest 72:2101−2114

18. Brown JP, Nishiyamau K, Hellstrom I et al. (1981) Structural characterization of human melanoma-associated antigen p97 using monoclonal antibodies. J Immunol 127:539−546

19. Brown JP, Hemwick RM, Hellstrom I et al. (1982) Human melanoma-associated antigen is structurally and functionally related to transferrin. Nature 296:171−173

20. Hellstrom I, Garrigues J, Cabasco L et al. (1983) Studies of a high molecular weight hu-man melanoma-associated antigen. J Immunol 130:1467−1472

21. DeNardo SJ, Erickson KL, Benjamini E (1980) Use of I-131 antibodies for radiation ther-apy. Clin Nucl Med 5:9 S

22. DeNardo SJ, Erickson KL, Benjamini E, Hines H, Scibeinski R (1981) Radio-immunotherapy for melanoma. Clin Res 29

23. DeNardo SJ, Erickson K, Benjamini E, Hines H, Scibienski R, DeNardo G (1982) Mono-clonal antibodies for radiation therapy of melanoma. In: Raynaud C (ed) Nuclear medi-cine and biology. Pergamon, Paris, pp 182−185

24. DeNardo SJ, Hines HH, Erickson KL, DeNardo GL (1983) Evaluation of radiolabeled monoclonal antibody parameters necessary for cancer immunotherapy. In: Chabner BA (ed) Rational basis for chemotherapy. Liss, New York, pp 379–387
25. Adams DA, DeNardo GL, DeNardo SJ (1984) In vivo monitoring of RIT in lymphoma by quantitation of phosphate metabolites with P-31 NMR. Clin Nucl Med 9(9S):P33
26. Epstein AL, Zimmer AM, Spies SM, Mills SL, DeNardo GL, DeNardo SJ (1984) Radio-immunodetection of human B-cell lymphomas with a radiolabeled tumor-specific monoclonal antibody (Lym-1). Proceedings of the 2nd International conference on malignant lymphoma. Nijhoff, Boston
27. Cole W, DeNardo SJ, Meares C, DeNardo G, O'Brien H (1983) Development of copper-67 chelate conjugated monoclonal antibodies for radioimmunotherapy. J Nucl Med 24(5):P30
28. DeNardo GL, DeNardo SJ, Peng J-S, O'Grady LF, Cardiff RD, Mills SL (1984) Effects of protein mass on the pharmacokinetics of monoclonal antibodies. Clin Nucl Med 9(9S):P37
29. Kassis AI, Adelstein SJ, Haydock C, Sastry KSR, McElvany KD, Welch MJ (1982) Lethality of auger electrons from the decay of bromine-77 in the DNA of mammalian cells. Radiat Res 90:362–373
30. Gullberg GT (1979) The attenuated Radon transfer: theory and application in medicine and biology. Ph. D. Thesis, University of California, Berkeley, LBL 7486
31. Macey DJ, Marshall R (1982) Absolute quantiation of radiotracer uptake in the lungs using a gamma camera. J Nucl Med 23:731–734
32. Epenetos AA (1984) Antibody-guided irradiation of malignant lesions: three cases illustrating a method of treatment. Lancet: 1441–1443
33. Barth RF, Johnson CW, Wei W-Z, Carey WE, Soloway AH, McGuire J (1982) Neutron capture using boronated monoclonal antibody directed against tumor-associated antigens. Cancer Detect Prev 5:315–323

Treatment of Pleural and Peritoneal Carcinosis with Radioactive Colloids

G. Riccabona[1]

The concept of treating effusions due to pleura or peritoneal carcinosis with radioactive colloids was introduced 40 years ago [2]. For this purpose, ^{63}Zn sulfide and later on ^{198}Au colloid have been used [2, 3]. Both cases involved the application of beta and gamma emitters, where the beta emission was almost exclusively responsible for the therapeutic effect. As the gamma radiation necessitated inconvenient precautions for radiation protection [1], radioactive colloids with pure beta emission have been developed since 1954 for intracavitary radionuclide therapy [4 – 7]. This concerned primarily ^{32}P chromium phosphate and ^{90}Y silicate; ^{169}Er citrate and ^{186}Re sulfate were also recommended. Whereas the two latter compounds were not applied on a large scale, the ^{90}Y colloid has for almost 30 years proved to be the most suitable substance for the treatment of malignant effusions in pleura and peritoneum.

In 1955 Weisberger et al. [8] introduced the intracavitary application of cytostatic drugs, which also proved to be very effective. In view of the lack of any radiation risk, they were frequently regarded as preferable. Both the application of radioactive colloids and that of cytostatic drugs represent a merely palliative treatment. However, over a long period this sometimes leads to the elimination of the uncomfortable and, because of the protein loss, weakening effusion, which is a considerable help for the patient.

On the basis of the now extensive experience, it can be ascertained that the radionuclide treatment is still indicated under certain conditions and retains its fixed place in the treatment of malignant effusions.

The dosage of ^{90}Y citrate is 100 – 120 mCi for the pleural cavity or the peritoneal cavity. The colloid is instilled in 250 ml saline after removal of the effusion. In the 1st h after application, the patient has to change position in order to guarantee sufficient distribution of the radioactive substance. The colloid is taken up in the cells of the pleura or the peritoneum by phagocytosis. The radioactivity appears in amounts of less than 10% in the circulation. The selective radiation effect on the tissues which produce the effusion significantly inhibits the production of fluid in the treated cavities.

The prerequisite for carrying out the radionuclide therapy is that malignant cells have been detected in the fluid, that the necessary interval for the removal of the fluid is less than 10 days, and that a life expectation of more than 4 weeks can be assumed. The radionuclide treatment is not indicated when effusions are encapsulated, or when the white cell count is less than 3000. To settle the ques-

---

1 Universitätsklinik für Nuklearmedizin, Anichstraße 35, A-6020 Innsbruck

Nuclear Medicine in Clinical Oncology
Ed. by C. Winkler
© Springer-Verlag Berlin Heidelberg 1986

Table 1. Results of intracavitary therapy of pleural and peritoneal carcinosis in comparison with other intracavitary therapy programs

	Source	n	Side effects (%)	Method	Objectively positive results (%)	Duration of remission ($\bar{x}$)
Intracavitary cytostatic drugs	Fracchia et al.	138	43 (3.6)[a]	Cycloph. thiotepa	27.5	8.8
	Weisberger et al.	88	?	Cycloph.	63.5	?
	Mark et al.	32	47 (6.2)[a]	Mechlorethamine	?	?
	Anderson et al.	60	50 (13.2)[a]	Cycloph.	47.0	3 m
	Anderson, Brincker	86	41	Thiotepa	37.0	?
Intracavitary tetracycline	Zaloznik et al. [9]	30	7.7	Tetracycline + chest tube	69.0	4.9 m
Intracavitary radioactive colloids	Emrich	131	5	^{198}Au coll. ^{32}P Cr phosph.	38.8	?
	Scheer et al.	239	?	198 Au coll.	46.9	?
	Own material	62	8.1	^{90}Y coll. (^{198}Au coll.)	68.5	4.5 m

[a] Severe side effects due to serious bone marrow damage

tion whether there is an encapsulated effusion, a test dose of ^{198}Au colloid or ^{99m}Tc colloid can be applied in order to check the distribution of the substance. For this purpose the scatter radiation of ^{90}Y can also be used.

Some groups consider the radionuclide therapy to be indicated only if a previous cytostatic treatment has been unsuccessful. Opinions differ on this subject. The cytostatic treatment is in the first place cheaper than intracavitary radionuclide therapy; however, through the application of cytostatics side effects can occur in the form of extensive lesions of the bone marrow. These can cause relatively high additional costs. Side effects are at least 5 times as rare in the case of radionuclide treatment (Table 1).

A certain problem sometimes arises during the nuclear medical treatment, namely, the necessity to remove an effusion which reappears relatively quickly following the instillation of the radioactive material. This has been observed more frequently after the application of ^{32}P chromium phosphate than in the case of ^{90}Y silicate. If an early removal of the radioactive contamination effusion must be carried out, the usual prerequisites of radiation protection must be carefully observed.

To summarize and in conclusion: It can be stated that the application of ^{90}Y colloid for the treatment of malignant effusions in the pleura and peritoneal cavities still represents today an important possibility for the palliative treatment.

As a precondition, the indication must be thoroughly examined; furthermore, it is necessary to check the regular distribution of the radioactive substance in the cavity. The mean interval of necessary evacuations of effusions can be extended to 10 weeks or more regardless of the general tumor progression. Serious side effects as have been observed in the use of intracavitary chemotherapy practicly never occur, and radiation necroses can always be avoided by correct and orderly application of the method.

References

1. Becker J, Scheer KE (1961) Die lokalisierte Applikation künstlich radioaktiver Isotope. In: Höfer K (ed) Künstliche radioaktive Isotope in Physiologie, Diagnostik und Therapie, vol 2. Springer, Berlin Göttingen Heidelberg, p 702
2. Müller JH (1945) Über die Verwendung von künstlich radioaktiven Isotopen zur Erzielung von lokalisierten biologischen Strahlenwirkungen. Experientia 1:199
3. Müller JH (1961) Interne Tumortherapie mit künstlich radioaktiven Isotopen. In: Künstliche radioaktive Isotope in Physiologie, Diagnostik und Therapie, vol 2. Springer, Berlin Göttingen Heidelberg, p 785
4. Riccabona G (1978) Intracavitäre Isotopentherapie, klinische Bedeutung in Diagnostik und Therapie. Nuc Med, p 698
5. Riccabona G (1983) Therapy with radionuclides − Actual state of the art. In: Nuclearmedicine, imaging of metabolism and organ function. Schattauer, Stuttgart, p 910
6. Root SW, Taylor MP, Andrews GA, Knisely RM (1954) Distribution of colloidal radioactive chromic phosphate after intracavitary administration. Radiology 63:251
7. Siegel EP, Hart HE, Brothers M, Spencer H, Laszlo D (1956) Radio-yttrium (^{90}Y) for the palliative treatment of effusions due to malignancy. JAMA 161:499
8. Weisberger AS, Levine B, Storaasli JP (1955) Use of nitrogen mustard in treatment of serous effusions of neoplastic origin. JAMA 159:1704
9. Zaloznik AJ, Oswald SG, Langin M (1983) Intrapleural tetracycline in malignant pleural effusions, a randomized study. Cancer 51:752−755

Treatment of Hepatic Malignancies by Intravascular Administration of Radioisotopes

R. V. P. Mantravadi[1], D. G. Spigos, E. D. Grady, W. S. Tan, S. G. Karesh, and V. Capek

Introduction

The blood supply to hepatic metastases varies depending on their stage of development. Established tumors derive their blood supply almost exclusively from hepatic arteries, whereas microscopic tumor deposits are nourished by the portal venous blood [1 – 3]. Treatment of liver metastasis with a hepatic arterial infusion of chemotherapeutic agents [4, 5] and radioisotopes [6 – 8] and with hepatic artery ligation [9] is based on their vascularity. Clinical trials testing the effectiveness of these treatment methods are currently in progress.

While the efforts continue in the treatment of documented hepatic metastases, attention is also directed towards the prevention of the development of micrometastatic disease in the liver in locally advanced colon cancer patients undergoing curative resection [7, 10 – 12]. Taylor et al. [12] employed continuous portal vein infusion with 5-fluorouracil during the first 7 days after surgery. They reported a decreased incidence of liver metastasis in 1 of 24 treated patients as compared with 6 of 26 patients in the control group. Grady administered ^{32}P chromic phosphate via both superior mesenteric and celiac arteries in similar patients with encouraging results [7].

This paper reports the results in 12 patients with established liver metastasis treated with intra-arterial injection of Yttrium-90 (^{90}Y) microspheres. We also report on the results of a pilot study on 31 patients treated with ^{32}P injected via the superior mesenteric artery in an attempt to prevent the development of liver metastasis following enbloc resection of colon cancer.

Materials and Methods

Intra-arterial ^{90}Y Therapy

Between December 1979 and December 1981, fifteen patients with documented liver metastases were submitted to ^{90}Y therapy. The primary tumor was located in the colon in six patients, stomach in three, lung in four, pancreas in one, and liver (hepatoma) in one. All patients received a variety of chemotherapeutic agents prior to ^{90}Y therapy.

---

1 Radiation Oncology Associates, P.C., 2200 Lake Avenue, Suite 230, Fort Wayne, IN 46805, USA

Nuclear Medicine in Clinical Oncology
Ed. by C. Winkler
© Springer-Verlag Berlin Heidelberg 1986

The isotope was made available by the Medical Research Foundation in Atlanta, Georgia, U.S.A., in the form of a sterile suspension of resin microspheres of 15 ± 5 microns diameter. It is a pure beta emitter with a half-life of 64.2 h and mean energy of 0.93 MeV.

At the outset, the weight of the liver in grams was determined by the body weight and/or body surface area as suggested by DeLand et al. [13]. Corrections to the liver weight were made depending on the extent of liver enlargement. Assuming uniform distribution of the isotope in the liver, the absorbed dose for each gram of liver tissue was calculated to be 182 rads per microcurie. The ^{90}Y activity required to deliver a 5000 rad does to the liver was estimated as follows:

$$\text{Isotope dose } (\mu\text{Ci}) = \frac{5000 \text{ rad} \times \text{liver weight (g)}}{182}$$

The arterial supply of the liver was catheterized percutaneously via transfemoral route in 12 of 15 patients. Selective catheterization of hepatic arteries was unsuccessful in 3 patients due to anatomical variations, tumor encircling the arteries, and tortuosity of the vessels. After confirming the satisfactory placement of the catheter tip in the hepatic artery, the isotope suspension in a shielded syringe was slowly injected via the catheter. The microspheres travel along the hepatic arterial blood and terminate in the end capillaries due to the difference in the size of microspheres and capillaries.

^{32}P Injection Via Superior Messenteric Artery

A total 31 patients who underwent complete resection of the primary tumor and regional lymph nodes were treated with ^{32}P injected via the superior mesenteric artery. Patient distribution according to the primary tumor location is shown in Table 1. The age range was between 32 and 64 years. Staging was done according to Astler-Coller modification of the Dukes System [14]. The extent of the tumor was determined to be B_2 (tumor extending through the entire bowel wall, including serosa; nodes negative) in 4 patients, C_1 (tumor limited to the bowel wall; nodes positive) in 12, and C_2 (tumor extending through the serosa; nodes

Table 1. Adjuvant ^{32}P therapy for colon cancer

Location	No. of patients
Cecum	5
Ascending Colon	4
Descending Colon	3
Sigmoid	8
Rectosigmoid	6
Rectum	5
Total	31

positive) in 11. In 4 patients isolated metastatic nodules found at the time of the laparotomy were completely resected. Postoperative isotope liver-spleen scan and computed tomography of the liver revealed the liver to be free of any metastatic disease in these patients.

The dosimetry was based on the liver weight calculated by the body surface area of each patient using the formula of DeLand and North [13].

$$\text{Liver weight (kg)} = 1.02 \times \text{body surface area (m}^2) - 0.22$$

The absorbed dose from uniformly distributed ^{32}P to each gram of liver tissue was calculated to be 730 rad per microcurie according to the standard beta dosimetry formula. Radiation dose of 4500 rad was prescribed and the activity needed to deliver this dose was calculated as follows:

$$^{32}\text{P activity (}\mu\text{Ci)} = \frac{\text{liver weight in grams} \times 4500 \text{ rad}}{730}$$

The superior mesenteric artery was catheterized via percutaneous transfemoral route. The calculated ^{32}P dose was withdrawn into a plastic syringe and diluted with normal saline to a total volume of 10 cc. The isotope was then slowly injected via the selectively placed catheter into the superior mesenteric artery. The injected isotope mixed with arterial blood rapidly passed through the wall of the small bowel in approximately 70 s into the superior mesenteric vein and then into the portal vein. Once the colloidal isotope reached the liver it was rapidly phagocytized by the kupffer cells and was localized to the liver. Less than 2% of the isotope escaped the liver into the systemic circulation after first pass through the liver as was reported previously [10]. Bremmsstrahlung scans were utilized initially to assess the isotope distribution. Currently, 0.5 mCi ^{99m}Tc sulfur colloid is added to ^{32}P for satisfactory imaging. Postoperative external radiotherapy to a dose of 4500–5500 rad over 5–6 weeks was given to operative bed in 24 patients with primary tumors in cecum, sigmoid, rectosigmoid, and rectum.

All patients are followed at two monthly intervals for 6 months, and at three monthly intervals subsequently with physical examination, complete blood counts, liver enzyme levels, blood coagulation profile, serum proteins, and carcinoembryonic antigen values. The follow-up in our patients ranged between 6 and 48 months, with a median of 24 months.

Results

^{90}Y Therapy

Eight of 12 treated patients died within 6 months due to progressive metastatic disease in the liver. Three patients died with tumor progression at 9, 10, and 13 months after treatment. One patient with extensive hepatoma is alive and ambulatory to date 5 years after treatment. Symptomatic hepatomegaly was present in only 1 of 12 patients and she experienced pain relief within 72 h of

[90]Y therapy. Five of 12 patients had elevated liver enzymes prior to therapy, and these values remained unchanged in two and worsened in the remainder. Follow-up liver scans were obtained in nine patients who survived longer than 3 months. Greater than 50% regression in the size of metastases was noted in three patients (33%) and near complete resolution of radiographically visible tumor in two patients (18%). Thus the overall response rate was 51%. In two patients with dual arterial supply, metastases remained stable in the treated region of the liver, whereas disease progression was evident in the untreated lobe of the liver.

There was no gastrointestinal toxicity or radiation hepatitis in any of the treated patients. With the exception of one patient, no hematopoietic suppression was noted in the treated patients. In this patient death occurred due to pancytopenia from bone marrow damage secondary to leaching of ^{90}Y from the microspheres. This resulted in termination of ^{90}Y microspheres production in December 1981 and is expected to resume soon.

[32]P Chromic Phosphate Therapy

Twenty-six of 31 patients treated with [32]P (or 84%) are alive to date without any evidence of tumor recurrence in the liver or at other sites. Two patients died of pelvic recurrence without liver metastases. Hepatic metastasis developed in three patients, and two of these had stage C_2 tumor. The third patient had isolated liver metastases resected initially.

Asymptomatic scattered fatty changes documented by needle biopsy were noted in two patients (6%). Radiation hepatitis was not noted in any of the treated patients. In one patient there was an elevation of serum bilirubin to 4.1 mg/dl 2 months after therapy which gradually returned to normal in 2 years. This patient is alive to date 4 years after therapy.

Table 2 shows the results of liver function tests during patient follow-up. Uncomplicated elevation of one or more liver enzymes was noted at 3 to 6 months in 11 patients (28%). The elevated levels did not exceed 50% of the normal range and returned to normal within 8 months. Elevation of SGOT levels was seen in all patients with abnormal liver enzymes.

Table 2. Liver function tests

Test	Frequency of abnormal results	
	n	%
One or more	11/31	28
LDH	1/31	3
SGOT	11/31	28
SGPT	6/31	19
Alk. phos.	7/31	22
Bilirubin	1/31	3

White blood cell count dropped to $2800-3200$ per mm^3 in four patients (13%) and in one patient (3%) platelet count fell to $85,000/mm^3$. Hematopoietic recovery was complete and spontaneous within 2 months. Acute or delayed gastrointestinal toxicity was not seen. However, temporary loss of appetite was observed in three patients.

Discussion

Results with hepatic arterial administration of ^{90}Y microspheres in this study are considered encouraging, since four of 12 treated patients survived longer than 12 months, with one 5-year survivor. The overall response rate was 51% as compared with 68% objective response rate in 25 patients reported by Grady [7]. Ariel reported 40% objective response and 60% subjective response in 40 patients treated with combined ^{90}Y and 5-fluoroacil [8]. The average duration of life in asymptomatic patients with liver metastases from colon cancers was 26 months and 12 months in symptomatic patients. Toxicity was acceptable in all these studies.

Blanchard et al. [2] demonstrated preferential localization of the microspheres by as much as 4 times that of normal hepatic parenchyma. Use of vasoconstrictors may further improve localization of the ^{90}Y microspheres in the tumors and spare the healthy liver tissue [15]. Our data also indicate that patients with well-vascularized metastases benefit most, as all the long-term survivors had such lesions. Because of sparing of hematopoietic tissues, ^{90}Y therapy would not contraindicate use of systemic chemotherapy.

The limitation of the use of intra-arterial ^{90}Y therapy is that vascular anomalies of hepatic arterial system may preclude catheterization of all of the arterial supply for microsphere infusion. Secondly, as the center of metastatic tumors exhibits decreasing blood flow with increasing tumor size, a tumoricidal radiation dosage may not be delivered leaving tumor cells viable in the core of the metastasis.

It is estimated that liver metastasis as the only site of surgical treatment of failure occurs in $25\%-30\%$ of patients with stage C_1 or C_2 colon carcinomas [16]. Thus, eradication of micrometastases in the liver following curative resections may improve survival. Furthermore, micrometastases are well oxygenated and are more radiosensitive. Thus far, attempts at preventing the development of hepatic metastases with adjuvant chemotherapy have been unsuccessful. Recently, the Gastrointestinal Tumor Study Group [17] reported disappointing results in 621 patients with colon cancer treated with adjuvant chemotherapy following curative surgical resection. They discouraged the use of fluorouracil alone or in combination with semustine for patients who have undergone curative surgical resection for colon carcinoma.

Animal studies [18, 19] have demonstrated that prophylactic radiation to the liver can significantly decrease the development of liver metastases in treated animals as compared with controls. Radiation dosages of 3000 to 5000 rads were utilized in these studies. It appears from our data that a 4500 rad dose with beta radiation can be given to the human liver without undue morbidity. With this prescribed dose the cumulative dose to the liver during the first two effective half-lives of ^{32}P (28.6 days) would be 3375 rad, which equals the suggested radiation tolerance dose to the liver with fractionated external radiation therapy [20]. However, long term effects of low-dose-rate continuous irradiation of liver with ^{32}P to 3375 rad in 28.6 days has yet to be established.

The advantages of ^{32}P injection via superior mesenteric artery are that 1) origin of the superior mesenteric artery is constant, and catheterization is relatively easy, 2) there is near complete localization of the isotope to the liver and 3) the isotope reaches the liver in the same pathway as colon carcinoma cells take to reach the liver via the mesenteric and portal veins from the colon cancers.

Though the long-term follow-up data are awaited, the results from the pilot study of 31 patients are optimistic. Only 10% of our patients have developed liver metastases, and more importantly, only 1 of 4 patients with initial liver metastases which were resected developed hepatic metastasis subsequently. The ability to localize the isotope into the liver with our technique, the lack of acute toxicity, and thus far absence of radiation hepatitis suggest that this treatment should be further investigated in randomized clinical trials.

References

1. Ackerman NB, Lien WM, Kondi ES, Silverman NA (1969) The blood supply of experimental liver metastases. 1. The distribution of hepatic artery and portal vein blood to "small" and "large" tumors. Surgery 66:1067–1072
2. Blanchard RJ, Grotenhuis I, LaFave JW, Perry JF Jr (1965) Blood supply to hepatic V2 Carcinoma implants as measured by radioactive microspheres. Proc Soc Exp Biol Med 118:465–468
3. Shibata HR, MacLean LD (1966) Blood flow to tumors. Prog Clin Cancer 2:33–47
4. Ansfield FJ, Ramirez A, Davis HL et al. (1975) Further clinical studies with intrahepatic arterial infusion with 5-fluorouracil. Cancer 36:2413–2417
5. Grage TB, Vasilopoulos PP, Shingleton WW et al. (1979) Results of prospective randomized study of hepatic artery infusion with 5-fluorouracil versus intravenous 5-fluorouracil in patients with hepatic metastases from colon rectal cancer: a central oncology group study. Surgery 86:550–555
6. Mantravadi RVP, Spigos DG, Tan WS, Felix EL (1982) Intraarterial Yttrium-90 in the treatment of hepatic malignancy. Radiology 142:783–786
7. Grady ED (1979) Internal radiation therapy of hepatic cancer. Dis Colon Rectum 22:371–375
8. Ariel I (1978) Treatment of metastatic cancer to the liver from primary colon and rectal cancer by the intra-arterial administration of chemotherapy and radioactive isotopes. In: Spencer RP (ed) Therapy in nuclear medicine. Grune and Stratton, New York, pp 357–366
9. Petrelli NJ, Barcewicz PA, Evans JT et al. (1984) Hepatic artery ligation for liver metastasis in colorectal carcinoma. Cancer 53:1347–1353
10. Mantravadi RVP, Spigos DG, Karesh SM et al. (1983) Intra-arterial P-32 chromic phosphate for prevention of postoperative liver metastasis in high risk colorectal cancer patients. Radiology 148:555–559
11. Mantravadi RVP, Grady ED, Spigos DG et al. (1985) Prevention of liver metastasis with 32P chromic phosphate in completely resected colon cancers. Proc Am Soc Clin Oncol 4:81
12. Taylor I, Brooman P, Rowling JT (1977) Adjuvant liver perfusion in colorectal cancer: initial results of a clinical trial. Br Med J 2:1320–1322

13. DeLand FH, North WA (1968) Relationship between liver size and body. Radiology 91:1195–1198
14. Astler VP, Coller FA (1954) The prognostic significance of direct extension of carcinoma of the colon and rectum. Ann Surg 139:846–851
15. Grady ED, Auda SP, Cheek WV (1981) Vasoconstrictors to improve localization of radioactive microspheres in the treatment of liver cancer. J Med Assoc Georgia 70:791–795
16. Axtell LM, Asire AJ, Myers M (eds) (1976) Cancer patient survival report no. 5. A report from the cancer surveillance, epidermiology, and end results (SEER) program. DHEW Publ (NIH) 77-992 Washington D.C., US Government printing office
17. Gastrointestinal study group (1984) Adjuvant therapy of colon cancer—results of a prospectively randomized trial. N Engl J Med 310:737–743
18. Ackerman NB, McFee AS, Loken MK (1964) Prevention of liver metastasis by intravenous radioisotopes. JAMA 187:826–828
19. Alfonso AE, Hasson A, Gardner B et al. (1978) Prevention of hepatic metastases by intravenous radioactive gold. Cancer Res 38:2740–2744
20. Ingold JA, Reed GB, Kaplan HS, Bagshaw MA (1965) Radiation hepatitis. AJR 93:200–208

Treatment of Local Prostatic Cancer by [125]Iodine Seeds

J. J. BATTERMANN[1]

Introduction

For treatment of localized prostatic cancer with a curative intent three possibilities are available, viz. radical prostatectomy, external irradiation, and interstitial radiation therapy. Radical prostatectomy is a major operation with a relatively high complication rate (urinary dysfunction). In experienced hands, however, the complication rate can be reduced [1]. Still, impotency will occur in all patients. As many of the patients suitable for radical therapy are relatively young and still sexual active, this could be a major problem.

Over the past 20 years it became clear that external radiation therapy can be curative in the treatment of localized prostatic cancer. Although the adenocarcinomas are relatively radioresistant, with the modern megavoltage armamentarium a high dose can be delivered in the target area and serious reactions from bladder and intestine reduced [2]. Still, about 10% complications will occur and in approximately 20%−40% of cases, the patient will lose his sexual functions.

Interstitial radiation therapy for prostatic carcinoma is already an old technique and different radionuclides have been used. Table 1 illustrates the physical data of these nuclides. The implantation with ^{125}I seeds was introduced in 1970 by Hilaris and Whitmore. Due to the low energy of the X-rays (between

Table 1. Radionuclides for interstitial therapy

	Photon energy in MeV	Half-life
Gold-198	0.42	2.70 days
Radon-222	0.76	3.83
Iodine-125	0.027	60.2
Iridium-195	0.35	74.2
Tantalum-182	0.59	115.0
Caesium-137	0.66	30 years
Cobalt-60	1.25	5.26
Radium-226	0.78	1604

1 Antoni van Leeuwenhoekhuis, Het Nederlands Kankerinstituut, Plesmanlaan 121, NL-1066 CX Amsterdam

Nuclear Medicine in Clinical Oncology
Ed. by C. Winkler
© Springer-Verlag Berlin Heidelberg 1986

27 and 35 keV) a very high dose can be delivered to a relatively small volume, and thus radiation reactions from the bladder and intestine can be avoided to a large extent in contrast to most interstitial radiation therapy. The implantation with ^{125}I seeds is permanent and with a half-life of about 60 days, doses of 120–200 Gy are admitted to the prostate. With this technique the anatomical and functional integrity of the lower urinary tract is preserved as are the sexual functions.

As was mentioned, the longest experience is gathered in the Memorial Sloan Kettering Cancer Center in New York [3]. In this paper our preliminary results are described and discussed.

Material and Methods

Since the introduction of this implantation technique in 1981 in the Antoni van Leeuwenhoek Hospital in Amsterdam, 32 patients have undergone surgery so that iodine seeds could be implanted. The careful selection of patients includes the following criteria:

1. Age under 75 years and good general health.
2. Stage $T_1 - T_2$ prostate cancer as determined by rectal examination. The volume of the prostate should be between 20 and 40 g. Patients who have undergone transurethral resection (TUR) of the prostate are excluded from this technique because many seeds are likely to be lost due to insufficient prostate tissue.
3. High or medium degree of differentiation as assessed by histology and aspiration cytology.
4. No evidence of regional or distant metastases assessed by bone scan, PSAP, and lymphangiography. If suspect glands are found on the lymphangiograms, aspiration cytology is done, and if positive, external irradiation or hormonal treatment is proposed.

The treatment procedure is started with a limited regional lymphadenectomy for further staging of the tumor. Frozen section examination is not done as a routine. The node dissection is performed via a midline incision from the pubis to the umbilicus. The seminal ducts are transected near the inguinal canal, thereby facilitating the removal of the peritoneal envelope from the pelvic wall and iliac vessels. All fatty tissue containing lymph nodes is now removed from the triangle between the iliac vein, hypogastric artery, and pelvic wall upwards from the obturator canal. Dissection should be meticulous to prevent as much lymph and blood leakage as possible. After completion of the lymphadenectomy on both sides, the prostate is freed from the endopelvic fascia, so that it can be palpated completely. Now it is possible to establish the exact measurements of the prostate, and the number of seeds to be introduced can be calculated. Under guidance of a finger in the rectum, the radiotherapist now places hollow needles in the prostate. Typically, 8–10 needles are introduced, carefully distributed over the prostate. The ^{125}I seeds are introduced through the needles into the prostate. This can be done either with a system of plastic tubes in which the seeds are placed interspaced by pieces of catgut, as described by Hilaris, or by the use of the Mick applicator. For reasons of radiation safety, the later method is preferred. During the introduction of the seeds in the prostate, the radiotherapist keeps his finger in the rectum to make sure that the needle remains in position and the rectum wall is not perforated. Typically, 24–40 seeds are placed in the prostate. Occasionally, there is some bleeding from the prostate after removal of the needle. Such bleeding should be stopped immediately so that the seeds are not washed out. After careful inspection and hemostasis, the wound is closed, leaving a drain in Retzius' space. The whole operating theater, with special attention to cloths and suction fluids, is now measured with a Geiger counter to identify seeds that might have been lost. The patient is isolated, but no special radiation shielding is needed because the energy of the irradiation is very low. The urine of the patient is collected and measured for loss of seeds. The urine catheter is usually removed after 2–3 days and the drain after 4–5 days. If a patient loses one or more seeds, this usually occurs after removal of the catheter. Most patients can leave the hospital within a fortnight of the operation.

Results

Of 32 patients considered suitable for this treatment technique, 31 patients were implanted. In one patient very large nodes were found, and so the patient was not implanted, but treated with hormones. The nodes were found to be positive in another 4 patients at microscopic examination. In 3 of 5 patients with positive nodes, the findings on lymphangiograms also suggested positive nodes. No false-negative lymphograms were observed. In 27 patients, the follow-up is 6 months or longer and the results of these patients are further analyzed.

The age of the patients varied from 53 to 73 (mean 63.9) years.

The initial complaints of the patients were nonspecific in 14 patients, light voiding problems in 6, and moderate to severe in another 7. The PSAP (radioimmunoassay method) was normal in all but 6 patients. Positive nodes were found in one of these six. Two patients died postoperatively of thromboembolic complications in spite of routine use of minidoses heparine subcutaneously. In another two these complications were not fatal. Further complications were serious infections in 4, hematoma in 1, delayed wound healing in 1 and (temporary) lymphedema of the lower extremities in 3 patients. No late complications were observed, although in 4 patients resection of the bladder neck was necessary in the follow-up period because of persisting voiding problems.

The duration of hospitalization varied from 7 to 36 (mean 14.7) days from the day of operation. The number of seeds implanted varied from 24 to 40. In many patients some seeds were lost, but always during the hospitalization period. This number varied from 0 (12 patients) to 14 in one patient. This patient received additional external radiation as a substitute for the loss of seeds. No relation was found between the number of seeds lost and the local result of the treatment. During the follow-up period one more patient died of heart failure 30 months after the implantation. In 3 of 4 patients with positive nodes, bone metastases were found during the follow-up period (respectively after 20, 23 and 26 months). Two had also a local recurrence of their cancer, found after transurethral resection of the prostate. In one more patient recurrent tumor was found in the true pelvis after 19 months. So, a total of 3 patients had a proven local recurrence and 2 patients had distant metastases as well, while one patient had distant spread only.

Discussion

The preliminary results of our series of patients are hopeful and in agreement with the data from the group of Hilaris and Whitmore [4]. However, we have to realize that only a very small number of patients with prostatic cancer was selected for this treatment procedure. The majority of the patients present already with distant metastases and only about 5% of patients will meet the criteria for ^{125}I seeds implantation. As stated before, patients after TUR of the prostate have to be excluded from this technique.

It is also our experience that the number of complications is negligible. However, it is often difficult to assess the preservation of sexual functions. In our group of patients only two patients had complaints of their potency.

The regional node dissection was positive in only 5 of 32 patients (15.5%). Although this dissection is not curative, it is very predictive for the prognosis. As the implantation after the node dissection does not substantially contribute to the morbidity of the treatment procedure, no frozen sections are taken during the operation, and all patients (except one) were implanted. Furthermore, no additional treatment (either external irradiation of the pelvis or hormonal intervention) is given to the patients with positive nodes, because one of the reasons for this treatment procedure is the preservation of the sexual functions.

Although we are optimistic about the results (see Table 2) we have to realize that adenocarcinomas of the prostate are relatively slowly growing and a long follow-up period is needed to establish the final results. Unfortunately, there are no strict criteria for the assessment of the local results. Aspiration cytology is done routinely after 6, 18, and 30 months (Table 3). A positive outcome of this cytology, however, still does not predict a fatal outcome and the meaning of cytology in the follow-up is still under discussion [5].

A longer follow-up period with more patients is needed to confirm the expectations from these preliminary data.

Table 2. Follow-up of patients (6–36 months)

Total analyzed	27
Alive and well	20
Intercurrent death	3
Local recurrence	1 (N−)
Local recurrence + bone metastases	2 (2 N+)
Bone metastases	1 (N+)

N−, nodes negative;   N+, nodes positive

Table 3. Follow-up aspiration cytology

	Positive	Negative
At 6·months	6	14
18 months	1	7
30 months	2	2

Summary

Interstitial radiation therapy for prostatic cancer is already an old technique. Different radionuclides have been used (e.g., ^{198}Au). Hilaris and Whitemore introduced the implantation with ^{125}I seeds in 1970. With this technique a very high dose (between 120 to 200 Gy) is given in the target area with a minimum involvement of bladder and intestinal mucosa. The anatomical and functional integrity of the lower urinary tract is preserved as is the potency.

Selection of patients includes the following criteria:

1. Stage $T_1 - T_2$ prostate cancer, as determined by rectal palpation and transrectal echography. The volume of the prostate should be between 20 and 40 g.
2. Medium or high degree of differentiation as assessed by histology and aspiration cytology.
3. No evidence of regional or distant metastases, assessed by bonescan, PSAP, and lymphangiography. If lymphangiography shows suspect glands, aspiration cytology is done. If cytology is positive, external irradiation or hormonal therapy is proposed.

The treatment procedure is started with a limited regional lymphadenectomy for further staging of the tumor. After completion of this node dissection, the prostate is brought into view and the endopelvic fascia incised to free the prostate from its surroundings. The radiotherapist takes over and measures again the prostate to determine the number of seeds to be implanted and the number of hollow needles to be placed. Usually 8 to 10 needles are placed and 24 to 40 seeds introduced into the prostate.

The catheter is usually removed after $2-3$ days and if no complications occur, the patient can leave the hospital in $7-10$ days. Postoperatively X-rays are made for localization of the seeds. With the use of a modified stereo-shift reconstruction method two images of each implanted seed are obtained in one radiographic film. A computer program was developed to combine the two isocentric images with an additional antero-posterior image. The information of these three images is sufficient to obtain the definitive localization of the seeds in a few minutes. After reconstruction, the dose distribution pattern can be derived. In general, a dose rate of $2.5-5$ cGy/h is achieved for the whole treatment volume. With a half-life of the ^{125}I of 60 days, this will result in an overall dose of $100-200$ Gy. Due to the low energy, the dose outside the treatment volume decreases very rapidly.

Since the introduction of this technique in our institute in 1981, 31 patients have been treated for T_1 and T_2 prostate cancers. Positive lymph nodes were found in 4 patients. In a fifth patient very large positive nodes were found, and so no implantation was done but hormonal treatment was given instead. Three patients died, two of heart failure postoperatively, one after 30 months. In none was a residual tumor manifest. In three patients bone metastases were diagnosed during the follow-up examination, all had positive nodes at the initial treatment. In one patient a local recurrence was found and treated with hormones.

Aspiration cytology is done routinely after 6 and 18 months. After 6 months positive cytology was found in 6 of 20 patients, after 18 months in 1 of 8. The meaning of this finding, however, is still under discussion.

Of course our data are still very preliminary, but they seem in good agreement with the extensive data from the Memorial Hospital in New York.

References

1. Paulson DF (1984) Treatment of locally confined prostatic cancer. Radiotherapy versus surgery, limits of curability. In: Kurth KH et al. (eds) Progress and controversies in oncological urology. Liss, New York, p 483
2. Pistenma DA, Ray FR, Bagshaw MA (1976) The role of megavoltage radiation therapy in the treatment of prostatic carcinoma. Semin Oncol 3:115
3. Whitmore WF (1984) Interstitial I-125 implantation in the management of localized prostatic cancer. In: Kurth KH et al. (eds) Progress and controversies in oncological urology. Liss, New York, p 513
4. Grossman HB, Batata M, Hilaris B, Whitmore Jr WF (1982) ^{125}I implantation for carcinoma of prostate; further follow-up of first 100 cases. Urology 20:591
5. Freiha FS, Bagshaw MA (1984) Carcinoma of the prostate: results of post-irradiation biopsy. Prostate 5:19

CT-Guided Stereotactic Implantation with Iridium-192 and Iodine-125 of Non-Resectable Intracranial Tumors

F. MUNDINGER [1]

From a total number of 1654 stereotactically irradiated cases (Table 1) treated by permanent interstitial implantation with radioisotopes of a low dose rate (Curietherapy), a series of 924 gliomas is reported on.

Survival probabilities after 3 and 5 years of patients treated with Curietherapy − 204 of them with iridium-192 (1965−1984) and 230 with iodine-125 − in comparison to exclusive biopsy are given (Table 2). Compared to the I-125-implantation, we observed better results with the Ir-192-implantation in the case of low-grade gliomas.

All stereotactic irradiation procedures were within the same session directly preceded by bioptic confirmation. Evaluations are subject to classification and dignity as well as localisation (hypothalamic, thalamic, mesencephalic, brainstem/pons and peripheral surroundings).

For the stereotactic brachy-Curie-therapy we use since 1964 the afterloading-iridium-192-contact radiation device "GammaMed" intraoperatively which is supplied with high dose rate source mainly in cases of malignant tumours of the hemispheres. Also afterloading temporary catheter implantation

Table 1. Radionuclides and number of stereotactic interstitial irradiation procedure 1952–31. 07. 85

Radionuclide	Number
P-32	6
Co-60	179
Y-90	44
Ta-182	21
Au-198	129
I-125	371
I-125 Brachy Curie	38
Ir-192 Gamma Med	293
Ir-192	573
Total	1654

1 Albert-Ludwigs-Universität, Abt. Stereotaxie und Neuronuklearmedizin, Hugstetter Straße 55, D-7800 Freiburg

Nuclear Medicine in Clinical Oncology
Ed. by C. Winkler
© Springer-Verlag Berlin Heidelberg 1986

Table 2. Survival rates – (life table-method)

Tumortype	Number of cases	3 years (%)	5 years (%)
Iridium-192-Implantation			
Astrocytoma I	60	76	54
Astrocytoma II	83	71	56
Astrocytoma III	21	53	41
Oligodendroglioma II + III	27	65	39
Glioblastoma	13	8 (2 y!)–	–
	204		
Iodine-125-Implantation			
Astrocytoma I	61	72	53
Astrocytoma II	98	67	56
Astrocytoma III	41	49	36
Oligodendroglioma II + III	12	58	31
Glioblastoma	18	8 (2 y!)	–
	230		
Biopsy only			
Astrocytoma I	75	69	51
Astrocytoma II	182	59	51
Astrocytoma III	112	51	40
Oligodendroglioma II + III	25	62	35
Glioblastoma	96	17 (2 y!)	–
	490		
Total	924		

Table 3. Indications of CT-stereotactic *low dose* rate Ir-192- or I-125-Curietherapy (Permanentimplantation)

	Biopsy obligatory
Primarily Curietherapy	– None resectable low grade tumors (WHO I, II) around the cerebral/cerebellar midline – Non resectable tumors (WHO II–III, III) followed by external irradiation
Secondary Curietherapy	– Resting low grade tumors (WHO I, II) after partially resection – High grade tumor recurrences after operation and external irrad. – After external irradiation only Brachy-Curie-Therapy not indicated

Table 4. Indications for CT-stereotactic *high dose* rate-Ir-192 or I-125 Brachy-Curie-Therapy (temporary implantation) of intracranial malign tumors

	Biopsy obligatory
Primarily Brachy-Curietherapy	– Small volume hemispheric tumors – Tumors in functional important region (central, temporal, parietal) – Non resectable deep seated tumors
Secondary Brachy-Curietherapy	– After operation and external irradiation – Recurrences after external irradiation Not indicated in processes around midline structures

Indications for non resectable deep seated malignomas around cerebral/cerebellar midline structures

	Biopsy obligatory
Grading WHO III	– Iridium-192 or Iodine-125-Curietherapy (permanent implantation)
Grading WHO IV	– External beam irradiation only Brachy-Curietherapy not indicated

of iodine-125-seeds has been carried out (since 1980) in cases of high-grade hemisphere tumours.

The intraoperative high-dose-rate with the Ir-192 "GammaMed" contact radiation device has proved better palliative results than the high-dose-rate radiation with I-125 using the after-loading techniques.

The Karnofsky scale rises after the implantation, indicating an improved quality of life which is maintained until shortly before death.

The indications for both techniques are shown in Tables 3 and 4.

IX. Experimental Approaches and Future Aspects

Radioimmunodetection of Hodgkin Tumors in Nude Mice

H. Burrichter[1], C. Rossbach, P. Gielow, M. Schaadt, H. Hundeshagen, and V. Diehl

Introduction

One of the major problems in clinical oncology is the detection of metastatic disease. As far as Hodgkin's disease is concerned, the selection of adequate stage-dependent treatment necessitates invasive techniques such as operative laparotomy including splenectomy and lower extremity lymphangiography, as well as computerized axial tomography (de Vita et al. 1965; Glatstein et al. 1970; Nicholson et al. 1970; Allison et al. 1982).

Several reports recently published have proved the value and applicability of monoclonal antibodies in detecting solid tumors of various origins in animal models and in man (Levine et al. 1980; Moshakis et al. 1981; Epenetos et al. 1982, 1982a; Farrands et al. 1982; Sears et al. 1982; Levy and Miller 1983; Smedley et al. 1983). The potential value for application of monoclonal antibodies in man needs to be assessed in model systems before clinical studies are attempted (Moshakis et al. 1981).

The localization of ^{131}I-labeled monoclonal antibody Ki 1 in an animal model is reported here.

Materials and Methods

Cell Lines

The Hodgkin derived cell lines L428 and L540 are described in detail elsewhere (Schaadt et al. 1980; Diehl et al. 1981). They represent in vitro counterparts of in vivo Hodgkin and Sternberg-Reed cells. In contrast to L428, the L540 cell line is tumorigenic in nude mice.

BJAB and Raji are Burkitt's lymphoma lines, Jurkat originates from a T-cell leukemia (Pulvertaft 1965; Klein et al. 1974; Schwenk and Schneider 1975).

Monoclonal Antibodies

The monoclonal antibody Ki 1 (Schwab et al. 1982) was produced against the Hodgkin cell line L428. Ki 1 reacts with Hodgkin and Sternberg-Reed cells in

---

1 Med. Universitätsklinik, Joseph-Stelzmann-Straße, D-5000 Köln 41

Nuclear Medicine in Clinical Oncology
Ed. by C. Winkler
© Springer-Verlag Berlin Heidelberg 1986

frozen sections of Hodgkin biopsies, but not with those of non-Hodgkin lymphomas of various types (Stein et al. 1982). Apart from that, Ki 1 reacts with a cell population in normal lymphoid tissue (Stein et al. 1982) and with a subpopulation of mononuclear cells (0.1%) in the peripheral blood of healthy donors (own observations).

H 141-31/2, a monoclonal antibody of the same subclass as Ki 1 (IgG 3), served as a control antibody (Lemke et al. 1979). It reacts with the private specificity of D^b.

Antibody Preparation

The ascitic fluid of hybridoma-bearing NMRI mice was precipitated with ammonium sulfate (45%), separated by ion exchange chromatography (FPLC, Mono Q column, Pharmacia) and the fractions tested for activity by immunofluorescence. The purity of the active preparation was confirmed by gel electrophoresis. The antibody was labeled using this preparation.

Iodination

Protein (150 µg) was iodinated with 100 MBq of Na^{131}-I (Amersham, Buckinghamshire, UK) by the lactoperoxidase method (Marchalonis 1969; Eckelmann et al. 1980). The enzyme was used in an immobilized form (Enzymobead Radioiodination Reagent; Biorad, Richmond, California). The reactants were incubated for 30 min and passed through a Sephadex G-50 column (Pharmacia, Sweden) that had been prewashed with 1 ml of human serum albumin (Behring, Marburg, FRG), followed by 30 ml of phosphate buffered saline (PBS). The eluate obtained with PBS was collected in fractions of $0.7-0.8$ ml, and the radioactivity and protein content were determined. The labeled protein was absorbed in several steps to mouse spleen cells to test reactivity to an aliquot of control tumor cells and to L540 cells. The antibody was injected into the mice on the same day that they were iodinated.

Antibody Administration

Mice were taken for the experiments when tumor size was about 0.5 cm in diameter. Each mouse was injected about 3 MBq of activity. The antibody preparation, containing about 10 µg of immunoglobulin, was taken up in 0.3 ml of 0.9% NaCl solution.

Iodine uptake by thyroid was blocked by adding sodium-perchlorate to the drinking water (100 µl/100 ml) 3 days prior to the experiments.

Imaging

Mice were anesthetized with ether gas and scanned for 5 min, 2, 24, 48, and 120 h after the injection of the labeled antibody. The imaging was performed with a ZLC 370 scintillation camera (Siemens, FRG) fitted with a 360 eV parallel collimator. The camera was linked to a computer with data display. The counts at different regions of interest were sequentially calculated.

In most experiments mice were exsanguinated 48 h after the antibody inoculation, since the most distinct accumulation could be achieved at this time. The tissues were removed, washed in 0.9% NaCl solution, dried, weighed, and the activity was determined with a gamma counter. The radioactivity was calculated for 1 g of tissue and is expressed as tumor tissue ratio (tissue = 1).

Results

Figure 1 shows the accumulation of activity 48 h after the injection of the labeled antibody Ki 1 in the gluteal region of a nude mouse bearing a Hodgkin tumor. No uptake is visible in the Jurkat tumor (BJAB and Raji tumors did not accumulate activity; pictures not shown). Increased activity is also to be seen in the thyroid gland of both animals, possibly due to insufficient blockade.

The antibody H 141-31/2 of the same subclass as Ki 1 (IgG3), was labeled and administered in the same way to prove that tumor detection with labeled Ki 1 was not a matter of perfusion but of constant uptake of the antibody, since gamma globulin injected into animals was described to accumulate unspecifically in subcutaneously transplanted tumors (Dewey 1959; Bale et al. 1980). No accumulation of activity in the tumors was seen during the observation period of 6 days when using the H 141-31/2 antibody. After this period labeled Ki 1 antibody was injected into the same mice and now a distinct localization of the Hodgkin tumors could be observed.

Pictures of a mouse scanned 3, 26, 50, and 120 h after inoculation are shown in Figure 2 and demonstrate an accumulation of activity in the Hodgkin tumor

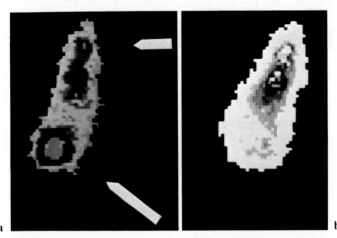

a   b

Fig. 1. Image of a nude mouse with transplanted Hodgkin tumor (**a**) and a Jurkat tumor (**b**) 48 h after intravenous injection of 3 MBq of ^{131}I-labeled Ki 1 antibody (*short arrow:* thyroid gland; *long arrow:* tumor)

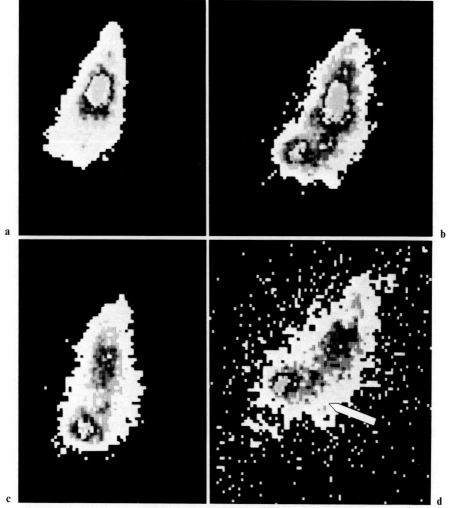

Fig. 2. Images of a nude mouse with transplanted Hodgkin tumor 3 h (**a**), 26 h (**b**), 50 h (**c**) and 120 h (**d**) after injection of the labeled Ki 1 antibody

area. This correlates well with the computerized determination of the count density having increased over the Hodgkin tumor area (Fig. 3) in contrast to continuously decreasing activity over the area of a Jurkat tumor and the thoracal regions of both animals.

Tumor tissue ratios of the removed tissues are shown in Table 1. The tumor to muscle activity ratio was 8.1, tumor to liver ratio 3.9, and spleen ratio 3.1. Activity ratios of control tumors (BJAB, Jurkat, Raji) show that, apart from tumor/muscle ratio, activity in liver and spleen is higher than in the tumors.

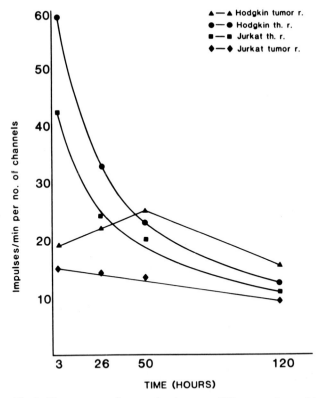

Fig. 3. Time course of count density over different regions of interest (tumors, central blood pool = lung, liver, spleen, heart) of Balb/c nude mice bearing tumors of Hodgkin and Jurkat origin. Count density was recorded 3, 26, 50 and 120 h after the injection

Table 1. Ratio of ^{131}I- concentration in tumor to that in muscle, liver and spleen (tissue = 1; n = 5, mean values; in brackets: standard deviation)

	Tumor:muscle	Tumor:liver	Tumor:spleen
Hodgkin tumors	8.10 (±2.46)	3.90 (±1.37)	3.10 (±0.83)
Control tumors (BJAB, Raji Jurkat)	2.10 (±1.77)	0.80 (±0.07)	0.90 (±0.21)

Discussion

The data presented here document the capacity of the radiolabeled monoclonal antibody Ki 1 to detect Hodgkin tumors in an animal model. The results were obtained without employing techniques of computerized background subtraction or other enhancement of visualisation (Deland et al. 1980). In every experiment the specific uptake of the antibody was higher in Hodgkin tumors than in the spleen or liver of the animals. Unspecific accumulation of the antibody was excluded by administration of an antibody of the same subclass which did not reveal specific uptake by Hodgkin tumors. Tumors of Burkitt's lymphoma and T-cell origin could not be visualized by Ki 1.

The size of the imaged tumors was about 0.5 cm in diameter and experiments are being carried out to scanning smaller deposits, since there are reports that smaller tumors show the highest degree of specific uptake (Moshakis et al. 1981). This would meet an oncologist's wish for a diagnostic system for detection of even small sites of involvement.

In our experiments we observed considerable activity in the thoracal region, probably due to contaminating proteins inspite of the applied purification procedures, but never did the background affect the visualisation of the tumors, because of a 2-cm distance between them and the central blood pool (lung, liver, spleen, heart). Another possibility for the background activity could be the reaction of the antibody with mouse Fc receptors, due to insufficient absorbtion to mouse spleen cells. Experiments in which Fab fragments are used are ongoing to elucidate this problem.

Should Ki 1 be employed in the detection of Hodgkin tumors in mediastinal and abdominal areas in man, a double isotope background subtraction technique for subtraction of the blood pool might become necessary. This might also be indicated because of the cross-reactivity of Ki 1 with a small subpopulation of mononuclear cells in the peripheral blood.

Ki 1 has already proved to be of value in detecting Hodgkin and Sternberg-Reed cells in frozen sections of lymphoid tissue (Stein et al. 1982). Ki 1 might also be promising as an additional, noninvasive tool for diagnosis of Hodgkin tumors in man.

Summary

The monoclonal antibody (moab) Ki 1, reacting with Hodgkin and Sternberg-Reed cells in culture and in frozen sections of Hodgkin (HD) biopsy material was labeled with iodine-131 by lactoperoxidase method and administered intraveneously into nude mice bearing tumors of Hodgkin, T-cell, or Burkitt's lymphoma origin.

A clearcut staining of the Hodgkin tumors was shown by the gamma scintillation camera 48 to 72 h after injection of the labeled antibody, whereas the control tumors were negative.

The specific activity of different tissues was measured in a gamma counter. The Hodgkin-derived tumors showed a significantly higher activity, whereas the uptake of the control tumors was in the range of the other organs.

Intravenous injection of a labeled unspecific moab of the same subclass as Ki 1 (IgG3) failed to stain any of the transplanted tumors.

We conclude from these data, that a specific radioimmunodetection of HD tissue is possible by using the ^{131}I-labeled moab Ki 1.

References

1. Allison JG (1982) Die Aufgabe der Chirurgie in der Lymphomtherapie. JAMA-D1 6:307–313
2. Bale WF, Contreras MA, Grady ED (1980) Factors influencing localization of labelled antibodies in tumors. Cancer Research 40:2965–2977
3. Deland FH, Kim EE, Simmons G, Goldenberg DM (1980) Imaging approach in radio-immunodetection. Cancer Research 40:3046–3049
4. Dewey WC (1959) Vascular-extravascular exchange of ^{131}I plasma proteins in the rat. Am J Physiol 197:423–431
5. Diehl V, Kirchner H, Schaadt M, Fonatsch C, Stein H, Gerdes J, Boie C (1981) Hodgkin's disease: Establishment and characterization of four in vitro cell-lines. J Cancer Res Clin Oncol 101:111–124
6. Eckelman WC, Paik CH, Reba RC (1980) Radiolabelling of antibodies. Cancer Res 30:3036–3040
7. Epenetos AA, Nimmon CC, Arklie J, Elliott AT, Hawkins LA, Knowles RW, Britton KE, Bodmer WF (1982) Detection of human cancer in an animal model using radiolabelled tumor-associated monoclonal antibodies. Br J Cancer 46:1–8
8. Epenetos AA, Britton KE, Mather S, Shepherd J, Granowska M, Papadimitriou JT, Nimmon CC, Derbin H, Hawkins LR, Malpas JS, Bodmer WF (1982a) Targeting of iodine-123-labelled tumor-associated monoclonal antibodies to ovarian, breast and gastrointestinal tumors. Lancet 2:999–1004
9. Farrands PA, Perkins AC, Pimm MV, Hardy JD, Embleton MJ, Baldwin PW, Hardcastle JD (1982) Radioimmunodetection of human colorectal cancers by an antitumor monoclonal antibody. Lancet 2:307–400
10. Glatstein E, Guernsey JM, Rosenberg SA (1969) The value of laparotomy and splenectomy in the staging of Hodgkin's disease. Cancer 24:705–718
11. Klein G, Giovanella B, Westermann A, Stehlin JS, Mumford D (1975) An EBV genome negative cell-line established from an American Burkitt lymphoma: receptor characteristics, EBV-infectability and permanent conversion into EBV positive sublines by in vitro infection. Intervirology 5:319–334
12. Lemke H, Hämmerling GJ, Hämmerling U (1979) Fine specificity analysis with monoclonal antibodies of antigens controlled by the major histocompatibility complex and by the Qa/TL region in mice. Immunological Rev 47:175–206
13. Levine G, Ballou B, Reiland J, Solter D, Gumerman L, Hakala T (1980) Localization of I-131 labelled tumor-specific monoclonal antibodies in the tumor-bearing BALB/C mouse. J Nucl Med 21:570–573
14. Levy R, Miller RA (1983) Tumor therapy with monoclonal antibodies. Federation Proceedings 42:2650–2656
15. Marchalonis JJ (1969) An enzymatic method for the tracer iodination of immunoglobulines and other proteins. Biochem J 113:299–305
16. Moshakis V, McIllhinney R, Raghavenan D, Neville AM (1981) Monoclonal antibodies to detect human tumors: an experimental approach. J Clinical Pathol 34:314–319
17. Nicholson WM, Beard MEJ, Crowther D, Stansfeld AG, Vartan CP, Malpas JS, Fairley GH, Scott RB (1970) Combination chemotherapy in generalized Hodgkin's disease. Br Med J 3:7–10
18. Pulvertaft RJV (1965) A study of malignant tumors in Nigeria by short-term tissue culture. J Clin Pathol 18:261–273
19. Schaadt M, Diehl V, Stein H, Fonatsch C, Kirchner HH (1980) Two neoplastic cell-lines with unique features derived from Hodgkin's disease. Int J Cancer 26:723–731
20. Schwab U, Stein H, Gerdes J, Lemke H, Kirchner H, Schaadt M, Diehl V (1982) Production of a monoclonal antibody for Hodgkin and Sternberg-Reed cells of Hodgkin's disease and a subset of normal lymphoid cells. Nature 299:65–67
21. Schwenk HU, Schneider U (1975) Cell-cycle dependency of a T-cell marker on lymphoblasts. Blut 31:299–306

22. Sears HF, Atkinson B, Mattis J, Ernst C, Herlyn D, Steplewshi Z, Hayry P, Koprowski H (1982) Phase 1 clinical trial of monoclonal antibody in treatment of gastrointestinal tumors. Lancet 1:762−765
23. Smedley HM, Finan P, Lennox ES, Ritson A, Takei F, Wraight P, Sikora K (1983) Localization of metastatic carcinoma by a radiolabelled monoclonal antibody. Br J Cancer 47:253−259
24. Stein H, Gerdes J, Schwab U, Lemke H, Mason DY, Ziegler A, Schienle W, Diehl V (1982) Identification of Hodgkin and Sternberg-Reed cells as a unique cell type derived from a newly-detected small cell population. Int J Cancer 30:445−459
25. de Vita VT, Maxley JH, Brace K, Frei E (1965) Intensive combination chemotherapy and X-irradiation in the treatment of Hodgkin's disease. Proc Am Assoc Cancer Res 6:15−19

Immunoscintigraphy of Human Pancreatic Carcinoma in Nude Mice with F(ab')₂ Fragments of Monoclonal Antibodies to CA 19-9 and CEA

R. SENEKOWITSCH [1], F. D. MAUL, R. P. BAUM, H. J. C. WENISCH, M. SCHNEIDEREIT, S. MÖLLENSTÄDT, H. KRIEGEL, and G. HÖR

Radiolabeled monoclonal antibodies directed against tumor antigens have been used to detect tumors in animals [1–6] and men by gamma imaging. Many of these studies used antibodies or their fragments reactive against colon carcinomas [7–9], melanomas [10, 11], and mammary carcinomas [12]. Most of the localization studies were performed using I-131 labeled antibodies. The detection of the tumor, however, is highly dependent on the concentration and distribution of the antigen recognized by the antibody.

Clinical investigations have recently been carried out using 19-9, a monoclonal antibody that reacts specifically with human gastrointestinal cancer [13] and anti-CEA antibodies for radioimmunodetection of colon carcinoma [14, 15]. The antigens recognized by the two antibodies are shed into the circulation where their serum levels can be detected by radioimmunoassays and can be used as tumor markers for gastrointestinal cancer [16, 17].

In the present study iodinated monoclonal antibody fragments to CA 19-9 and CEA were evaluated for their ability to localize specifically in human pancreatic carcinoma xenografts hosted in nude mice by scintigraphy and tissue uptake measurements [18].

Materials and Methods

A human pancreatic adenocarcinoma was passaged by s.c. implantation of slices of tumor tissue (diameter 1.5 mm) into the right flank of nude mice. Mice bearing tumors 200–400 mg in weight were given an intravenous injection of 1.8 MBq of iodinated antibody fragments (specific activity 55 MBq/mg) approximately 5–6 weeks after implantation of the tumor. Thyroid uptake of free iodine was blocked by adding perchlorate to the drinking water 48 h before activity injection and throughout the experiment.

The study in nude mice was performed in three parts. Distribution, tumor uptake, and the whole body retention of a) 19-9 F(ab')₂ fragments and an unspecific IgG of the same subclass, b) 19-9 F(ab')₂ fragments and anti-CEA F(ab')₂ fragments, and, c) whole anti-CEA antibody and its F(ab')₂ and Fab fragments were compared.

---

1 Gesellschaft für Strahlen- und Umweltforschung, Dept. Nuclearbiology, D-8042 Neuherberg

Nuclear Medicine in Clinical Oncology
Ed. by C. Winkler
© Springer-Verlag Berlin Heidelberg 1986

In one group of animals the CA 19-9 levels in blood were detected by radio-immunoassays before and after injection of the 19-9-antibody.

The whole body clearance of the injected antibodies was determined by whole body counting of the animals immediately after injection of the activity (100% retention) up to 6 days. For scintigraphic imaging the animals were anesthetized by an intraperitoneal injection of 100 mg ketamine (Ketanest) and 10 mg xylazine (Rompun) per kg body weight. Serial scintiphotos were obtained 6 and 12 h after injection of the antibodies and subsequently every 24 h up to 6 days. Imaging studies were performed with a Philips gamma camera equipped with a 2 mm pinhole collimator. At least 30,000 counts per image were collected. Images were recorded from the I-131 peak (365 keV with a 20% window) and the data were stored with a digital computer into a 64×64 pixel matrix (Philips NPS with DEC PDP-11/34).

The biodistribution data were obtained by killing and dissecting animals in groups of at least 4 at 24, 48, 72, 96, and 144 h after injection. Blood, tumors, heart, lungs, liver, kidneys, spleen, stomach, large intestine, pancreas, thyroid, muscle, and femur (bone marrow) were removed and weighed. The radioactivity was measured in a gamma counter and expressed as percentage of injected dose per gram of tissue.

Results

The tissue distribution of 19-9 F (ab')$_2$ fragments at 1, 2, 4, and 6 days after activity injection compared to that of an unspecific IgG is shown in Fig. 1. The highest activity concentration for 19-9 was found in the tumor between 48 and 144 h post injection (p.i.). Only at 24 h p.i. the concentration in the blood was higher. The activity in blood declined from 2.5% per gram at 24 h to 0.08% at 96 h and 0.03% at 144 h.

The radioactivity in the tumor revealed a high variability in uptake. The mean value was found 2.1% per gram at 24 h and dropped to 0.6% at day 4 and 0.09% at day 6 p.i. Of all other tissues excised only the lung showed an activity concentration higher than that found for the blood. The faster clearance of radioactivity from the blood pool and normal tissue than from the tumor leads to increasing tumor-to-blood ratios over a 4-day period after activity injection. The maximum tumor-to-blood ratio was 7.8 (range $4.1 - 14.2$) on day 4 p.i. and declined to 3 (range $2.4 - 6.0$) at day 6 probably because of the release of radioactivity from the tumor.

Scintigraphic images obtained at 6 and 12 h after injection of I-131-labeled 19-9 F (ab')$_2$ fragments primarily showed the activity in the areas of heart and lungs (Fig. 2). At this early phase of the study a bladder activity was seen in many cases, too. Imaging permitted tumor detection at 12 h p.i., but optimum tumor localization was reached at day 4 after injection of the labeled antibody fragments. At that time almost only tumor radioactivity was seen, as the activity in the area of heart and lungs significantly decreased. The weight of the implanted tumor in Fig. 2 was 310 mg at dissection 96 h p.i. The tumor-to-blood ratio was 14.2:1.

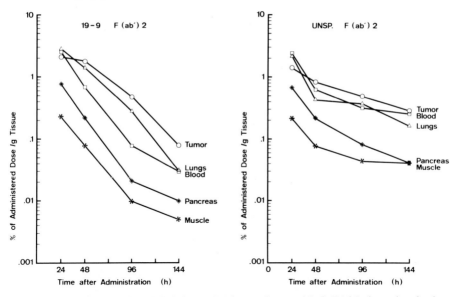

Fig. 1. Biodistribution of ^{131}I labeled 19-9 F (ab')$_2$ and control IgG F (ab')$_2$ in nude mice hosting a human pancreatic carcinoma shown as function of time after antibody injection (% inj. dose/g; mean; $n = 6$)

The serum levels of CA 19-9 determined in a group of mice bearing a human pancreatic carcinoma ($n = 10$), demonstrated elevated values of 57 U/ml (range 32–81) in 4 animals. In a control group without tumors no measurable CA 19-9 levels were found. After injection of the 19-9 fragments in tumor-bearing animals no elevated serum levels of CA 19-9 could be detected.

To assess the immunological specificity of 19-9 F (ab')$_2$ tumor uptake we compared this uptake with that of an unspecific IgG F (ab')$_2$.

As seen in Fig. 1 the unspecific IgG fragments cleared slower from the blood and other tissues between 48 and 144 h p.i. than the 19-9 fragments, resulting in a higher whole body retention for the unspecific IgG. The maximum tumor-to-blood ratio for this antibody was also reached at day 4 p.i., but it was only 1.8, indicating the preferential tumor uptake of 19-9 F (ab')$_2$.

The tumor uptake of anti-CEA F (ab')$_2$ was not as high as for 19-9 F (ab')$_2$. The tumor-to-blood ratio increased from 0.7 at 24 h p.i. to only 3.2 at day 3 compared to 7.8 for 19-9. The tumor-to-blood ratio, however, was higher for anti-CEA F (ab')$_2$ than for the unspecific IgG F (ab')$_2$.

A comparison of tumor uptake and blood levels between intact anti-CEA and its fragments from 24 to 72 h p.i. is given in Table 1. The highest tumor and blood levels were found for the intact antibody. Because of the very slow blood clearance of intact antibodies tumor-to-blood ratios of only 0.72 were reached during the time interval of 72 h p.i. Compared to F (ab')$_2$ fragments, Fab cleared to fast from the circulation to yield an appreciable tumor uptake. At 72 h p.i. nearly the same blood levels are detected for both fragments. At 24 h, however, the blood level for F (ab')$_2$ is 3 times higher than for Fab, which en-

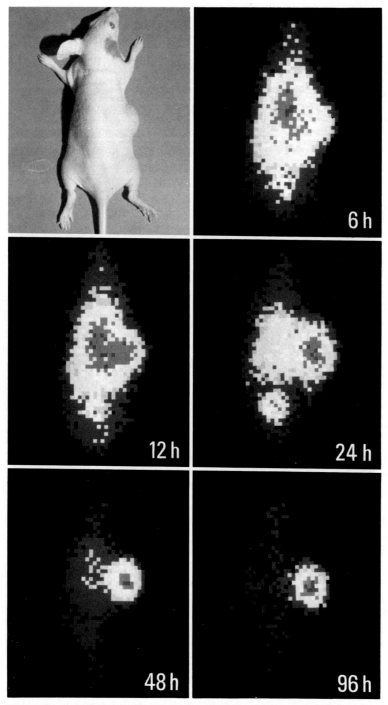

Fig. 2. Photograph and gamma images of a nude mouse grafted with a humanic pancreatic carcinoma in the right flank. Images obtained at 6, 12, 24, 48, and 96 h after i.v. injection of 60 μCi of ^{131}I labeled 19-9 F(ab′)$_2$ fragments. Tumor weight at dissection 310 mg; tumor-to-blood ratio at 96 h p.i. 14.2:1

Table 1. Blood levels and tumor uptake of ^{131}I labeled intact anti-CEA antibody and its F(ab')$_2$ and Fab fragments in nude mice bearing a human pancreatic carcinoma (% inj. dose/g; mean; $n=4$)

	Whole MAB		F(ab')$_2$		Fab	
	Tumor	Blood	Tumor	Blood	Tumor	Blood
24 h	3.2	6.1	1.6	2.3	0.54	0.70
48 h	3.3	5.5	1.1	0.56	0.26	0.23
72 h	3.1	4.3	0.63	0.20	0.31	0.16

ables a higher tumor uptake of F (ab')$_2$. For that reason a higher tumor-to-blood ratio of 3.2 for F (ab')$_2$ was found compared to 1.8 for Fab.

Whole body retention was determined in an animal whole body counter. It revealed a $T_{1/2}$ of approximately 7 days for the intact anti-CEA antibody compared to 12 h for the F (ab')$_2$ and 6 h for Fab.

Discussion

The antibody 19-9 first reported by Koprowski [13] recognizes a monoganglioside antigen of gastrointestinal cancer. It is shed into the circulation where it can be detected by radioimmunoassay and can be used as a tumor marker. The specificity of I-131 labeled 19-9 F (ab')$_2$ accumulation in a human pancreatic carcinoma heterotransplanted in nude mice was demonstrated by immunoscintigraphy and tumor uptake measurements. Compared to F (ab')$_2$ of an unspecific IgG the tumor uptake of 19-9 F (ab')$_2$ was almost 4 times higher. The rapid blood clearance of the F (ab')$_2$ leads to tumor-to-blood ratios up to 14.2 at 96 h p.i. At this time interval, best tumor localization was obtained by scintigraphic imaging. The wide range of antibody uptake in the tumor reflects at least in part the heterogeneity of tumor antigenic expression. The decrease of the CA19-9 levels of mice bearing a human pancreatic carcinoma after injection of the antibody fragments suggests that CA19-9/19-9 immunocomplexes were formed as already described for CEA by Mach [1]. The comparison between intact anti-CEA and its fragments in this tumor model demonstrates the superior biokinetic characteristics of F (ab')$_2$ in respect to tumor imaging as stated by Wahl [6].

The uptake of anti-CEA F (ab')$_2$ in the pancreatic carcinoma used in our study ranged between that of 19-9 and the unspecific IgG. These results support the demand for antibody cocktails to improve imaging of pancreatic carcinoma.

References

1. Mach JP, Carrel S, Forini M, Ritschard J, Donath A, Alberto P (1930) Tumor localization of radiolabeled antibodies against carcinoembryonic antigen in patients with carcinoma. A critical evaluation. N Engl J Med 303:5 – 10

2. Ballou B, Levine G, Hakala TR, Solter D (1979) Tumor location detected with radioactively labeled monoclonal antibody and external scintigraphy. Science 206:844–847

3. Buchegger F, Haskell CM, Schreyer M, Scazzig BR, Randin S, Carrel S, Mach JP (1983) Radiolabeled fragments of monoclonal antibodies against carcinoembryonic antigen for localization of human colon carcinoma grafted into nude mice. J Exp Med 158:413–427

4. Colcher D, Zalutzky M, Kaplan W, Kufe D, Austin F, Schlom J (1983) Radiolocalization of human mammary tumors in athymic mice by a monoclonal antibody. Cancer Res 43:736–742

5. Herlyn D, Powe J, Alavi A, Mattis JA, Herlyn M, Ernst C, Vaum R, Koprowski H (1983) Radioimmunodetection of human tumor xenografts by monoclonal antibodies. Cancer Res 43:2731–2735

6. Wahl LR, Parker CW, Philpott GW (1983) Improved radioimaging and tumor localization with monoclonal F (ab′)$_2$. J Nucl Med 24:316–325

7. Mach JP, Chatal JF, Lumbroso JD, Buchegger F, Forni M, Ritschard J et al. (1983) Tumor localization in patients by radiolabeled antibodies against colon carcinoma. Cancer Res 43:5593–5600

8. Keenan AM, Colcher D, Larson SM, Schlom J (1984) Radioimmunoscintigraphy of human colon cancer xenografts in mice with radioiodinated monoclonal antibody B72.3. J Nucl Med 25:1197–1203

9. Colcher D, Keenan AM, Larson SM, Schlom J (1984) Prolonged binding of a radiolabeled monoclonal antibody (B72.3) used for the in situ radioimmunodetection of human colon carcinoma xenografts. Cancer Res 44:5744–5751

10. Larson SM, Brown JP, Wright PW, Carrasquillo JA, Hellström I, Hellström KE (1983) Imaging of melanoma with I-131-labeled monoclonal antibodies. J Nucl Med 24:123–129

11. Larson SM, Carasquillo JA, McGuffin RW, Krohn KA, Ferens JM, Hill LD, Beaumier PL, Reynolds JC, Hellström KE, Hellström I (1985) Use of I-131 labeled, murine Fab against a high molecular weight antigen of human melanoma: Preliminary experience. Radiology 155:487–492

12. Khaw BA, Strauss HW, Cahill SL, Soule HR, Edgington T, Cooney J (1984) Sequential imaging of Indium 111-labeled monoclonal antibody in human mammary tumors hosted in nude mice. J Nucl Med 25:592–603

13. Koprowski H, Steplewski Z, Mitchell K, Herlyn M, Herlyn D, Führer P (1979) Colorectal carcinoma antigens detected by hybridoma antibodies. Somatic Cell Genet 5:957–971

14. Chatal J-F, Saccavini J-C, Fumuleau P, Douillard J-Y, Curtet C, Kremer M, Le Mevel B, Koprowski H (1984) Immunoscintigraphy of colon carcinoma. J Nucl Med 25:307–314

15. Baum RP, Maul FD, Klapdor R, Senekowitsch R, Lorenz M, Hottenrott C, Montz R, Happ J, Kriegel H, Chatal JF, Hör G (1985) Immunszintigraphie kolorektaler Tumoren mit ^{131}J-markierten monoklonalen Antikörpern (19-9/anti-CEA). Nuc Compact 16:121–128

16. Klapdor R, Lehmann U, Bahlo M, Greten H, v. Ackeren H, Dallek M, Schreiber HW (1983) CA 19-9 in der Diagnostik und Differentialdiagnostik des exkretorischen Pankreaskarzinoms. Tumor Diagn Ther 4:197

17. Klapdor R, Lehmann U, Bahlo M, Schmiegel W, Guthoff A, Schreiber HW, Greten H (1984) CA 19-9 and CEA in the follow-up of exocrine pancreatic cancer disease. Gastroenterology 86:1137

18. Senekowitsch R, Maul FD, Wenisch HJC, Kriegel H, Hör G (1985) Immunoscintigraphy of human pancreatic carcinoma in nude mice with I-131-F (ab′)$_2$-fragments of monoclonal antibodies. J Nucl Med 26:110

Physico-chemical Properties and Biokinetics
of Tumor-Affine Metal (M)-Ligand-Complexes

K. Schomäcker[1], W.-G. Franke, A. Gottscheck, C. Hartwig, A. Richter, and G.-J. Beyer

M-ligand-complexes with a radioactive central ion are significant for positive tumor imaging. Best known representative is ^{67}Ga-citrate, introduced by Edwards and Hayes in 1969 [1]. Since then numerous papers have been published on the biological behaviour of ^{67}Ga. Nevertheless, no satisfactory and non-contradictory theory about the biokinetics of tumor localization of ^{67}Ga as well as other M-ligand-complexes could yet be worked out.

Following the application of the citrate complex ^{67}Ga is stored not only in tumor tissue but also in muscles, in the liver, bones, and other organs. Because of this fact as well as through the presence of radioactivity in blood the applicability of ^{67}Ga-citrate for tumor diagnostics is restricted to cases in which the ratio of the radioactivity concentration in tumor and background (blood, muscles, adjacent tissue) is sufficiently high.

Searching for M-ligand-complexes, allowing a higher tumor/background ratio resulted in the application of ^{167}Tm-citrate, next to others. ^{167}Tm shows, compared to ^{67}Ga, a quicker blood clearance and a slower elimination from the tumor and in this way higher tumor/background ratios, which allow tumor imaging already 5 h p.i. [2, 3]. Influencing the biological behaviour (speeding up of the blood clearance and elimination from the body of the applied radionuclids as M-ligand-complexes) appeared a further possibility for improving the tumor/background ratios. Hereby the balance between the applied M-ligand-complexes and the M-protein-complexes formed in blood is of special significance. By exogeneous influence of the balance the supply of free diffusible M-compounds in the organism is altered. This is important for the change of the biodistribution of radionuclides in dependence on time and thus responsible for the achievable tumor/background ratio.

Our own investigations [4, 5] showed that the balance between M-ligand-complexes and M-protein-complexes can be influenced, for example, by varying the binding capacity of proteins acting as reaction partners in blood. Therefore, the biodistribution and biokinetics of ^{67}Ga-, ^{59}Fe- and ^{167}Tm-citrate after application of stable gallium, iron and thulium were investigated.

Iron application resulted in an increase of the ^{67}Ga-tumor/background ratio. The intratumoral accumulation of gallium is smaller after increasing the iron concentration in blood, than in normal concentration, but it proceeds distinctly slower than in blood and muscles. In case of gallium and iron a transferrin-con-

---

1 Medizinische Akademie „Carl Gustav Carus", Abt. für Nuklearmedizin, Fetscherstr. 74, X-8019 Dresden DDR

Nuclear Medicine in Clinical Oncology
Ed. by C. Winkler
© Springer-Verlag Berlin Heidelberg 1986

trolled mechanism of intratumoral uptake should be discussed. We have further established that ^{167}Tm, in contrast to ^{67}Ga and ^{59}Fe, is obviously not transported bound to transferrin. After application of ^{167}Tm-citrate, compared to Ga or Fe, the highest tumor/background ratios were found. This radio-nuclide is possibly bound to albumine and transported into the tumor.

The balance between M-ligand-complexes and M-protein-complexes in blood depends on the stability of the applied complexes as well as on that of the complexes built up in blood. The complex stability changes either in de-pendence on the size and charge of the central ion or in dependence on the type of ligand. As a further step, we therefore investigated the biodistribution in de-pendence on the time after injection of ^{67}Ga-, ^{59}Fe- and ^{169}Yb as differently stable complexes.

The main interest was thereby the relationship between the complex chemi-cal parameters of the compounds and the achievable tumor/background ratios. These investigations can be briefly described as follows.

Materials and Methods

We investigated the radioactivity concentration of ^{67}Ga, ^{59}Fe, and ^{169}Yb after application of the radionuclide as chloride (Cl$^-$), α-hydroxyisobutyrate (HIB), citrate (CIT), nitrilotriacetate (NTA), hydroxyethylethylenediaminetriacetate (HEDTA), ethylenediaminetetraacetate (EDTA) and diethylenetriamine-pentacetate (DTPA) in tumor, blood, muscles and in a series of organs 40 min, 2 h, 5 h, 24 h and 48 h p.i.

The complex stability altered as follows:

Cl$^-$ ◀ ◀ HIB ◀ CIT ◀ NTA ◀ HEDTA ◀ EDTA ◀ DTPA

The injection solutions had the following properties:

Radiochemical concentration:	37 MBq/ml
pH:	6.0
Ligand concentration:	10^{-2} mol/l

Each experimental animal was injected with 50 μl of the solution. The ani-mals were mice of the XVII-Bln-inbreeding strain, bearing a mamma car-cinoma (carcinoma solidum medullare partim adenomatosum) transplanted in-to the hind upper limb.

Results

The ^{67}Ga and ^{59}Fe concentrations in tumor and blood 24 h p.i. were only slight-ly dependent on the stability of the applied complexes.

^{67}Ga, ^{59}Fe, and ^{169}Yb were most strongly accumulated after application as relatively unstable complexes (Cl$^-$, HIB, CIT) in tumor. As a result, the highest tumor/background ratios were achieved after application of the radionuclides as relatively unstable complexes (Fig. 1, 2). The highest ^{67}Ga tumor/blood ra-

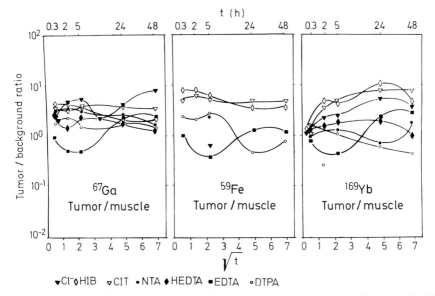

Fig. 1. Course of the tumor/muscle radioactivity ratios after i.v. application of different radioactive M-ligand complexes

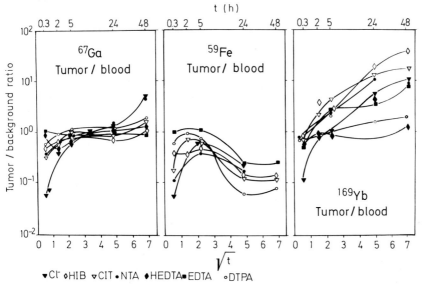

Fig. 2. Course of the tumor/blood radioactivity ratios after i.v. application of different radioactive M-ligand complexes

tios ($\sim$ 7) occurred after application of ^{67}Ga as NTA and Cl$^-$ 48 h p.i. The ^{59}Fe tumor/blood ratios were about three times lower in dependence on the complex stability. The highest ^{67}Ga tumor/muscles ratios were found after application of ^{67}GaCl$_3$ ($\sim$ 10, 48 h p.i.) and of Ga-CIT ($\sim$ 6, 48 h p.i.). The highest ^{59}Fe tumor/muscles ratios were about 7 at 48 h p.i. after application of ^{59}Fe-CIT and about 6 at 48 h after application of ^{59}Fe-HIB. The highest ^{169}Yb tumor/blood ratio ($\sim$ 30!) and tumor/muscles ratio ($\sim$ 26!) were observed 24 h after application of ^{169}Yb-HIB.

Discussion

The behavior of ^{67}Ga and ^{59}Fe is significantly determined by the building of highly stable complexes with transferrin in blood.

Except for ^{67}Ga-DTPA, which has a higher stability than ^{67}Ga-transferrin, all ^{67}Ga- and ^{59}Fe-ligand complexes should react to the corresponding transferrin complexes in blood. After application of relatively unstable complexes, the highest radioactivity concentrations in tumor and the highest tumor/background ratios were found. These results correlate with the observations of Rayundu et al. [6]. On the other hand, it is obvious that the balance between M-ligand complexes and M-protein complexes in blood is shifted towards the applied complexes with increasing stability of the applied M-ligand complexes.

Therefore the conclusion is that radionuclides which are applied as M-ligand complexes will be accumulated in the tumor in the form of protein complexes, i.e., protein mediated.

In case of ^{67}Ga and ^{59}Fe a transferrin-controlled uptake mechanism is discussed [7]. According to our own unpublished results, ^{169}Yb will be probably transported into the tumor as Yb-albumine-complex.

Our results show that the application of radioactive, relatively unstable lanthanoid-ligand-complexes with favourable radiophysical properties of the central ion (^{167}Tm-HIB) could strongly improve nuclear medical tumor diagnosis.

Summary

In animal experiments with tumor bearing (carcinoma solidum medullare pertim adenomatosum) mice (XVII-Bln) the radioactivity concentration of ^{67}Ga, ^{59}Fe and ^{169}Yb in tumor, blood, and organs 40 min, 2 h, 5 h, 24 h and 48 h p.i. was investigated, after injection of these radionuclides as cloride (Cl$^-$), α-hydroxiisobutyrate (HIB), citrate (CIT), nitrilotriacetate (NTA), hydroxiethylethylenediaminetriacetate (HEDTA), ethylenediaminetetraacetate (EDTA) and diethylenetriaminepentacetate (DTPA).

The complex stability changed as follows:

Cl$^-$ ◀ ◀ HIB ◀ CIT ◀ NTA ◀ HEDTA ◀ EDTA ◀ DTPA

The results may be interpreted in a way such that the application of radioactive unstable lanthanoid-ligand complexes with favorable radiophysical properties of the central ion (^{167}Tm-HIB) may be suitable for a significant improvement of tumor diagnosis.

References

1. Edwards CL, Hayes RL (1969) Tumor scanning with ^{67}Ga-chloride. J Nucl Med 10:103–105
2. Ando A, Hisida K, Hiraki T, Ando I, Sanada S (1974) The mechanism of the tumor affinity of ^{169}Yb, ^{67}Ga and ^{111}In (I). Distribution of ^{169}Yb, ^{67}Ga and ^{111}In in the short term after i.v.-injection and the form of chemical bond in the tumor tissue. Radioisotopes 23:161–166
3. Beyer GJ, Münze R, Fromm W-D, Franke W-G, Henke E, Khalkin VA, Lebedev NA (1981) Spallation produced thulium-167 for medical application. In: Medical radionuclide imaging 1980, vol 1. International Atomic Energy Agency, Vienna 1981, IAEA-SM-247/60
4. Franke W-G, Henke E, Maka G, Schomäcker K, Beyer G-J, Fromm WD, Lebedev NA, Novgorodov AF, Khalkin VA, Kljutschnikov AA (1984) Investigations on the relationship between the protein binding of trivalent metal (M 3$^+$) citrate complexes and their biokinetics. Work in Progress Poster of European Nuclear Medicine Congress, 14–17 August 1984, Helsinki
5. Franke W-G, Henke E, Maka G, Schomäcker K, Beyer G-J, Fromm WD, Lebedev NA, Novgorodov AF, Khalkin VA, Kljutschnikov AA (1984) Beeinflussungsmöglichkeiten der Biokinetik von Metall (M 3$^+$)-Zitratkomplexen und deren Bedeutung für eine verbesserte Tumordarstellung. In: Höfer R, Bergmann H (eds) Radioaktive Isotope in Klinik und Forschung, vol 16, part 2. International Symposium Gastein (1984)
6. Rayundu GVS, Abril ME, Fordham EW (1984) ^{169}Yb-complexes versus ^{67}Ga-citrate in tumor localization. Abstracts of the vth International symposium on radiopharmaceutical chemistry. Science University of Tokyo, Tokyo, Abstracts 48–49
7. Larson SM, Grundbaum Z, Rasey IJ (1981) The role of transferrins in gallium uptake. Int J Nucl Med Biol 8:257–266

Iodoazomycin Riboside [1-(5′-iodo-5′-deoxyribofuranosyl)-2-nitroimidazole], a Hypoxic Cell Marker In Vivo Evaluation in Experimental Tumors

L. I. Wiebe[1], D. C. Jette, J. D. Chapman, R. J. Flanagan, and B. E. Meeker

Introduction

Radiosensitizers labelled with nuclides which emit gamma rays have been proposed to have clinical value in the detection of radioresistant hypoxic cell populations in tumors [1]. Such a diagnostic procedure would be of value for radiation and/or chemotherapy treatment planning in oncology, and could aid the study and treatment of ischemic tissue in the myocardium and in the brain. However, the sensitizers 4-[^{82}Br]-bromomisonidazole (BrMISO) [2] and 1-[2-(2-[^{131}I]iodophenoxy)-ethyl]-2-nitroimidazole (IPENI) [3] failed to undergo selective uptake in experimental tumor models. In both cases, and especially with IPENI, the test substances were more lipophilic than hypoxic cell markers used previously [4]. Recent efforts with tritiated misonidazole to label hypoxic cell fractions in human tumors have provided clinical data which support the concept that hypoxic cells may be detected by scintigraphic methods [5].

5′-Iodo-5′-deoxyazomycin riboside (5′-IAZR) is a novel, effective and moderately-toxic sensitizer of hypoxic cells in vitro [6]. It binds to hypoxic tumor cells in vitro at rates which are 20 − 30 times higher than the rates of binding to normal cells. Its relatively low lipophilicity, combined with its properties as a potential substrate for the cell membrane nucleoside transporter [7], make it a suitable candidate for further investigation in experimental clonogenic tumors in vivo.

Materials and Methods

Azomycinriboside (AZR) was obtained from Terochem Laboratories Ltd., Edmonton, Alberta. 5′-Iodo-5′-deoxyazomycinriboside (5′-IAZR) was prepared using triphenylphosphine and iodine as described previously [6]. The more lipophilic 2′,3′-diacetoxy derivative (5′-IAZRAc$_2$) of 5′-IAZR was synthesized from 5′-IAZR according to standard procedures using acetic anhydride and pyridine.

Silica gel microplates (Whatman MK6F; 40 mm, with fluorescent indicator; 2.5 × 7.5 cm) were developed to 6.0 cm in methanol/chloroform (1:9). AZR,

---

1 Faculty of Pharmacy and Pharmaceutical Sciences, University of Alberta, Edmonton, Canada, T6G 2N8

Nuclear Medicine in Clinical Oncology
Ed. by C. Winkler
© Springer-Verlag Berlin Heidelberg 1986

5-IAZR and 5'-IAZRAc$_2$ were visualized under UV light. The radiochemical purity of 5'-IAZR and 5'-IAZRAc$_2$ was determined by scraping the appropriate areas and counting in a gamma well-counter.

HPLC on a C-18 reverse phase column, eluted with 30% methanol in water (flow rate 1.0 ml/min), was used to purify the radioiodinated compound as well as to analyze plasma and urine samples. Plasma samples were passed through Ultrafilters (Amicon, YMT) to separate free metabolites. A methanol extract of plasma was used to analyze for protein-bound metabolites.

Radiolabelling

5'-IAZR was radiolabelled by exchange with no-carrier-added [^{131}I]- or [^{125}I]-iodide in DMF as described previously [6]. The radiochemical yield obtained under these conditions was typically 85%.

Animal Studies

Male BDF$_1$ mice (23–30 g) bearing subcutaneously implanted Lewis lung tumors, received bolus injections of iodinated sensitizer via the dorsal tail vein. The chemical dose (25 µg; 0.1 µmole; 77.7 kBq of ^{131}I) was dissolved in 0.1 ml of physiological saline. Animals were sacrificed with CO_2 at various times after injection. Blood and tissues were excised and radioassayed using a gamma well-counter (Beckman 8000).

Female BALB/c mice, 8–12 weeks old and weighing 18–20 g, were also used for quantitative tissue distribution studies. EMT-6 tumors were transplanted as a cell suspension into the right flank of recipient mice. These mice were used when the tumor was approximately 6–7 mm in diameter. The 5'-[^{131}I] IAZR (178 kBq) was administered in 5 fractions of 0.1 ml each, given intraperitoneally at 30 min intervals. In protocols for this animal model, 5'-[^{131}I] IAZR or Na^{131}I (178 kBq) were given by multiple i.p. injection, using normal or NaI-pretreated animals. Tissue distribution data were obtained as described above.

Dunning R3327-H and R3327-AT tumors were implanted, one on each flank, into Copenhagen × Fisher F$_1$ rats for scintigraphic studies. Tumor weights ranged from 400 to 2000 mg in rats which weighed between 300 and 450 g at the time of the study. These animals were injected either i.v. or i.p. with 37 MBq (1.5 mg) of radiolabelled sensitizer. Scintigrams were obtained with a Tracor phoGamma scintillation camera. The data obtained was analyzed on an ADAC computer system.

Results

Injected radioactivity was rapidly cleared from the blood stream and eliminated from the body after i.v. injection of 5'-[^{131}I]IAZR or i.p. injection of 5'-[^{131}I]IAZRAc$_2$ into the BDF$_1$/Lewis lung tumor model. Within 30 min, less than

5% of the injected dose remained in the blood, and about half of the dose was excreted via the urine within 1 h. Tissues of interest, including brain, myocardium, spleen and lung acquired only very low concentrations of radioactivity. High concentrations measured at early times in both liver and kidney tissue were indicative of hepatobiliary and renal clearance respectively. Prolonged high levels in the intestinal tract, compatible with a model of hepato-biliary clearance, were observed. Although this tumor has an appreciable hypoxic cell faction [8], tumor:blood ratios of radioactivity ranged erratically from 1.5 to 3.0 over 2−24 h in after injection, and the radioactivity in tumor represented less than 0.2% of the injected dose. Selected tissue uptake data for longer time intervals are presented in Table 1.

HPLC analysis of blood and urine after injection of either 5′-[^{131}I]IAZR or 5′-[^{131}I]IAZRAc$_2$ was used to characterize and quantify free [^{131}I]iodide and 5′-[^{131}I]IAZR (Table 2). In the case of 5′-[^{131}I]IAZRAc$_2$, up to 11% of this lipophilic derivative was present in the urine.

Tissue distribution studies were repeated using BALB/c mice bearing EMT-6 tumors, since this tumor model is known to contain a large population of hypoxic cells. Tumor:blood ratios of radioactivity after multiple dose i.p. injection of 5′-[^{131}I]IAZR were consistently near 5 over the 3−48 h period after i.p. injection. Tumor:blood ratios were greater at earlier time intervals when Na^{131}I alone was injected, and the radioactivity was cleared more rapidly from the tumor at late times after Na^{131}I. These results, compared with 5′-[^{131}I]AZR, were consistent with the concept of metabolic trapping of 5′-[^{131}I]IAZR through adduct formation. Tissue distribution data after injection of either 5′-[^{131}I]

Table 1. Percent of injected dose per g of tissue in the BDF$_1$/Lewis lung model. Data are mean values ± standard deviation, $n = 5$, for 5′-[^{131}I]IAR (1), 5′-[^{131}I]IAZRc$_2$ (2) and Na^{131}I (3)

Tissue		Time after injection (h)			
		2	6	24	48
Blood	1	0.19±0.02[a]	0.23±0.05	0.03±0.01	0.01±0.01
	2	0.41±0.06	ND	ND	ND
	3	3.6 ±1.8	ND	0.21±0.15	0.04±0.01
Tumor	1	0.28±0.15[a]	0.23±0.04	0.08±0.08	0.01±0.01
	2	0.04±0.00[a]	ND	ND	ND
	3	2.6 ±1.0	ND	0.14±0.11	0.01±0.01
Stomach	1	1.3 ±0.4[a]	2.18±0.47	0.16±0.01	0.06±0.04
	2	3.8 ±4.3	ND	ND	ND
	3	4.6 ±2.6	ND	2.4 ±2.3	0.13±0.11
Kidney	1	0.38±0.11[a]	0.26±0.04	0.04±0.01	0.03±0.01
	2	3.5 ±4.1	ND	ND	ND
	3	3.0 ±1.4	ND	0.06±0.03	0.11±0.05
Liver	1	0.19±0.03[a]	0.18±0.08	0.04±0.02	0.02±0.01
	2	0.40±0.07[a]	ND	ND	ND
	3	1.8 ±1.1	ND	0.03±0.01	0.04±0.01

ND, not determined
[a] Significantly different from Na^{131}I at the 99% confidence limit

Table 2. Radioactive constituents of plasma and urine of mice given single i.v. doses of 5′-[^{131}I]IAZR. Data represent the percent composition as determined by HPLC

Sample	Time after injection (h)	% as radioiodide	% as 5′-[^{131}I]IAZR
Plasma	0.5	51	28
	1.5	56	34
	3.0	50	27
	6.0	60	28
	24	56	29
Urine	0.5	90	7
	1.5	89	7
	3.0	76	18
	2.4	68	18
	48	85	7

Table 3. Tissue:blood radioactivity ratios in BALB/c mice bearing EMT-6 tumors, after i.v. injection of [^{131}I]IAZR (group 1), [^{131}I]IAZR after NaI pretreatment (group 2), Na^{131}I (group 3) and Na^{131}I after NaI pretreatment (group 4)

		3 h	6 h	24 h	48 h
Tumor	1	5.5 ±0.5[a]	5.4 ±1.0[a]	5.5 ±1.1	3.4 ±2.8
	2	5.7 ±2.5	4.8 ±1.2	4.7 ±1.1[a]	4.3 ±1.4[a]
	3	9.5 ±1.7	8.3 ±1.8	5.6 ±2.9	1.6 ±0.3
	4	4.8 ±3.3	7.4 ±2.6	1.00±0.17	0.70±0.20
Stomach	1	9.9 ±2.4[a]	7.4 ±1.3	2.2 ±0.6[a]	5.5 ±1.6[a]
	2	6.7 ±1.5[a]	7.5 ±4.2	5.7 ±1.8[a]	3.1 ±1.7[a]
	3	14.3 ±2.8	10.0 ±2.3	6.8 ±6.7	2.0 ±0.3
	4	15.2 ±4.9	7.7 ±4.1	0.50±0.14	0.40±0.08
Kidney	1	1.6 ±0.2[a]	1.4 ±0.2	3.1 ±0.4[a]	2.1 ±0.4
	2	1.3 ±0.3	1.2 ±0.1	2.6 ±0.8[a]	2.4 ±1.2[a]
	3	0.81±0.05	0.76±0.04	1.1 ±0.3	1.2 ±0.3
	4	0.91±0.05	0.75±0.47	0.44±0.03	0.36±0.04
Liver	1	1.03±0.12[a]	1.3 ±0.12[a]	2.5 ±0.5	2.0 ±0.5
	2	1.01±0.6	0.9 ±0.1	1.8 ±0.4[a]	1.3 ±0.6[a]
	3	0.35±0.02	0.36±0.03	1.05±0.48	0.90±0.22
	4	0.38±0.04	0.56±0.21	0.39±0.05	0.31±0.02

[a] Significantly different at the 99% confidence limit (group 1 vs group 3; group 2 vs group 4).

IAZR, 5′-[^{131}I]IAZR with NaI pretreatment, Na^{131}I, or Na^{131}I with NaI pretreatment are presented in Table 3.

Scintigraphic evaluation of tumor radioactivity in Copenhagen × Fisher rats which carried both implanted Dunning prostatic tumors, also showed a preference for the rapidly-growing, anaplastic R3327-AT tumor which has a significant hypoxic cell fraction [9]. Although quantitative data were not obtained, region-of-interest values from the scintigrams indicated a two-fold higher radioactivity content in the R3327-AT tumor.

Discussion

The rapid renal clearance of 5'-[^{131}I]IAZR, combined with appreciable deiodination and perhaps other metabolic catabolism such as the decoupling of the riboside moiety, presents a severe limitation to the use of 5'-IAZR as an in vivo marker of hypoxic tissue in these animals models. Attempts to delay renal excretion by making the compound more lipophylic through the acetylation of the ribose hydroxy groups on 5'-[^{131}I]IAZR proved to be ineffective, probably because of high levels of esterase (acetylase) activity in blood. Although the tumors appeared to take up free iodide as well as or better than 5'-[^{131}I]AZR, and although there was physiological (stomach uptake) and chemical (HPLC) evidence for deiodination of 5'-[^{131}I]AZR, clearance patterns for Na^{131}I- and 5'-[^{131}I]IAZR-derived radioactivity were different. The slower loss of radioiodide from tumor after 5'-[^{131}I]AZR supported the concept of metabolic trapping of the radiosensitizer through adduct formation. Uptake of free radioiodide by the tumors, and its subsequent wash-out, are rapid and concentration-dependent without evidence for metabolic trapping.

The utilization of gamma-emitting radiosensitizers such as 5'-[^{131}I]AZR for the noninvasive detection/quantification of hypoxic cells in tumors in vivo has remained an elusive goal in spite of the range of compounds tested to date. However, the effective application of principles developed through this and previous studies leave room for optimism that a radiochemically stable nitroimidazole radiosensitizer with acceptable biological properties will be developed as an effective diagnostic tool.

Summary

5'-Iodoazomycin riboside (5'-IAZR) is a novel iodine-containing radiosensitizer. Its tissue uptake, catabolism and excretion have now been tested in vivo in four experimental tumor models. Three of the tumor lines are known to have significant hypoxic cell populations (EMT-6 and Lewis lung carcinoma in mice and the Dunning R3327-AT in rats) whereas the fourth (Dunning R3327-H in rats) has a small or non-existent hypoxic cell fraction. Distribution studies were characterized by rapid urinary excretion (90% within 6 h) of a bolus i.v. dose of 5'-[^{131}I]IAZR, with concomitant high renal radioactivity. The tumor:blood ratios of radioactivity after 24 h were 5.5 ± 1.1 in the EMT-6 model, approximately double that of other tissues which showed radioactivity accumulations. The relative concentration of radioactivity in tumor in the Lewis lung model was lower than in the stomach. Region of interest measurements on scintigrams of similarly-sized R3327-AT and R3327-H tumors growing in the same rat indicated a nearly two-fold higher uptake by the hypoxic-cell containing R3327-AT tumor. Rapid excretion of 5'-IAZR resulted in only a small percentage (< 5% after 1 h) of the injected dose remaining in the blood. About 50% of the injected radioactivity was excreted via the urine in one hour. Attempts to reduce renal clearance by injecting the lipophilic 3',5'-diacetate derivative (5'-[^{131}I]IAZRAc$_2$) were ineffective in reducing renal clearance and in improving distribution characteristics in other tissues.

References

1. Chapman JD, Franko AJ, Sharplin J (1984) A marker for hypoxic cells in tumors with potential clinical applicability. Br J Cancer 43:546
2. Jette DC, Wiebe LI, Chapman JD (1983) Synthesis and in vivo distribution and metabolism of the radiosensitizer 4-(^{82}Br) bromomisonidazole in tumor-bearing and normal mice. Int J Nucl Med Biol 10:205–210
3. Wiebe LI, Jette DC, Chapman JD (1984) Electron-affinic compounds for labelling hypoxic cells: the synthesis and characterization of 1-[2-(2-iodophenoxy)-ethyl]-2-nitroimidazole. Nuklearmedizin 2:63–67
4. Chapman JD, Baer K, Lee J (1983) Characteristics of the metabolism-induced binding of misonidazole to hypoxic mammalian cells. Cancer Res 43:1523–1528
5. Chapman JD et al. Unpublished work in progress
6. Jette DC, Wiebe LI, Lee J, Flanagan RJ, Chapman JD (in press) Iodoazomycin riboside [1-(5'-iodo-5'-deoxyribofuranosyl)-2-nitroimidazole], a hypoxic cell marker. 1. In vitro characterization. Rad Res
7. Jarvis SM, Chapman JD, Ngan-Lee J, Rutledge KA, Barr PJ, Paterson ARP (1982) Azomycin riboside, a sugar homologue of misonidazole with favorable radiosensitizing properties. Cancer Res 42:4358–4363
8. Moulder JE, Rockwell S (1984) Hypoxic fractions of solid tumors: Experimental techniques, methods of analysis and a survey of existing data. Int J Radiat Oncol Biol Phys 10:695–712
9. Thorndyke C, Meeker BE, Thomas G, Lakey WH, McPhee MS, Chapman JD (1985) The radiation sensitivities of R3327-H and R3327-AT rat prostate adenocarcinoma. J Urol 134

The Potential Use of Alpha and Auger-Electron Emitting Radionuclides for Therapy

S. J. Adelstein[1], W. D. Bloomer, A. I. Kassis, and K. S. R. Sastry

A number of investigations have demonstrated the extreme radiotoxicity of alpha particle and Auger-electron emitting radionuclides in cell culture and model tumor systems. These experiments also show that Auger-electron emitting agents are more demanding in their localization than those emitting alpha and beta particles. Therefore, the choice of a radionuclide for therapy depends, in part, on the degree of specificity provided by its carrier. When the radionuclide can be transported only to the vicinity of the cells to be irradiated, beta particles are employed (hopefully to provide a homogeneous radiation field). When the radionuclide can be brought within one or two cell diameters of the target cells, alpha particles can be used. If the radionuclide can be delivered very close to or incorporated into the genome, Auger-electron emitting labels can be employed. Conversely, Auger-electron emitters generate the least damage to surrounding normal tissues, while the toxicity of the other radionuclides to surrounding tissues is in direct relation to the range of their emitted particles.

Alpha Particle Emitters

Among the currently available alpha emitting radionuclides, astatine-211 appears the most promising. Astatine (from the Greek *astatos* meaning unstable) was discovered in 1940 [9] when bismuth was bombarded by alpha particles in the 60-in. Berkeley cyclotron. Despite its being the fifth halogen element, astatine appears to have considerably different chemical properties from iodine, its nearest halogen neighbor [16]. [211]At decays by a complex double-branched pathway to lead-207 directly by alpha emission (42%) and indirectly through electron capture (58%) to polonium-211 which almost spontaneously decays by alpha emission. The physical half life is 7.2 hours, the average alpha particle energy is 6.8 MeV, the range in water 60 μm ($\sim$ 6 cell diameters) and the linear energy transfer is $\sim$ 113 keV/μ. Clonogenic survival assays in V-79 Chinese hamster cells exposed to ionic [211]At yield a linear dose response relationship with no shoulder in the low dose region; furthermore, the oxygen enhancement ratio of $\sim$ 1.5 is close to that of other densely ionizing (high LET) particles [11].

We studied the therapeutic efficacy of [211]At colloid in experimental malignant ascites and reported that the radiocolloid can be curative with minimal normal tissue toxicity [2]. Under the experimental conditions, the therapeutic

---

1 Harvard Medical School, Building A, 25 Shattuck Street, Boston, MA 02115, USA

Nuclear Medicine in Clinical Oncology
Ed. by C. Winkler
© Springer-Verlag Berlin Heidelberg 1986

ratio is favorable because the colloid represents a form of directed administration that physically separates and protects the sensitive mucosal lining of the intestine. Finely ground elemental tellurium was chosen as the colloid because of its strong affinity for astatine at neutral and acidic pH. Single graded doses of [211]At colloid were administered by intraperitoneal injection 24 h after the intraperitoneal inoculation of 10^6 tumor cells. Mice treated with $< 50\,\mu$Ci of the [211]At colloid demonstrated a dramatic increase in median survival that was proportional to dose. Doses of 25 and 50 μCi were curative in all animals; although there was some acute morbidity at these doses, there were no acute deaths.

The therapeutic efficacy of [211]At colloid was compared with the beta particle emitters ^{32}P, [165]Dy, and ^{90}Y prepared as radiocolloids. Unlike radio-astatine, none of the beta emitters were curative but relatively large doses did substantially prolong median survival [6]. Dose-survival curves also showed a threshold for cell killing not seen with the astatine-211 colloid.

For the present, the most obvious applications of alpha emitting radiocolloids are in the therapy of ascites and surface spreading abdominal and pelvic malignancies, but other uses are worthy of exploration.

Auger-Electron Emitters

[125]I decays by electron capture and undergoes internal conversion in 93% of disintegrations. These electron vacancies are filled by outer shell electron rearrangements and ionizations which continue until the valance shell is reached (Auger effect). The number of Auger electrons released per ^{125}I disintegration is substantial and the electrons most frequently produced have a subcellular range [8]. Assuming homogeneous distributions of ^{125}I within spherical volumes whose diameters approximate those of the DNA helix and an idealized tumor cell, there is at least an order of magnitude increase in energy deposition within the genome. Consequently one would expect the biological toxicity to be critically dependent on subcellular localization.

Regardless of the assay system used, ^{125}I accumulation within nuclear structures is singularly damaging [10]. Much of the supporting data has been obtained from studies where the thymidine analogue [125]IUdR is incorporated into the DNA backbone. The process is highly efficient — nearly every ^{125}I disintegration produces a double strand break in coliphage and mammalian DNA [15]. The extent to which toxicity is dependent upon specific molecular or nuclear localization is less well understood. Considerable evidence exists to suggest that the molecular lesion(s) produced by [125]IUdR differ from those created by photon irradiation. [125]IUdR decay leads to marked molecular fragmentation; by comparison, external gamma radiolysis of nonradioactive IUdR results almost exclusively in simple dehalogenation [20]. Recent studies using ^{125}I-labeled deoxycytidine located at a single position within a DNA fragment of defined sequence have shown that most radiochemical damage occurs within five nucleotides or 15 to 20 Å of the site of decay [17]. Despite possible mechanistic differences, ^{125}I shares a common lethal expression in chromatin with other radiations, at least in terms of morphologically observable phenomena [7].

Other Auger-electron emitters behave similarly and, when incorporated into DNA, in proportion to the energy deposited in very small (subcellular) spheres. In terms of cell survival, iodine-123 and bromine-77 have been compared with iodine-125 [4]. ^{77}Br emits 7 electrons per decay on average, ^{123}I 11 and ^{125}I 20; the average energy (eV) deposited per 5-nm sphere is 300, 560, and 1000 respectively; the mean lethal dose is 4.8, 2.6, and 1.5 mBq/cell.

The use of ^{125}IUdR in vivo raises a number of potential difficulties: Rapid hepatic dehalogenation, S-phase specificity, and high growth fraction are necessary for efficacy. Despite these obstacles, therapeutic doses of carrier-free ^{125}IUdR can be administered by intraperitoneal injection to mice bearing ascites tumor cells without producing overt signs of normal tissue toxicity [1]. Under these circumstances, tumor cells are exposed directly to ^{125}IUdR in the peritoneal cavity before the drug enters the systemic circulation and is degraded. A survival fraction of 10^{-5} can be obtained with 7 injections of 20 μCi each over a 24-h period.

Alternatives to the use of DNA precursors as carriers of ^{125}I are steroid hormones or their analogues, which are translocated from the cytoplasm to the nucleus of cells that contain specific hormone receptors. Although steroids enter all cells by passive diffusion at a rate proportional to concentration, retention involves binding to two types of sites — one group with limited number but high affinity and marked specificity, and a second group with low affinity but large capacity [13]. Once formed, the specific receptor-hormone complex is translocated from the cytoplasm to the nucleus. Although the site of action of the translocated receptor-hormone complex within the nucleus is not known, much of the nuclear estradiol-receptor complex is associated with nucleosomal subunits of chromatin [19].

Tamoxifen is a nonsteroidal antiestrogen that competes with 17-β-estradiol for the estrogen receptor and is translocated to the nucleus [10]. Carrier-free ^{125}I-tamoxifen (^{125}ITAM) can be synthesized by the chloramine-T reaction using the tri-N-butyltin tamoxifen intermediate [18]. An in vitro line of human breast cancer cells (MCF-7) derived from a malignant pleural effusion contains biologically active estrogen receptor and is well-suited to investigate ^{125}I cytotoxicity. The specific cytosol estrogen receptor levels for MCF-7 (receptor-rich) and Chinese hamster V-79 (receptor-poor) cell lines are 60 and 4 fmol/mg protein, respectively. When survival is expressed in terms of cellular uptake, ^{125}ITAM is differentially cytotoxic to MCF-7 cells [4]. There is a two decade difference in surviving fraction between the two cell lines at the highest doses tested. Although ^{125}ITAM is heterogenously distributed throughout the cell, only a small fraction being associated with nuclear structures. Trichloroacetic acid ethanol precipitable radioactivity (^{125}ITAM$_{ppt}$) will isolate ^{125}ITAM associated with nucleic acid and protein, specifically or nonspecifically bound, from that associated with the whole cell. ^{125}ITAM$_{ppt}$ is just about as toxic as ^{125}IUdR localized within the DNA backbone [3, 5]. The fact that the two survival curves cannot be superimposed probably reflects contributions of extranuclear ^{125}ITAM bound nonspecifically to cytoplasmic protein as well as differences in genome associations and nuclear retention time.

Conclusion

We have devised several therapeutic strategies in model systems to demonstrate that Auger and alpha emitting radionuclides, when affixed to appropriate carriers, hold great promise for selectively destroying tumor cell populations. Auger emitters must be localized within the genome to manifest maximal toxicity. Such localization requirements are less precise but no less exacting for alpha emitters where the mean path length is several cell diameters. Further development of therapeutic radiopharmaceuticals will require the concentrated efforts of chemists and biologists to identify selectively localized carriers and design labeled compounds that retain biological specificity.

References

1. Bloomer WD, Adelstein SJ (1977) 5-^{125}I-Iododeoxyuridine as prototype for radionuclide therapy with Auger emitters. Nature 265:620−621
2. Bloomer WD, McLaughlin WH, Neirinckx RD, Adelstein SJ, Gordon PR, Ruth TJ, Wolf AP (1981) Astatine-211-tellurium radiocolloid cures experimental malignant ascites. Science 212:340−341
3. Bloomer WD, McLaughlin WH, Weichselbaum RR, Hanson RN, Adelstein SJ, Seitz DE (1981) The role of subcellular localization in assessing the cytotoxicity of iodine-125 labeled iododeoxyuridine, iodotamoxifen and iodoantipyrine. J Radioanal Chem 65:209−221
4. Bloomer WD, McLaughlin WH, Weichselbaum RR, Tonnesen GL, Hellman S, Seitz DE, Hanson RN, Adelstein SJ, Rosner AL, Burstein NA, Nove JJ, Little JB (1980) Iodine-125-labeled tamoxifen is differentially cytotoxic to cells containing estrogen receptors. Int J Radiat Biol 38:197−202
5. Bloomer WD, McLaughlin WH, Milius RA, Weichselbaum RR, Adelstein SJ (1983) Estrogen receptor-mediated cytotoxicity using Iodine-125. J Cell Biochem 21:39−45
6. Bloomer WD, McLaughlin WH, Lambrecht RM, Atcher RW, Mirzadeh S, Madara JL, Milius RA, Zalutsky MR, Adelstein SJ, Wolf AP (1984) ^{211}At radiocolloid therapy: further observations and comparison with radiocolloids of ^{32}P, ^{165}Dy and ^{90}Y. Int J Radiat Oncol Biol Phys 10:341−348
7. Chan PC, Lisco E, Lisco H, Adelstein SJ (1976) The radiotoxicity of iodine-125 in mammalian cells. II. A comparative study on cell survival and cytogenetic responses to ^{125}IUdR, ^{131}IUdR and ^{3}HTdR. Radiat Res 67:332−343
8. Charlton DE, Booz J (1981) A Monte Carlo treatment of the decay of ^{125}I. Radiat Res 87:10−23
9. Corson DR, MacKensie KR, Segre E (1940) Artificially radioactive element 85. Physiol Rev 57:1087
10. Halpern A, Stöcklin G (1977) Chemical and biological consequences of β-decay. Radiat Environ Biophys 14:167−183, 257−274
11. Harris CR, Adelstein SJ, Ruth TJ, Wolf AP (1978) Loss of reproductive capacity of cultured mammalian cells irradiated by emissions from an alpha emitting radionuclide (^{211}At) in solution. Radiat Res 74:590
12. Heel RC, Brogden RN, Speight TM, Avery GS (1978) Tamoxifen: a review of its pharmacological properties and therapeutic use in the treatment of breast cancer. Drugs 16:1−24
13. Jensen EV, Jacobson HI (1962) Basic guides to the mechanism of estrogen action. Recent Prog Horm Res 18:387−411
14. Kassis AI, Adelstein SJ, Haydock C, Sastry KSR, McElvaney KD, Welch MJ (1982) Lethality of Auger-electrons from the decay of bromine-77 in the DNA of mammalian cells. Radiat Res 90:362−373

15. Krish RE, Sauri CJ (1975) Further studies of DNA damage and lethality from the decay of iodine-125 in bacteriophage. Int J Radiat Biol 27:553–560
16. Lavrukhina AK, Pozdnyakov AA (1976) Analytical chemistry of technetium, promethium, astatine and francium. Humphrey Science, Ann Arbor, pp 227–260
17. Martin RF, Haseltine WA (1981) Range of radiochemical damage to DNA with decay of iodine-125. Science 213:896–898
18. Seitz DE, Tonnesen GL, Hanson RM, Hellman S, Adelstein SJ (1980) Iododestannylation: position-specific synthesis of iodotamoxifen. J Organomet Chem 186:C33–C36
19. Senior MB, Frankel FR (1978) Evidence for two kinds of chromatin binding sites for the estradiol-receptor complex. Cell 14:857–863
20. Stöcklin G (1979) Chemical and biological effects of β-decay and inner-shell ionization in biomolecules: a new approach to radiation biology. In: Okada S, Imamura M, Teroshima T, Yamaguchi H (eds) Proceedings of the 6th International congress of radiation research. Tappan, Tokyo, pp 382–391

Studies on the In Vivo Stability of ^{211}At Labelled Albumin Particles in Mice

G. Wunderlich[1], E. Henke, B. Iwe, W.-G. Franke, S. Fischer, and R. Dreyer

Introduction

From the group of known α-emitters, ^{211}At appears to be one of the most suitable representative for radiotherapy owing to its excellent physical properties (i.e. a short physical half-life of 7.2 h and a decay of almost 100% α-particles). The short pathway of the α-particles of ^{211}At ($60-70$ µm in aqueous medium) should mean in the case of radiotherapeutical application that the tissue surrounding the tumor are protected to a large extent. Experiments with cell cultures and animals delivered some clues for a successful therapy of malignant tumors with ^{211}At [1–3]. The main problem not yet solved for such a radionuclide therapy is the temporally limited selective accumulation of At-labelled carrier molecules at the desired activity-accumulating site (the tumor). A further problem is the distinguished deastatization in vivo in most of the At compounds tested up to now. One possibility is the i.v. injection of radiopharmaceuticals with a specific accumulation behaviour, another is to achieve a high radionuclide concentration by application of substances whose transport away from the application site is hindered (e.g. β-emitters are already used in therapy). As shown in animal experiments, ^{211}At-labelled Tl-colloid has a substantially higher therapeutical effect than β-emitters labelled particles [5]. Human serum albumin particles (HSA-microspheres) are used for lung scanning and imaging of the hepatobiliary tract. We have succeeded in labelling HSA microspheres with ^{211}At in an advantageous manner. We shall report about experimental animal studies on the stability of the At bend to the HSA particles.

Materials and Methods

Labelling of the Microspheres

Highly pure ^{211}At (contents of ^{210}At $< 10^{-5}$%) was obtained in the $(\alpha, 2n)$ reaction of 28 MeV α-particles on natural Bi in the Rossendorf cyclotron U-120. The separation of the ^{211}At isotope was performed thermochromatographically as described earlier [6]. Microspheres produced from denatured HSA (e.g. ROTOP-B20 particles, diameter $15-25$ µm) were prepared as patented [7]. Labelled microspheres in saline solution were used for injection.

---

1 Medizinische Akademie „Carl Gustav Carus", Abt. für Nuklearmedizin, Fetscherstr. 74, X-8019 Dresden DDR

Nuclear Medicine in Clinical Oncology
Ed. by C. Winkler
© Springer-Verlag Berlin Heidelberg 1986

Animal Experiments

Healthy white mice were available as experimental animals. The animals received 0.5 ml of the saline solution of labelled microspheres injected into the tail vein.

In the case of the microspheres B20, more than 95% of the particles stick fast in the lung capillaries. After previously determined time intervals p.i. the animals were killed. The organs were removed and their radioactivity content measured in a well-type scintillation counter, which registered the 79 keV X-rays emitted during the electron capture decay of ^{211}At.

The radioactivity content in the lungs was determined at different times p.i. and compared with the At concentration in other organs. This gives a measure for the in vivo stability of ^{211}At-labelled HSA microspheres.

Results and Discussion

There is only a very slow decrease in the radioactivity in the lungs (Fig. 1). At 20 h p.i. we found in the region of the lungs about 40% of the injected At. Since after three physical half-lives only about 12% of the originally applied radioactivity could still be utilized for the exposure, the achieved labelling stability is considered to be sufficient. In contrast, an increase in radioactivity could be observed outside the lungs, i.e. in the thyroid and in the gastrointestinal tract. The At set free during the slow deastatization of the microspheres is accumulated predominantly in the unblocked thyroid (Fig. 2). Still the uptake proceeded much more slowly than we saw in former investigations after application of ^{211}At in the form of At$^-$ or At $\times$ H$_2$O [4]. Therefore the uptake in the thyroid 3 h p.i. was much lower after application of labelled microspheres (2%) than the uptake after application of At$^-$ or At $\times$ H$_2$O (11%).

Incubation of At-labelled particles in human serum for 2 h (room temperature) showed only 5% free At in the supernatant solution after centrifugation.

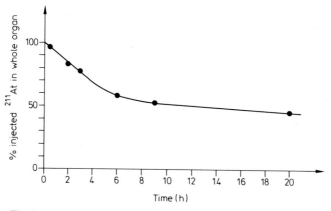

Fig. 1. Retention of ^{211}At in the lungs after i.v. application of ^{211}At microspheres ROTOP B 20 in healthy mice (measurements corrected to the time of injection)

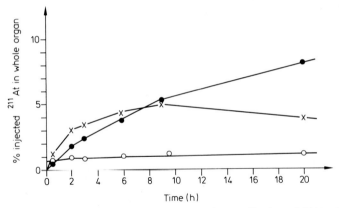

Fig. 2. Retention in selected organs after i.v. application of ^{211}At microspheres ROTOP B 20 in healthy mice. Measurements corrected to the time of injection; $--$x$--$, stomach; $--\bullet--$, thyreoid, $--$o$--$, liver

The ^{211}At-labelled microspheres appear quite stable in vivo compared with a series of other biomolecules and so give a potential possibility for using the excellent radiophysical features of ^{211}At in endogeneous therapy of malignant tumors.

References

1. Smit JA, Myburh JA, Neirinckx RD (1972) Clin Exp Immunol 14:107
2. Aay L, Tschroots WRJM, Lindner L, Feltkamp TEW (1975) Int J Appl Radiat Isot 26:25
3. Brown J, Carpenter RN, Mitchell JS (1984) Int J Appl Radiat Isot 35:843
4. Wunderlich G, Henke E, Rösch F, Franke WG, Dreyer R (in press) Radiobiol Radiother (Berl)
5. Bloomer WD, McLaughlin WH, Lambrecht RM, Atcher RW, Mirzadeh S, Madara JL, Milius RA, Zalutsky MR, Adelstein SJ, Wolf AP (1984) Int J Radiat Oncol Biol Phys 10:341
6. Beyer GJ, Dreyer R, Odrich, Rösch F (1981) Radiochem Radioanal Lett 47:63
7. Wunderlich G, Henke E, Iwe B, Franke WG, Fischer S, Dreyer R (in press) Nucl Med Comm

Subject Index